Richard O'Kennedy

Immunoassays

Immunoassays

Development, Applications and Future Trends

edited by

Richard O'Kennedy
Caroline Murphy

Pan Stanford Publishing

Published by

Pan Stanford Publishing Pte. Ltd.
Penthouse Level, Suntec Tower 3
8 Temasek Boulevard
Singapore 038988

Email: editorial@panstanford.com
Web: www.panstanford.com

British Library Cataloguing-in-Publication Data
A catalogue record for this book is available from the British Library.

Immunoassays: Development, Applications and Future Trends

ISBN 978-981-4669-97-9 (Hardcover)
ISBN 978-1-315-20654-7 (eBook)

MIX
Paper from responsible sources
FSC® C011748

Printed in Great Britain by Ashford Colour Press Ltd

Contents

Preface xv
Glossary xvii

1 An Overview of Immunoassays **1**
Caroline Murphy, Sarah Gilgunn, and Richard O'Kennedy
1.1 Introduction to Antibodies and Immunoassays 1
1.1.1 Polyclonal Antibody Production 3
1.1.2 Production of Monoclonal Antibodies 4
1.1.3 Recombinant Antibody Fragments 5
1.1.3.1 Production of recombinant antibodies by phage display technology 6
1.2 Types of Immunoassays 7
1.3 Choosing a Suitable Immmunoassay Technique 9
1.3.1 Detection of Target Analyte: An Immunometric Approach 9
1.3.1.1 Direct immunoassay 9
1.3.1.2 Indirect immunoassay 10
1.3.1.3 Sandwich immunoassay 11
1.3.2 Detection of Small Molecules Using a Competitive Approach 12
1.4 Signal Generation in Immunoassays 14
1.4.1 Signal Generation 14
1.4.1.1 Colourimetry as a method of immuno-detection 14
1.4.1.2 Luminescence as a method of immuno-detection 18
1.4.2 Nanomaterials, for Signal Generation and Immobilisation 21

1.5 Next Generation Signal Transduction Systems 23
1.5.1 Electrochemical Transducers for Immunoassay Applications 24
1.5.2 Nanomechanical Sensors/Piezoelectric Mass Sensors 24
1.5.3 Optical Signal Transduction 27
1.6 Conclusions and Key Issues 27

2 Recombinant Antibodies for Diagnostic Applications: Design Considerations and Structural Correlates 37
Stephen Hearty and Richard O'Kennedy
2.1 Diagnostic Antibodies: Co-opting Natural Immunity 38
2.2 Harnessing Natural Diversity 38
2.3 Affinity 41
2.4 Exploiting Synthetic Diversity in vitro 43
2.4.1 Introducing Diversity 44
2.4.2 Introducing Diversity: Affinity Maturation 46
2.5 Paradigms Challenged 47
2.6 Single-Domain Antibodies 49
2.7 Conclusion 53

3 Surfaces and Immobilisation Strategies for Use in Immunoassay Development 59
Chandra K. Dixit and Paul Conroy
3.1 Introduction 60
3.2 Tailoring Immunoassay Surfaces 63
3.2.1 Surface Designing/Modulation and Customisation for Antibody Immobilisation and Immunoassay Development 64
3.2.1.1 Precursor modulation and post-manufacture treatments for controlling the surface properties 64
3.2.1.2 Grafting functional groups by physical and chemical methods 69
3.3 Antibody Immobilisation 71
3.4 Antibody Conjugation to Quantum Dots 75

3.5 Aspects and Case Studies of Antibody Immobilisation 76
3.6 Conclusions and Future Perspectives 80

4 Immunoassay Validation **89**
Paul Leonard
4.1 Why Is Validation Necessary? 90
4.2 Assay Validation Overview 90
4.2.1 Planning 'It Takes Time to Save Time' 91
4.3 Assay Development 92
4.3.1 Immunogen for Antibody Production and Screening 95
4.3.2 Antibody Production 96
4.3.3 Assay Format 96
4.4 Pre-validation 97
4.4.1 Select Assay Reagents 97
4.4.2 Evaluate Assay Conditions 97
4.4.3 Define Calibration Model 98
4.4.4 Evaluate Selectivity and Specificity 99
4.4.5 Preliminary Estimates for LLOQ and ULOQ 100
4.4.6 Preliminary Estimates of Precision and Accuracy 101
4.4.7 Estimation of the Assay Limit of Detection (LOD) 104
4.4.8 Reference Method 107
4.4.9 Validation Samples and Method Definition 108
4.4.10 Evaluate Extraction Efficiency/Effects 108
4.5 Pre-study Validation 110
4.5.1 Stability 110
4.5.2 Evaluate Dilutional Linearity 111
4.5.3 Evaluate Assay Robustness and Ruggedness 112
4.5.4 Assay Validation Report and Documentation 112
4.6 Summary 113

5 Lab-on-a-Chip Immunoassay Systems **117**
Barry Byrne and Louise M. Barrett
5.1 Introduction 118
5.2 Substrates Used for Microfluidic Chip Design 119

5.3 Microfluidic Channel Design and Fabrication 122
5.4 Analyte Delivery, Mixing and Washing 125
5.5 Antibody Integration 128
5.6 Lab-on-a-Chip–Based Immunodetection: Applications 132
5.6.1 Bacterial Pathogens and Toxins 132
5.6.2 Marine and Fungal Toxins 140
5.7 Disease Markers and Their Detection Using Microfluidics-Based Devices 145
5.8 Conclusions 148

6 Clinical Applications of Immunoassays 161
Karen Lawler and Gregor Kijanka
6.1 Clinical Specimen Analysis 162
6.2 Cardiovascular Disease 165
6.2.1 Ischemic Heart Disease and Cardiac Enzymes 165
6.2.2 Heart Failure and Brain Natriuretic Peptide 166
6.2.3 Serum Lipids and Lipoproteins 167
6.3 Respiratory Disease 168
6.3.1 Bacterial Respiratory Infections 168
6.3.1.1 *Streptococcus pneumonia* 168
6.3.1.2 Legionella species 169
6.3.1.3 *Mycoplasma pneumonia* 169
6.3.1.4 *Haemophilus influenzae* 170
6.3.1.5 *Chlamydia pneumonia* 170
6.3.2 Fungal Respiratory Infections 170
6.3.2.1 Aspergillus 170
6.3.3 Viral Respiratory Infections 171
6.3.3.1 Influenza A and B 171
6.3.4 Cystic Fibrosis 171
6.3.5 Pulmonary Embolism and D-Dimers 172
6.4 Endocrinology 173
6.4.1 Type 1 Diabetes Mellitus 173
6.4.2 Thyroid Disease 173
6.4.3 Adrenal Hormone and Cushing's Syndrome 174
6.5 Rheumatology 175
6.5.1 Rheumatoid Arthritis 175
6.5.2 Systemic Lupus Erythematosus 176
6.5.3 Systemic Sclerosis 177

6.5.4 Sjögren's Syndrome 177
6.5.5 Vasculitis 178
6.5.6 Dermatomyositis and Polymyositis 178
6.6 Oncology 179
6.6.1 Alpha-Fetoprotein 179
6.6.2 Prostate-Specific Antigen 180
6.6.3 Carbohydrate Antigens 181
6.6.3.1 CA 125 181
6.6.3.2 CA 15-3 and CA 27-29 181
6.6.3.3 CA 19-9 181
6.6.4 Carcinoembryonic Antigen 181
6.6.5 Beta-Human Chorionic Gonadotrophin 182
6.6.6 Antibody-Associated Paraneoplastic Disease 182
6.7 Conclusion 183

7 Immunoassay-Based Detection of Infectious and Parasitic Diseases 191
Paul J. Conroy
7.1 Introduction 192
7.2 Current Technologies for the Detection of Infectious Diseases in Humans 193
7.2.1 Appropriate Technologies 196
7.2.2 Human Immunodeficiency Virus (HIV) 197
7.2.3 Tuberculosis 198
7.2.4 Malaria 199
7.2.5 Rapidly Spreading Infectious Agents 200
7.3 Challenges in Detecting Infectious and Parasitic Diseases 202
7.3.1 Current Research into New Platform Development 202
7.3.2 Current Antibodies for Infectious Disease Agents 205
7.4 Future Trends 207
7.4.1 Rapid Assay Development: Antibodies 207
7.4.2 Rapid Assay Development: Microfluidics and Nanotechnology and Their Relevance to Infectious Disease Detection 209
7.5 Conclusion 212

8 Detection of Food, Agricultural and Aquatic Contaminants 221
Marie Le Berre, Caroline Viguier, Caroline Murphy, and Niamh Gilmartin
8.1 Immunoassays Used in the Detection of Contaminants in Food 222
8.1.1 Foodborne Pathogens 222
8.1.2 Foodborne Toxins 227
8.2 Immunoassays in the Agricultural Environment 228
8.2.1 Immunoassays in Animal Feedstuffs 228
8.2.2 Immunoassays for Agricultural Veterinary Infections 232
8.2.3 Immunoassays Used to Assist in the Management of Reproduction in Animals 233
8.3 Immunoassays in Aquatic Environments 235
8.3.1 Detection of Marine Toxins 235
8.3.2 Detection of Freshwater Algal Toxins 239
8.4 Conclusion 242

9 Next-Generation Immunoassays 255
Valerie Fitzgerald and Paul Leonard
9.1 History of the Immunoassay 255
9.2 Evolution of the Immunoassay 256
9.3 Improvements in Antibody Development 258
9.3.1 Antibody Engineering 259
9.3.1.1 Phage display 260
9.3.1.2 Cell display methods 261
9.3.1.3 In vitro display technologies 263
9.3.2 Mutagenesis Strategies 264
9.4 Improvements in Platform and Detection Methods 266
9.4.1 Nanomaterials 266
9.4.2 Nucleic Acid–Based Signal Amplification 269
9.4.2.1 Immuno-PCR 269
9.4.2.2 Hybridisation chain reaction 271
9.4.2.3 Loop-mediated isothermal amplification 272
9.4.3 Optical Detection Methods 273
9.5 Current Immunoassay Trends 275
9.5.1 Point-of-Care (POC) Diagnostics 275

9.5.2 Microfluidics 276
9.6 Commercially Available Novel Immunoassays 278
9.7 Conclusion 282

10 Recent Trends and the Future of Electrochemical Immunoassay Systems 291
Frank Davis and Seamus Higson
10.1 Introduction to Electrochemical Immunoassays 292
10.2 Electrochemical Immunoassays 294
10.2.1 Principle of Electrochemical Immunoassay 295
10.2.2 Labelled Immunoassay Methods 296
10.2.3 Label-Free Methods 298
10.3 Use of Nanomaterials 301
10.3.1 Metal Nanoparticles 301
10.3.2 Carbon Nanotubes 303
10.3.3 Other Nanomaterials 306
10.4 Microarrays and Nanoarrays 307
10.5 Multiple Target Detection 310
10.6 Imaging of Arrays and Scanning Electrochemical Microscopy (SECM) 312
10.7 Conclusions and Future Prospects 314

11 Optical Signal Transduction with an Emphasis on the Application of Surface Plasmon Resonance (SPR) in Antibody Characterisation 327
Caroline Murphy, Aoife Crawley, Hannah Byrne, Kara Moran, Jenny Fitzgerald, and Richard O'Kennedy
11.1 The Fundamentals of Optical Signal Transduction 328
11.2 Description and Evaluation of the Use of Surface Plasmon Resonance in Immunoassays 330
11.2.1 Optical Platforms Used in SPR 333
11.3 Fundamental Steps in SPR-Based Analysis 335
11.4 Surfaces Used in SPR Immunoassay Development 336
11.4.1 Dextran-Coated Sensor Chips: The Carboxymethylated Series 337
11.4.2 Sensor Chip with Pre-immobilised Surfaces: Capture Applications 337
11.4.3 Sensor Chips for Specialised Applications 340

11.4.4 Functionalisation of SPR Surfaces 341
11.4.5 The Use of Reference/Control Surfaces in SPR Immunoassays 343
11.5 Determination of Kinetic Parameters between Binding Partners Using SPR 344
11.6 Immobilisation of Ligands onto Sensor Surfaces 347
11.6.1 Electrostatic Pre-concentration of the Protein onto the Sensor Chip 348
11.7 Regeneration of Surfaces 348
11.8 Advances in SPR Immunoassays 349
11.9 Conclusions 353

12 Protocols for Key Steps in the Development of an Immunoassay 361
Caroline Murphy and Richard O'Kennedy
12.1 Introduction: Immunoassay Protocols 361
12.2 Preparation of Sample Analyte from Complex Matrices 363
12.3 Purification of Antibodies 364
12.3.1 Purification of Antibodies by Chromatography 366
12.3.2 Antibody Storage Considerations 371
12.3.3 Antibody Conjugation 372
12.3.3.1 Conjugation of quantum dots to antibodies 376
12.3.4 Preparation of Biotinylated Antibodies 379
12.4 Protein Aggregation 382
12.4.1 Prevention of Protein Aggregation 382
12.5 Immunoassay Optimisation 384
12.5.1 Immunoassay Buffers 384
12.5.2 Decreasing Background Signal 384
12.5.3 Coating Buffer 385
12.5.4 Inclusion of Wash Steps 386
12.5.5 Blocking of Non-specific Reaction Sites 386
12.5.6 Checkerboard Titration for Optimisation of ELISA Components 388
12.5.7 Introduction of Appropriate Positive and Negative Controls into the Assay Protocol 390

12.5.7.1 Use of a spiked control 391
12.5.7.2 Standard curve 391
12.5.8 Immobilisation Strategies for Biomolecules onto Solid Surfaces 391
12.6 What Type of Immunoassay to Choose? 395
12.6.1 Enzyme-Linked Immunosorbent Assay (ELISA) 395
12.6.1.1 Binding of capture protein/antibody to the surface 395
12.6.2 Commonly Used ELISA Protocols 396
12.6.3 Fluorescence-Linked Immunosorbent Sandwich Assay (FLISA) 405
12.6.4 Time-Resolved Fluorescence Immunoassay 406
12.6.5 Fluorescence Polarisation Immunoassay (FPIA) 408
12.6.6 Fluorescence Resonance Energy Transfer (FRET) Immunoassay 410
12.7 Surface Plasmon Resonance Protocols 411
12.8 Trouble Shooting 418
12.8.1 Binding of Protein to Surfaces 418
12.8.2 ELISA Trouble Shooting 419
12.9 Summary 420

Index 425

Preface

Immunoassays are analytical tests that utilise antibodies to measure the amount, activity or identity of an analyte. The concept behind this book is to provide a detailed and practical overview of the development and use of immunoassays in many different areas. It is designed to provide a critical and helpful insight into the subject and to give the user practical information that may be of assistance in assay format selection, antibody generation/selection and choice of appropriate detection strategies. This book comprises 12 chapters written by highly experienced researchers in the fields of antibody-based research, immunoassay development, assay validation, diagnostics and microfluidics.

Chapter 1 is a comprehensive survey of antibodies, immunoassay formats and signalling systems. Chapter 2 elucidates key topics related to the development of an antibody-based sensor. Chapter 3 focuses on the important topic of surface modification and explores key parameters in the immobilisation of antibodies onto solid surfaces. Chapter 4 provides a detailed account of what is involved in immunoassay validation. Chapter 5 discusses the move to 'lab-on-a-chip'-based devices and investigates the key parameters necessary for their development. Chapters 6, 7 and 8 are dedicated to the areas of clinical diagnostics, infectious disease monitoring and food security, where immunoassay-based applications have become highly valuable tools. The future of immunoassays and electrochemical-based detection systems are discussed in Chapters 9 and 10. Chapter 11 concentrates on the use of optical detection systems (with a focus on surface plasmon resonance) in immunoassays. Finally, Chapter 12 is a compilation of important, routinely used, immunoassay protocols and addresses problems that may be encountered during assay development.

We would like to sincerely thank all the authors involved, the Applied Biochemistry Group for their help reviewing the chapters and Garvan Doherty, from the Biomedical Diagnostics Institute, for his help in developing the images used in the book.

The support of the publishers and their staff in relation to the initiation, evolution and execution of the text and their patience is gratefully acknowledged.

The financial support of Dublin City University, the Biomedical Diagnostics Institute and Science Foundation Ireland through Grant No. 10/CE/B1821 and 14/IA/2646 was vital for the completion of this work.

Finally, Caroline would like to thank her family, Mary, Claire, Aisling, Rosemary, Pauric, Dicky, her husband George and her daughter Fia for all their support, and Richard would like to thank his family, Kristina, Molly and Jack, for their support and enduring patience during the preparation of this book.

Caroline Murphy
Richard O'Kennedy
January 2017

Glossary

If words are not explained at first sight in the book, they are highlighted in bold and are explained in the glossary.

AC impedance Alternating current impedance is a measure of the opposition to the flow in an AC electrical current.

Accuracy Accuracy is a measure of the closeness of agreement of a test result obtained by an analytical method to its theoretical true value, or the accepted reference/standard value.

Affinity The affinity of an antibody refers to its ability to bind to the target antigen. It is a function of how well the antigen fits the binding site of the antibody.

Affinity ceiling Antibody recognition is thought to have an upper boundary for optimal affinity under natural biological conditions. This is called an affinity ceiling. Natural equilibration dissociation constant (K_D) is considered to be in the order of 10^{-8} to 10^{-10}.

Amino acids Amino acids are organic compounds that are composed of an amine ($-NH_2$) group and carboxyl ($-COOH$) group. They are the building blocks of proteins. In proteins, specific amino acids are linked together as if in a chain, and when folded, the tertiary structure makes up a protein.

Amperometric Amperometric analytical signalling systems operate when a current is created as a result of redox reactions at a sensor surface. They rely on either the release or consumption of electrons during these reactions.

Analyte Any chemical or substance under analytical scrutiny.

Anthelmintics Anthelmintics are a class of drugs used to treat infections with parasitic worms (helminths) from the body. Tapeworms, roundworms and flukes are classified as helminths.

Antibacterials See **antibiotics.**

Antibiotics Antibiotics are also known as antibacterials and are types of medication that destroy or slow down the growth of bacteria.

Antibody An antibody, also known as immunoglobulin, is an important part of the immune system. Most antibodies are Y-shaped molecules that recognise the presence of invading species such as viruses, bacteria, fungi, parasites and many more. Antibodies recognise these invasive agents through their antigen binding sites and signal to initiate an immune response via their fragment crystallisable (Fc) regions.

Antibody-based latex particle agglutination test (LAT) LAT utilises latex particles coated with antibodies or antigens to detect their counterparts through immunoagglutination of the latex particles to form quantifiable aggregates in the presence of the analyte in the sample.

Anti-idiotype This is an antibody that binds to the antigen-combining site of another antibody.

Assay An assay is a qualitative or quantitative scientific test to measure the amount, functional activity or identity of an analyte. An **immunoassay** incorporates antibodies into key steps for the quantitation of the target analyte.

Autoantibody An antibody produced by the immune system targeting the body's own proteins as opposed to proteins originating from external pathogens. Autoantibodies are involved in the pathogenesis of autoimmune diseases and are also found in sera of cancer patients.

Autoantigen A 'self' antigen; any host component that evokes an immune response by the host.

Batch Synonymous with 'run'. A set of standard curve calibrators, validation samples, and/or quality control samples, and/or study samples that are analysed in a single group.

Bias Systematic difference between a measured test result and the theoretical true value (nominal). Bias is expressed either as a relative error (%RE) or as a ratio (%recovery).

Biomarker The term biomarker refers to a broad subcategory of molecules indicative of the presence of a disease (examples of which include proteins, genes or other molecules). They provide objective indications of a medical state, which can be measured with a high degree of accuracy and reproducibility. They help to identify the presence or progress of disease or the effects of treatment.

Calibration curve A functional relationship between the analyte concentration in the standards (calibrators) and the measured response. The calibration curve is used to estimate the analyte concentration in test samples by dose interpolation. A calibration curve is synonymous with a standard curve.

Calibrator A volume of matrix spiked with the analyte of interest at a predetermined concentration using a well-characterized reference material.

Carbon nanotubes Are tube shaped molecules composed of carbon atoms that have a diameter on a nanometer scale. They can have either 'metal or semiconductor-like' properties and can be generated as single-walled nanotubes (SWNTs), multi-walled nanotubes (MWNTs) or double-walled nanotubes (DWNTs).

Coefficient of variation (CV) A quantitative measure of precision expressed relative to the mean result (also referred to as the relative standard deviation).

Competitive immunoassay A competitive immunoassay is one in which free analyte competes with immobilised analyte for antibody binding or where antibody in the matrix competes with labelled antibody for binding to an immobilised cognate antigen.

Confirmation assay A secondary assay, following a screening assay, which confirms the result (and may include assessment of **specificity** and/or **titre**).

Cross-validation Validation that utilises the use of two or more bioanalytical methods within the same study.

Cut-off point The cut-off point of the assay is the level of response of the assay at or above which a sample is defined to be positive and below which it is defined to be negative.

Diagnostic A diagnostic is a tool used to identify/characterise a particular disease from its signs and symptoms.

Dialysis/dialyse Dialysis is a diffusion-based process whereby larger soluble molecules are separated from smaller ones. It generally employs a differentially permeable membrane that achieves the separation based on size.

Diffraction grating Can separate light into its constituent wavelengths.

Dilutional linearity A condition in which dilution of a spiked sample does not result in biased measurement of the analyte concentration. For example, when a spiked sample is serially diluted to give a set of samples having analyte concentrations that fall within the quantitative range of the assay, the entire set of dilutions can be measured with acceptable accuracy.

Direct antigen testing (DAT) A rapid antibody-based test that utilises direct antigen binding to identify pathogens such as *Mycobacterium tuberculosis* or influenza virus antigens.

EC50 An abbreviation for the 'concentration necessary to produce a response of 50%'. For a competitive assay, the EC50 is the concentration of the analyte that is necessary to produce a 50% displacement of the tracer. For a non-competitive assay, the EC50 is the concentration of analyte necessary to produce a response of 50% or one-half of the observed maximum of binding.

Electrochemistry/Electrochemical reaction Electrochemistry is the production of an electric current during a chemical reaction. The most common type of electrochemical reaction used in biotechnology is the reduction/oxidation reaction or redox reaction during which electrons are transferred between two interacting species.

Enzyme immunoassay (EIA) Synonymous with ELISA; used for the detection and quantification of specific antigens or antibodies in a given sample through enzymatic colour or fluorescence changes.

Enzyme-linked immunosorbent assay (ELISA) An enzyme-linked immunosorbent assay (ELISA) uses the basic immunological concept of an antigen binding to its specific antibody, allowing for the detection of antigens such as proteins, peptides, hormones or antibodies in a fluid sample or in tissue. ELISAs are commonly used as **diagnostic** tools in medicine and as quality control measures in various industries; they are also used as analytical tools in biomedical research for the detection and quantification of specific antigens or antibodies in a given sample.

Epitope An epitope is an area on an antigen that is recognised by antibodies of the immune system. An epitope can be either conformation-based (on the three-dimensional structure of the antigen's antigenic region) or linear (where an antibody recognises a continuous length of **amino acids** or other constituent components).

Evanescent wave An evanescent wave is an electrical wave that decays exponentially away from the surface interface where it was formed.

Factorial experiments A multivariate approach where two or more variables are varied simultaneously to achieve an optimal solution after taking into account the interaction between these variables. This approach is typically more efficient than one-factor-at-a-time for optimising assays and/or when analysing multiple variables of an assay that are interdependent.

False negative Negative test result from a truly positive sample.

False positive Positive test result from a truly negative sample.

Fluorometric assay An assay that relies on the presence of increased fluorescence or a change in the amount present as a means of quantification.

Four-parameter logistic (4PL) A versatile function that is recognized as the 'reference standard' for function fitting the mean concentration response for immunoassays. The function is defined by the equation $E(Y) = D+(A-D)/[1+(X/C)^B]$ where $E(Y)$ is the expected response; X, concentration; A, response at zero concentration; D, response at infinite concentration; C, concentration resulting in a response halfway between A and D (ED_{50}); and B, slope parameter that is typically near 1.0.

Fractional factorial experiments A type of multi-factorial experiment in which only a subset of factor-level combinations is tested. These experiments are very useful for screening a large number of factors prior to optimising the most important factors.

Full validation A validation that includes the evaluation of accuracy, precision, curve-fitting (model assessment), sensitivity, specificity, stability, etc.

Functionalisation (surface modification) Functionalisation, also known as surface modification, is the act of changing the surface of a material by altering its chemical characteristics, generally to enhance its ability to bind biomolecules or resist fouling.

Gold nanoparticles Gold nanoparticles (GNPs) or colloidal gold are nano-sized (1–100 nm) particles of gold that are in suspension. Depending on their size, shape, surface chemistry and aggregation properties they produce different optical and electrical properties; as a result of this, they are widely used in sensors.

Gravimetric sensors These are a type of sensor that can detect changes in analyte concentration on the basis of changes in mass.

Hapten A hapten is a small molecule that is of itself incapable of stimulating an immune response (i.e. it is not immunogenic). To overcome this, it is tightly linked to a carrier molecule (most often a protein) by a covalent bond. When used for immunisation purposes, this hapten carrier complex stimulates the immune system and subsequently the production of antibodies.

Hook effect Describes an artefact seen when an analyte is present in very high concentration, beyond the dynamic range of the method. This excess amount cannot be measured accurately and generates spuriously low results.

Hybridoma technology Antibody-producing B-lymphocytes are fused to continuously multiplying cancer cells (myelomas) to generate a hybrid cell or hybridoma. It is used for the continuous production of monoclonal antibodies.

Immunoassay See **assay.**

Immunodepletion Refers to the removal of a target using anti-target antibodies.

Immunodepletion assay A form of confirmation assay wherein the target (anti-product antibody) is specifically depleted by inhibition of reactivity during a pre-incubation step with an excess of product. It demonstrates the presence of antibodies that bind to the product.

Immunosensor An immunosensor is an analytical device that incorporates an antibody as a biological recognition element and links the binding event that occurs between an antibody and an antigen with a physiochemical detector that signals the presence of a target molecule.

Incoupling This is a resonance phenomenon that occurs at a precise angle of incidence. It is dependent on the refractive index (RI) of the medium covering the surface of a waveguide.

Interference Presence of entities in samples that prevent the target analyte from being detected or accurately quantified. It is a significant bias in the measured analyte concentration due to the effect of another component or properties of the specimen or matrix.

Intermediate precision Precision of repeated measurements within a laboratory, taking into account all relevant sources of variation affecting the results (runs, days, analysts, equipment, reagents, etc.). Intermediate precision is also termed inter-assay or inter-batch precision.

Isoelectric point The isoelectric point of a protein or molecule is the point, where at a certain pH, the protein or molecule has no net charge. In a buffer with a pH less than the pI of the protein or molecule under consideration, the net charge of the protein will be positive. In a buffer with pH greater than the pI, the net charge of the protein will be negative.

Lab-on-a-chip Such devices integrate a panel of laboratory functions on a single microfluidic device, permitting for example, immunoassays to be performed using reduced sample volumes, and without the requirement for multiple platforms.

Ligand-binding assay A type of assay format that depends on the specific binding of an analyte to another molecule, usually a macromolecule (biopolymer). This format typically involves reversible non-covalent interactions governed by the laws of mass action.

Limit of detection (LOD) Lowest concentration of analyte for which the response can be reliably distinguished from background noise.

Linearity Ability of the analytical method within a specified concentration range to obtain test results that are proportional to the concentration of the analyte in the test sample.

Lower limit of quantitation (LLOQ) The lowest concentration of analyte that has been demonstrated to be measurable with acceptable levels of accuracy (mean bias) and precision.

Macromolecule Macromolecules are commonly biopolymers that have the potential to provoke an immune response. Due to their inherent molecular complexity, macromolecules are generally more difficult to characterize than conventional small molecules.

Magnetoresistance Refers to a change in electrical resistance in metal or a semiconductor when it is subjected to a magnetic field.

Mass spectrometry (MS) An analytical method used to identify small molecules, proteins, lipids and others substances through changes in their mass-to-charge ratios which are introduced by an ion source and analysed in a mass analysis detector.

Matrix The type of environment (e.g. serum, plasma or other biological fluid) in which the target (antibody or analyte) is present.

Matrix effect Interference in an assay that is caused by adding the sample matrix. Commonly refers to analytical interference produced by factors other than those that have physicochemical similarity to the analyte.

Microarray Microarrays are two-dimensional high-throughput tests used to identify binding partners to a sample of interest. They are composed of multiple microscopic spots that can be made of, for example, DNA, tissues, cells, proteins or antibodies to formulate the respective microarrays. A biological sample of unknown content is applied to the microarray and binders can be identified using dyed probes or tagged antibodies.

Microfluidics This is a multidisciplinary research field, which integrates biomedical engineering, physics, chemistry, biology and biotechnology. Microfluidic applications focus on the implementation of these disciplines in developing systems accommodating microlitre volumes of fluid as analytical samples.

Nanoarray A nanoarray is an array in which nano-sized objects such as proteins or cells are spotted onto a solid surface. They can use picolitre volumes of liquid. (See **microarray**.)

Nanomaterials These are materials that have at least one dimension in the nanometer scale (1–100 nm). Engineered nanomaterials have unique optical, magnetic and electrical properties. One such example is graphene; it is a lattice-based structure that is composed of carbon atoms. Graphene is being increasingly used in the area of biological sensors.

Nanoparticle A nanoparticle has all three dimensions in the nanoscale range (1–100 nm).

Negative control A negative control is one in which the sample is known to be devoid of a particular substance. By not including this substance it can be shown that the experimental conditions used would generate a negative result.

Nominal concentration A stated or theoretical concentration that may or may not differ from the true concentration.

Nonparametric methods A statistical approach that makes no assumptions about a distribution. Nonparametric methods are a class of methods that are used for a broad non-parameterized set of underlying distributions. Mean, median and percentiles of a sample are nonparametric estimates of the corresponding population quantities.

Nonspecific non-specificity Analytical interference caused by factors other than those that are related physicochemically to the analyte of interest, but which nevertheless affect the in vitro binding reaction. This type of non-specificity is commonly referred to as matrix effects.

Optimisation The process of developing an assay, prior to validation, wherein the variables affecting the assay are elucidated (e.g. antibody concentration, incubation time, wash cycles).

Parallelism A condition in which the dilution of test samples does not result in biased measurements of the analyte concentration. Thus, when a test sample is serially diluted to result in a set of samples having analyte concentrations that fall within the quantitative range of the assay, there is no apparent trend toward increasing or decreasing estimates of analyte concentration over the range of dilutions.

Parametric methods Parametric methods are a class of methods that assume a particular parameterized set of underlying distributions for the data (e.g. normal distribution). These methods may use mean or robust estimates such as median within the framework of the assumed underlying parametric distribution such as the normal distribution.

Pathogen A pathogen is defined as a microorganism that causes, or can cause, disease. That is, a microbe that can cause damage in a host.

Photobleaching Photobleaching (also referred to as fading) is the photochemical alteration of a dye or a fluorophore molecule such that it permanently is unable to fluoresce.

Plasmons A plasmon is a quantum of plasma oscillation. A plasmon is a collective excitation of the electronic 'fluid' in a piece of conducting material and can be considered a quasiparticle (like ripples on the surface of a pond are a collective mode of the water molecules of the liquid).

Point-of-care Point-of-care is a form of medical testing that is performed at or near the site of patient care.

Polymerase chain reaction (PCR) An enzymatic method for the amplification of DNA that relies on melting and enzymatic replication of DNA through a series of thermal cycles.

Positive control Experiments have two major groups: the test subject and the control subject. A positive control is usually what researchers expect from the test, so it gives them something to compare. Hence, positive controls are used to validate the assay and demonstrate legitimacy of the test data.

Potentiometric A potentiometric immunosensor can be defined as a device incorporating a biological sensing element connected to an electrochemical potential transducer.

Precision The closeness of agreement (degree of scatter) between a series of measurements obtained from multiple sampling of the same homogeneous sample under the prescribed conditions. Precision may be considered at three levels: repeatability, intermediate precision and reproducibility.

Pre-study validation Procedures used prior to the analysis of study samples to establish that an analytical method is suitable for its intended application.

Pre-validation Assay development experiments conducted prior to formal validation in order to enhance immunoassay performance.

Quality controls A set of negative and positive controls included in each assay run to monitor, and maintain consistency of assay performance (system suitability).

Radioimmunoassay (RIA) An immunoassay that utilises radioactive substances as markers/labels for measurement. Either an antibody or an antigen may be labelled depending on the assay format. RIA is a very sensitive method, however, it is less frequently used due to safety issues.

Radioreceptor assays Radioreceptor assays are used to quantify receptor proteins present in tissue specimen through the addition of radiolabelled ligands specific to the receptor.

Range The interval between the upper and lower concentrations (amounts) of analyte in the sample for which it has been demonstrated that the analytical procedure has a suitable level of accuracy (mean bias), precision and linearity.

Recovery A measurement of the closeness of an observed result to its theoretical true value. Recovery is generally expressed as the percentage of the observed to the nominal (theoretical) concentration. 'Spike recovery' relates to cases where the theoretical concentration corresponds to the concentration of analyte added to a sample by the analyst.

Reference interval Values set for a clinical test defining a positive or negative meaning of a test result in terms of clinical decision making.

Reflection Reflection is the change in direction of a wavefront (such as light, sound or water waves) at an interface between two different media so that the wavefront returns into the medium from which it originated.

Refraction The change of direction of a wavefront in passing obliquely from one medium into another in which its wave velocity is different.

Regeneration (in terms of its use in surface plasmon resonance (SPR)) Regeneration of the surface of a chip used in SPR is carried out using a solution (which will be identified following a regeneration scout) that will remove all bound analyte while maintaining a fully functional surface.

Regression model A statistical model relating a dependent variable to one or more independent variables.

Relative error (RE) A quantitative measure of the closeness of an observed result to its theoretical true value, expressed as a percent relative difference from the nominal (theoretical) concentration %RE = [(Observed/Nominal) – 1] × 100.

Relative standard deviation A quantitative measure of precision (also referred to as the coefficient (RSD) of variation) expressed relative to the observed or theoretical (nominal) mean value %RSD = (SD/Mean) × 100. For repeatability, the SD is computed from replicate analyses within a single validation run. For intermediate precision, the SD is computed from replicate analyses over multiple validation runs within the same laboratory.

Repeatability Repeatability is the precision of repeated measurements within the same analytical run under the same operating conditions over a short interval of time. It is also termed intra-assay precision.

Reproducibility Precision of repeated measurements between laboratories; also termed inter-laboratory precision. Usually applies to collaborative studies that involve the standardisation of a bioanalytical method across multiple laboratories.

Resonant mirror A resonant mirror is an optical sensing system that probes the sensing surface to which an evanescent wave has been applied.

Response error relationship (RER) The relationship between the SD in replicate response values (e.g. counts per minute) and the mean response.

Robust estimates Robust estimates are estimates that down-weight the influence of extreme values in summarising the data via the use of median, trimmed mean, median absolute deviation, etc.

Robustness of the assay A measure of the capacity of an assay to remain unaffected by small changes in test conditions. Robustness provides an indication of the ability of an assay to perform under normal usage. Studies of the robustness of an assay measure the effect on the assay output of deliberate changes in assay inputs (incubation time, temperature, sample preparation, buffer pH) that can be controlled through specifications in the assay protocol.

Ruggedness The robustness/ruggedness of an analytical procedure is a measure of its capacity to remain unaffected by small, but deliberate variations in method parameters and provides an indication of its reliability during normal usage.

Run A run represents a set consisting of standard curve (calibrators) and validation samples and/or quality control samples and/or study samples that are analysed together as a single group using the method to be validated. Run is synonymous with 'batch'.

Screening assay The primary assay that differentiates study samples into potential negatives or positives for the presence of anti-product antibodies.

Sedatives Sedatives are central nervous system (CNS) depressants, a category of drugs that work by slowing down brain activity resulting in drowsiness or relaxation.

Selectivity The extent to which a bioanalytical method can measure particular analyte(s) in a complex mixture without interference from other components of the mixture.

Sensitivity The ability of an assay to discriminate small changes in analyte concentration.

Solid-phase extraction (SPE) SPE is a basic sample preparation process by which compounds that are dissolved or suspended in a liquid mixture are separated from other compounds in the mixture according to their physical and chemical properties.

Specific nonspecificity Analytical interference that is caused by substances in the test sample that have physicochemical similarity to the analyte of interest. Examples of such substances include metabolites, degraded forms of the analyte, isoforms, precursors and structural variants that differ with regard to post-translational modification.

Specificity The ability to unequivocally measure the analyte in the presence of other components (often very closely related in terms of structure) that may be expected to be present in the biological specimen, including impurities, metabolites and endogenous matrix components.

System suitability System suitability comprises quantitative or qualitative criteria which ensures that a validated assay performs as expected in day-to-day assay runs. System suitability tests are used to verify that the reliability of the system is adequate (in other words, remains in a validated state) for the analysis to be performed. This quality control system alerts the analyst when the assay is out of specification and ensures that the results obtained in a given run are meaningful.

Titre It is the reciprocal of the highest dilution of the sample that tests positive in the method. It is a common practice to express titer as the common logarithm of the highest dilution of the sample that tests positive in the method. This dilution must be clearly discernible above background.

Total error A concept that expresses the closeness of agreement between a measured test result and its theoretical true value. The term total error describes a combination of systematic (mean bias) and random (precision) error components. In other publications, the term total error is also referred to as accuracy, e.g. ISO definition.

Total internal reflection (TIR) When polarised light is shone through a prism onto a metal surface at a certain angle, light is reflected. By altering the angle at which the light passes through the prism, at a certain angle, total internal reflection (TIR) occurs.

Toxin A toxin is a poisonous substance. It is a specific product of the metabolic activities of a living organism and is harmful when introduced into biological tissues.

Tracer A tracer molecule is a labelled version of the target analyte. The tracer is frequently labelled with an enzyme or fluorophore which is capable of generating a detectable signal.

Upper limit of quantitation The highest concentration of analyte that has been demonstrated to be measurable with stated levels of accuracy (mean bias) and precision.

Validated range The interval of analyte concentrations over which the assay method has been validated. This interval includes concentrations from **LLOQ** to **ULOQ**.

Validation It is the confirmation, via extensive laboratory investigations, that the performance characteristics of an assay are suitable and reliable for its intended analytical use. It describes in mathematical and quantifiable terms the performance characteristics of an assay.

Validation samples Biological matrix samples spiked with the analyte of interest at predetermined concentrations. Alternatively, the analyte may be present endogenously in the biological matrix. A set of validation samples is used during pre-study validation to assess accuracy (mean bias) and precision.

4-6-20 QC rule A batch (run) acceptance criterion widely used in the pharmaceutical industry, which requires that 4 out of 6 QC results be within ±20% of their respective nominal value. Recently, this rule was modified for small-molecule chromatographic-based assays to require 67% (4 out of 6) of QC results to be within 20% of their respective nominal values; 33% of the results (not all replicates at the same concentration) may be outside the ±20% of the nominal value. In this book, this rule has been modified for the bioanalysis of macromolecules to require 4 out of 6 of QC results to be within ±30% of their respective nominal value with at least 50% of the QC results in range at each concentration level.

Chapter 1

An Overview of Immunoassays

Caroline Murphy, Sarah Gilgunn, and Richard O'Kennedy

School of Biotechnology and Biomedical Diagnostics Institute, Dublin City University, Collins Avenue, Dublin 9, Ireland

caroline.s.murphy@dcu.ie

The aim of this chapter is to provide a detailed and practical introduction to immunoassays and set the overall context for the other detailed chapters on specific key elements of immunoassays. The production of antibodies, various antibody structures and their fundamental role in immunoassays is outlined. Comprehensive guides to different immunoassay formats ranging from direct to competitive are provided, and subsequently, important signalling systems, including colourimetric and fluorescence-based approaches, are examined. Finally, electrical, mechanical and optical signal transduction mechanisms that are used in the next generation of immunoassays are described.

1.1 Introduction to Antibodies and Immunoassays

Immunoassays are biochemical tests that utilise immunoglobulins (Ig) (antibodies) as high sensitivity binders to detect the presence

Immunoassays: Development, Applications and Future Trends
Edited by Richard O'Kennedy and Caroline Murphy

ISBN 978-981-4669-97-9 (Hardcover), 978-1-315-20654-7 (eBook)
www.panstanford.com

of molecules that are present at low concentrations. Antibodies are an integral part of the humoral immune system and are nature's major recognition devices. They are found on the surface of B-cells (B-lymphocytes) and recognise the presence of foreign antigens. The B-cell can detect and signal the presence of an extensive range of antigens, consisting of molecules ranging from prions to viruses, drugs, toxins and aberrant biomolecules that invade our bodies. Immunoglobulin proteins exist in many different formats, the five main isotypes of immunoglobulin are IgG (shown in Fig. 1.1), IgM, IgD, IgA and IgE.

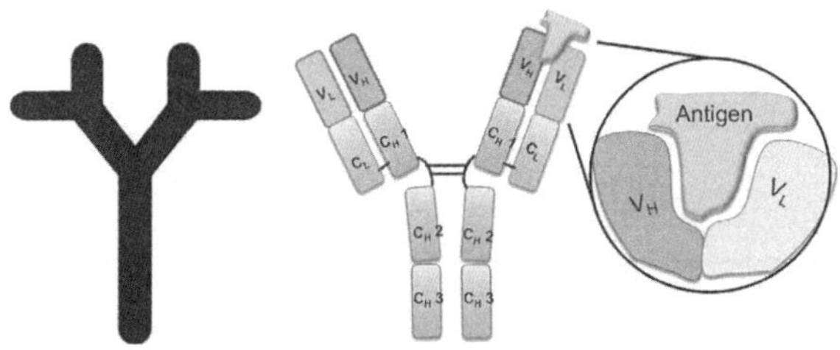

Figure 1.1 Structure of immunoglobulin G (IgG). IgG is made up of two heavy chains (composed of constant domains C_{H1}, C_{H2} and C_{H3} and variable heavy domain, V_H), and two light chains (composed of the constant light domain, C_L and the variable light domain, V_L), connected by disulphide bonds. The antigen-binding region is composed of a variable heavy chain and a variable light chain, which recognises the epitope (specific area where binding occurs) of the antigen.

Antibodies are at the forefront of targeted therapeutics and diagnostics due to their natural high affinities and excellent half-lives. They can be readily manipulated using standard molecular biological techniques into customised antibodies that are tailored to perform efficiently in their chosen end-point application. The biopharmaceutical industry has heavily invested in antibody-based diagnostics and therapeutics, and the latter currently represents the largest and fastest growing class of biopharmaceuticals [1, 2].

Antibodies are generally represented in three forms: (i) polyclonal (produced from a mixture of various B-cell clones), (ii) monoclonal (secreted from a single clone of B-cells) and (iii) recombinant antibodies (the product of the genetic manipulation of antibody genes) [3, 4].

1.1.1 Polyclonal Antibody Production

Polyclonal antibody production involves the immunisation of animals with an antigen and adjuvant (immune system stimulating material) mixture, resulting in the activation of multiple B-cells targeting different antigen epitopes. This produces a vast number of antibodies with different specificities and epitope affinities [3]. These polyclonal antibodies are purified from the serum of immunised animals. Polyclonal antisera can be obtained relatively quickly (6–12 weeks for highly immunogenic antigens) but the time may be antigen-dependent. Methods of purification are generally associated with the antibody type and the intended application(s) for the antibody. These are listed in Table 1.1 [5] and are discussed in detail in Chapter 12.

Several key steps need to be considered for the production of polyclonal antibodies, including (i) preparation/availability of antigen, (ii) choice of host species, (iii) injection regime, (iv) monitoring antibody response to **immunogen** and (v) collection/purification of antibodies. The choice of host is of particular importance when developing polyclonal antibodies against human derived targets, as a large number of proteins are highly conserved throughout mammalian evolution, and, are, therefore, common to many mammalian species. Hence, immunisation of such proteins into rabbits and mice, may generate a limited immune response [6]. The use of a species more phylogenetically distant from humans such as chickens (that diverged from mammalian genomes some 310 million years ago [7]) is an ideal alternative for immunisation and selection of antibodies against highly conserved human proteins [6, 8].

Table 1.1 Polyclonal antibody purifiation methods [5]

Purification type	Methodologies involved in the purification
Crude	Precipitation of a subset of total serum proteins that includes immunoglobulins.
General	Affinity purification of certain antibody classes (e.g. IgG).
Specific	Affinity purification of only those antibodies in a sample that bind to a particular antigen molecule.

1.1.2 Production of Monoclonal Antibodies

The development of 'hybridoma technology' won Georges Köhler and César Milstein the Nobel Prize in Physiology or Medicine in 1984. They created an immortal cell line capable of producing an endless supply of identical antibodies with known specificity called 'monoclonal antibodies' signifying the fact that they were derived from a single hybrid cell [9]. The production of monoclonal antibodies is shown in Fig. 1.2 [3].

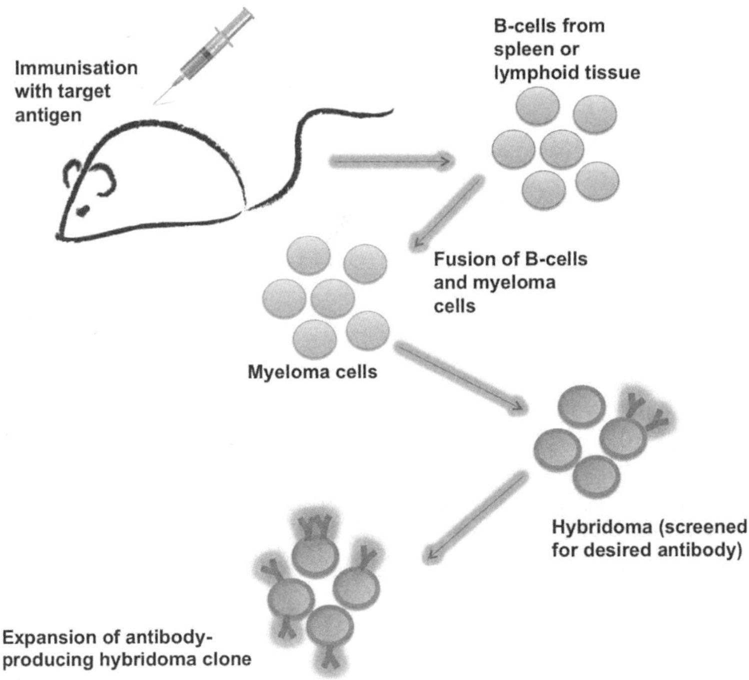

Figure 1.2 Production of monoclonal antibodies by hybridoma technology. B-cells from an immunised mouse are isolated and fused with a myeloma cell line creating hybridomas (generally mediated by the addition of polyethylene glycol (PEG)). Cloning and selection of a specific hybridoma is carried out by **'limiting dilution'**. The clones are screened for reactivity and specific antibody-producing clones are further characterised and expanded for generation of the desired antibody.

1.1.3 Recombinant Antibody Fragments

Recombinant antibodies are highly attractive for customised antibody development as genetic manipulations can be easily employed to precisely tailor their specificity and biophysical properties [10–14]. The ability to readily generate bulk quantities of recombinant proteins, with low production costs in *Escherichia coli,* has fuelled the emergence of an assortment of distinct antibody constructs that can be employed in a wide variety of applications. Some common recombinant antibody constructs are shown in Fig. 1.3.

The smallest antibody fragment that retains the full monovalent antigen binding capabilities of a human IgG is the variable fragment (Fv) and it is comprised of the variable heavy (V_H) and variable light (V_L) domains held together by non-covalent interactions [12, 13].

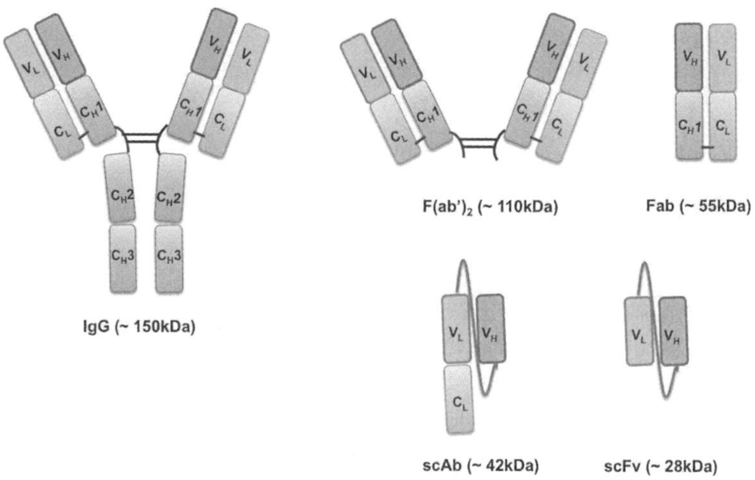

Figure 1.3 Antibody fragment constructs. The mammalian IgG construct (150 kDa) consists of two heavy and two light polypeptide chains linked together by disulphide bonds. The heavy chain consists of variable heavy (V_H) and three constant (C_{H1}, C_{H2}, and C_{H3}) regions. The scFv consists of the V_H and V_L chains joined together by a flexible linker. A single chain antibody (scAb) fragment consists of a scFv with an additional constant chain (either heavy or light). The Fab (antigen-binding fragment) contains the full light chain with V_H and C_{H1}. F(ab')$_2$ is comprised of two Fab fragments held together by disulphide bonds.

The single chain fragment variable (scFv) is more stable than the Fv (which is more prone to aggregation than the scFv) and typically, a flexible 15 residue glycine/serine ($(Gly_4Ser)_3$) linker is incorporated to link the chains together and aid antibody folding and stability during bacterial expression [14].

The antigen-binding fragment (Fab) is a larger, more stable fragment of approximately 50 kDa. The Fab fragment consists of the variable heavy, variable light, constant heavy and constant light chains (V_H & C_{H1} and V_L & C_L). An interchain disulphide bond exists between the C_{H1} and C_L (Fig. 1.3) [15].

There are various advantages and disadvantages associated with the different types of recombinant antibody structures that can be engineered. It should also be noted that antibody fragments can be relatively easily reformatted for improved characteristics such as expression [16], reduction in non-specific binding [17] and enhanced specificity [18]. The selection of superlative antigen-specific recombinant fragments can be achieved using a process known as phage display technology.

1.1.3.1 Production of recombinant antibodies by phage display technology

When George P. Smith first demonstrated in 1985, that the link between phenotype and genotype could be established in filamentous bacteriophage, the advent of phage display technology emerged [19]. Over the last few decades an increased understanding of antibody structure and function has allowed phage display to become one of the most powerful tools in the controlled selection of unique antibodies with properties unattainable from conventional hybridoma methods [20, 21]. Phage display can be used with naïve, immunised or synthetic repertoires [22] and allows for the controlled selection and screening of antibodies against defined antigen conformations from a highly diverse combinatorial library of antibody fragments [23]. Selection involves subjecting the phage library to successive rounds of antigen exposure, allowing antigen-specific phage-displayed antibodies to bind to their targets, in a process known as 'panning'. The antigen-specific phage are recovered and subsequently infected into bacteria for re-amplification

[21]. Ideally, a high affinity antibody would be selected for in the initial round. However, non-specific binding of phage confines the enrichment that can be achieved during each round. Hence, 2–5 rounds of panning are necessary to identify high affinity binders [23]. One round of panning is outlined in Fig. 1.4.

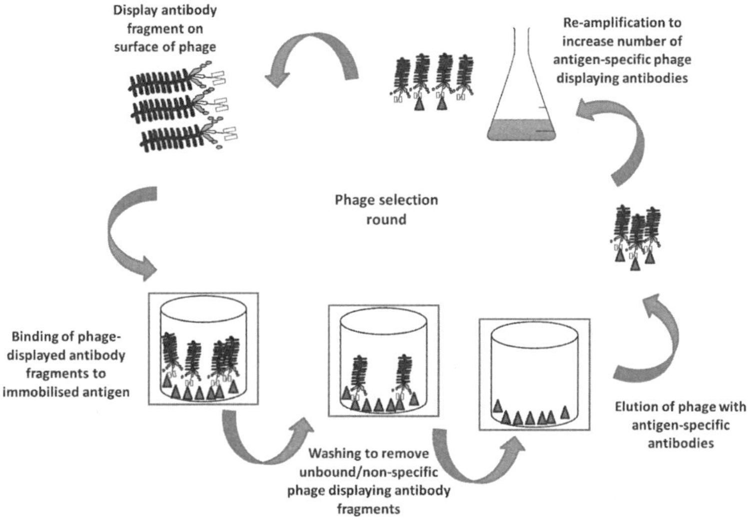

Figure 1.4 Selection of antibodies by phage display. The process of 'panning' is a means of selection of defined clones through binding of the phage library to the target, washing to remove unbound phage and elution of the target-specific phage. This process is repeated for a number of 'rounds' to enrich for a high affinity binder.

1.2 Types of Immunoassays

Following the production of the antibody of choice, the most ideal immunoassay format must be selected. Immunoassays can be divided into homogenous and heterogeneous formats. A homogenous immunoassay does not require the physical separation of the antibody bound to the **analyte** from free analyte. An example of a homogenous immunoassay is a fluorescence polarisation immunoassay (FPIA) (Section 12.6.5 in Chapter 12 of this book). A heterogeneous immunoassay involves the separation of free analyte from antibody-bound analyte, an example of which is an enzyme-linked immunosorbent assay (ELISA) (Section 12.6.1).

Immunoassay methods can be further subdivided into 'immunometric' and 'competitive' immunoassays (Fig. 1.5). Immunometric assays require the use of two specific detection molecules (normally antibodies) and are also referred to as sandwich assays. The immobilised antibody captures the analyte by binding to one of its epitopes. A second labelled antibody then binds and the amount of signal generated, due to the label, is directly proportional to the concentration of the analyte in the sample (Fig. 1.5).

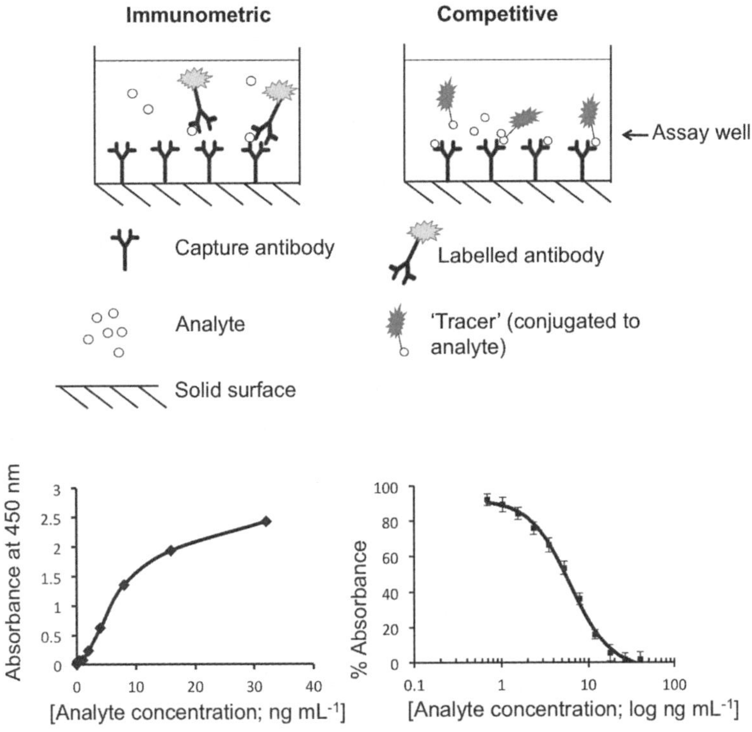

Figure 1.5 Schematic representation of immunometric and competitive immunoassay systems. An example of a typical response curve for each assay format is also shown.

In the competitive assay, labelled ('**tracer**') antigen and free antigen (from the sample to be analysed) compete for binding to the immobilised antibody. The greater the level of analyte in the sample, the smaller the amount of labelled antigen available for binding. Hence, the signal generated is inversely proportional to the concentration of the free antigen, as demonstrated by the curve in Fig. 1.5.

Immunometric immunoassays are commonly used for the detection of molecules such as proteins and viruses, as these entities have the capacity to facilitate the binding of two or more antibodies.

Competitive immunoassays are commonly used to detect small molecules such as drugs and toxins. Competitive immunoassays use an analyte-specific detection antibody and a '**tracer**' molecule, which is a labelled version of the target analyte. The **tracer** is frequently labelled with an enzyme or fluorophore which is capable of generating a detectable signal.

1.3 Choosing a Suitable Immmunoassay Technique

In order to determine the concentration of analyte present in a sample, a number of basic techniques can be used. Each technique has its own unique properties, which renders it suitable for recognising different types of analyte, ranging from bacteria to endogenous proteins to viruses and toxins. The nature of analyte to be detected (size, structure, and whether cytoplasmic, periplasmic or membrane bound) must also be considered.

1.3.1 Detection of Target Analyte: An Immunometric Approach

There are a number of different immunometric immunoassay formats that can be used and these are outlined in the following sub-sections.

1.3.1.1 Direct immunoassay

A direct antibody immunoassay involves coating analyte either passively or actively onto a solid surface, as shown in Fig. 1.6. Antigen standards of known concentration are serially diluted and added to the plate, which is then incubated for a set time and

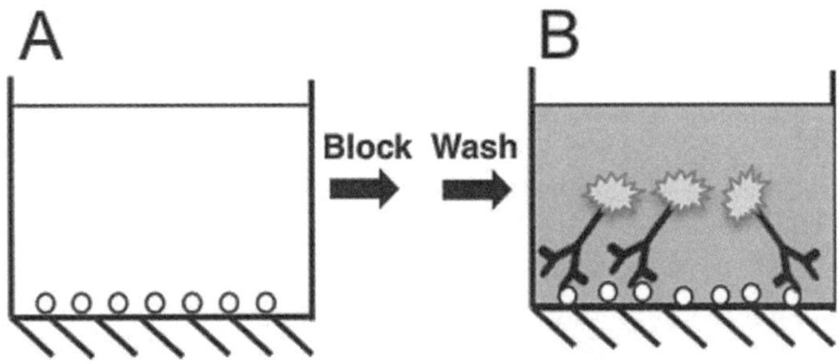

Figure 1.6 Direct immunoassay. (A) Sample analyte is applied and binds to the solid surface. Following blocking and washing steps, (B) a specific detection antibody is introduced which produces a signal.

temperature (e.g. 4°C overnight, room temperature for two hours or 37°C for one hour). The surface is blocked and washed to eliminate non-specific binding and any unbound analyte is removed. Antigen-specific-labelled antibodies are added and the signal produced is measured.

1.3.1.2 Indirect immunoassay

Indirect immunoassays may be used to detect antibodies in a sample that bind to a particular antigen (Fig. 1.7). Target antigen is first coated onto a solid surface. Appropriately diluted serum samples are applied to the coated antigen and any antigen specific antibodies present in the sample will bind. A wash step (e.g. 3 washes with phosphate buffered saline (PBS)) is incorporated to remove any unbound antibody and any non-specific antibody-antigen interactions. A species-specific enzyme-linked antibody is then applied, the enzyme's substrate is added, the enzyme converts the substrate into coloured or fluorescent product and the signal is measured.

For example, the indirect immunoassay has been used to detect the presence of antibody to human immunodeficiency virus (HIV) [24]. Since the 1980s, the indirect ELISA was employed to detect anti-HIV antibodies. In 2015, a modern version of the indirect immunoassay called a 'reverse-indirect' immunoassay was developed by Jeong and Ahn using DNA-encoded gold-nanoparticles

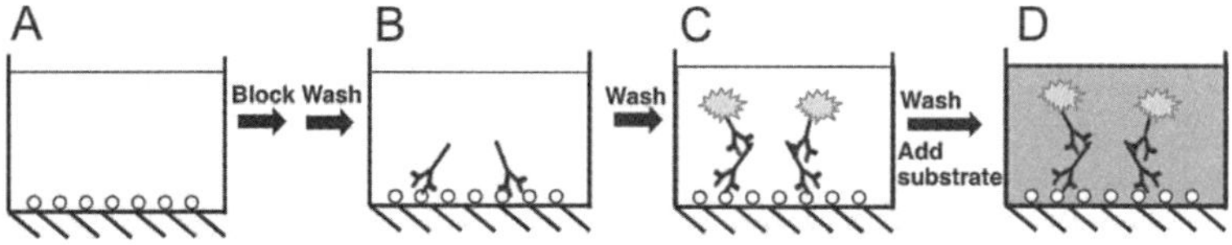

Figure 1.7 Indirect immunoassay. (A) The analyte of interest is first bound to a solid surface (e.g. to the well of a microtitre plate), followed by blocking and washing steps. (B) Serum containing the antibody of interest is diluted in a suitable buffer. This is followed by a second wash step and non-specifically bound antibodies are washed away. (C) Enzyme-labelled species-specific antibody is added to detect serum antibodies. (D) The plate is washed again, an enzyme substrate is added and a signal is generated and measured.

(GNPs) to detect multiple viral analytes [25]. Their system is called a 'gold nanoparticle-enhanced oligo-nucleotide-linked immunosorbent assay' (GNP-OLISA). DNA strands surround the GNP and bind to antigen from HIV, hepatitis C virus (HCV) and hepatitis B virus (HBV), yielding Ag-GNP-DNA particles. Spiked human serum samples (containing antibodies against HIV, HCV and HBV) were added to the multiplex assay. Meanwhile, a 96-well plate was coated with anti human-IgG and the samples were added to the wells for capture. Three different RNA fluorogenic probes were used and cleavage by RNAse H generated a fluorescent signal that was linearly proportional to the amount of antibody to the respective virus present. Nanoparticles (which will be discussed in more detail later in this chapter) were incorporated for increased screening efficiency and greater detection sensitivities.

1.3.1.3 Sandwich immunoassay

The key principle of the sandwich immunoassay is the use of an antibody that captures antigen, followed by the addition of a detection antibody that binds to a separate **epitope**. In order for efficient measurement to occur, the antigen must be large enough to contain two antigenic sites (epitopes) where each antibody has sufficient unimpeded access. It allows both the detection and the quantitation of sample analyte (Fig. 1.8) [26]. For quantification, a standard curve composed of standards of known concentration of

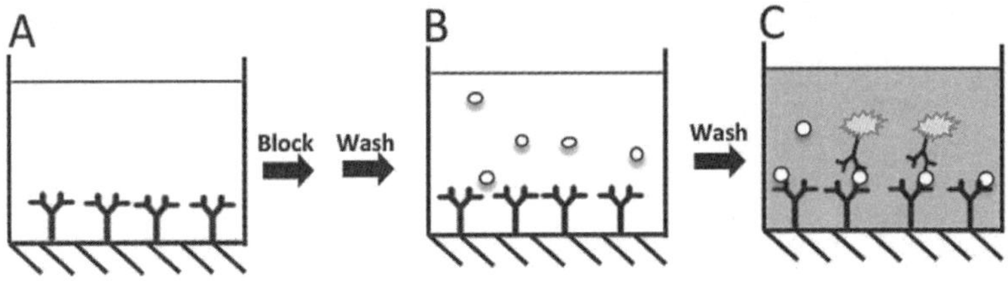

Figure 1.8 Sandwich immunoassay. (A) A capture antibody is applied and binds to the solid surface. The surface is blocked and washed to remove any non-specifically bound antibody and to prevent non-specific binding. (B) Sample analyte is applied and incubated, followed by a second wash step. (C) An enzyme-labelled specific detection antibody is introduced and a substrate is added which produces a measurable signal.

the analyte to be measured must be included. A range of at least eight analyte dilutions and a negative control should be included and each determination should be performed in triplicate.

The fundamental steps of a sandwich immunoassay include firstly, the surface immobilisation of analyte-specific antibody, followed by blocking and washing steps. The sample analyte is applied for a suitable length of time and is detected using an enzyme-linked detection antibody. If sample analyte is present, the detection antibody binds, the enzymic substrate is introduced and a signal is produced and measured.

1.3.2 Detection of Small Molecules Using a Competitive Approach

Competitive immunoassays are commonly used to measure the presence and concentration of small molecules such as drugs, hormones and toxins [27–29]. They require the use of only one specific antibody. This is beneficial, as small molecules do not have sufficient **epitopes** to facilitate binding of more than one detection antibody. Competitive assays require a '**tracer**', which is composed of the analyte in question conjugated to either a signal generating enzyme, a fluorophore, a nanoparticle or a radiolabel. Competitive assays are effective in determining cross-reactivity to other antigens. In a competitive immunoassay, the analyte competes with a pre-titrated '**tracer**' of known concentration. A competition curve is generated. The higher the concentration of analyte in the sample the lower the signal generated. Conversely, the lower the concentration of analyte the higher the signal generated, thus the intensity of signal generated is inversely proportional to the concentration of analyte present. A competitive immunoassay approach was utilised to measure the presence of a small (<1 kDa) algal-toxin molecule called microcystin-LR [30]. Due to the diminutive size of the algal-toxin a competitive immunoassay was chosen as microcystin-LR could only facilitate the binding of one specific antibody to a single epitope.

Figure 1.9 outlines the fundamental steps in a competitive immunoassay. A predefined optimised concentration of antigen is coated onto the surface of a 96-well plate and the plate is washed and blocked using appropriate blocker. Sample analyte of unknown concentration and a pre-defined amount of antibody are mixed together, incubated and added to the plate. The plate is incubated for a defined length of time. Following washing, an enzyme-conjugated secondary antibody may be added and, following the addition of chromogenic or fluorescence substrate, a signal is generated and measured [31].

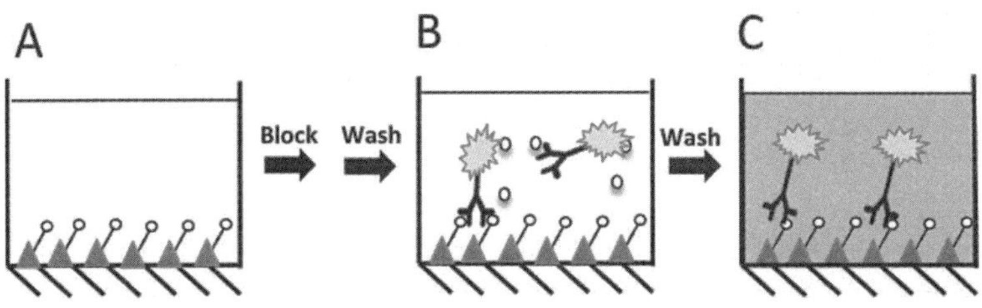

Figure 1.9 Competitive immunoassay. (A) Conjugated small molecules are applied at an optimal concentration onto a solid surface. The assay surface is blocked and washed to reduce non-specific binding. (B) A mixture of sample analyte (to be detected) and pre-titrated enzyme-labelled antibody are applied and incubated. The free analyte (small molecule) competes with surface bound analyte for antibody binding. This is followed by a second wash step. (C) Unbound antibody is washed away. The substrate for the enzyme label is added and the signal produced is measured and is inversely proportional to the concentration of analyte present.

1.4 Signal Generation in Immunoassays

Detection approaches can be divided into 'labelled' and 'label-free' signalling systems. Immunoassays that use an antibody linked to either an enzyme, fluorescent label, radiolabel, colourimetric marker or nanoparticle are classified as 'labelled' (Table 1.2 and Table 1.3).

1.4.1 Signal Generation

The first ever antibody detection systems employed the use of radiolabels [32]. Rosalyn Yalow and Solomon Aaron Berson reported the first use of radiolabels in an assay to detect insulin in the 1950s [32, 33]. The hazardous working conditions, waste disposal and potential health issues associated with working with radioactivity lead to the accelerated development of alternative detection systems. Current technologies are safer, do not pose major health risks to the user and waste generated can be disposed of with minimal inconvenience. Today, radiolabels have been substantially replaced with detection methodologies that provide high sensitivities using much safer methodologies and these will be discussed in greater detail in the following subsections.

1.4.1.1 Colourimetry as a method of immuno-detection

Colourimetry is a technique that is used to measure coloured compounds in a solution. Upon enzymatic action, chromogenic substrates produce coloured compounds. Peroxidase is a small enzyme (approximately 40 kDa), which can be used to produce a readable signal in the presence of its substrate and the oxidising agent, hydrogen peroxide. Peroxidase can be used to aid generation of both chromogenic substrates (using 3,3′,5,5′-tetramethylbenzidine (TMB) or 2,2′-azino-bis(3-ethylbenzothiazoline-6-sulphonic acid (APTS)) or light (using enhanced chemiluminescence (ECL) substrate). Peroxidase enzymes exist in many isoforms and the most commonly used in biotechnological and biochemical applications are plant peroxidases e.g. horse radish peroxidase (HRP) and soybean peroxidase (SRP). To further enhance the utility of

Table 1.2 Immunoassay signalling systems

Labels	Examples	Ref.
Radioactive labels	Iodine 125 (^{125}I); tritium (^{3}H)	[32, 33]
Enzyme labels	Alkaline phosphatase (AP); glucose oxidase; horse radish peroxidase (HRP); soybean peroxidase (SBP); glucose-6-phosphate dehydrogenase and xanthine oxidase.	[34–36]
Chemiluminescence	Acridinium sulphonamides; acridinium esters; luminol; HRP; coelenterazine; dioxetanes and peroxyoxalic acid.	[37, 38]
Enhanced chemiluminescence	HRP, in presence of its substrate H_2O_2; in the presence of enhancer molecules, phenols or naphthalines.	[38–40]
Fluorescence	Fluorescein iosothiocyanate (FITC); lanthanide cryptates; rhodamine; Texas red; semiconductor nanocrystal quantum dots; ethidium bromide and Alexa fluor dyes.	[41]
Bioluminescence	Aequorin (from Jellyfish, *Aquoria victoria*); luciferase (from firefly and sea pansy, *Renilla reniformis*)	[42–47]
Phosphorescence	Phosphors–Europium-activated yttrium oxisulphide	[48, 49]
Time-resolved fluorescence	Dissociation - Enhanced Lanthanide Fluorescent Immunoassay (DELFIA®) from Perkin Elmer. Europium (lanthanide)-conjugated antibodies or antigen in sandwich or competitive immunoassays	[50, 51]
Nano- and microparticle labels	Fluorescent quantum dots - typically 2–8 nm in size and coated in a layer of organic material to facilitate functionalisation, e.g. Quantum dots (QDS) Qdots® available from Invitrogen Hydrophilic magnetic beads (2.8 μm) coated with amine, carboxyl, epoxy or tosyl groups – e.g. Dynabeads from Invitrogen. Polystyrene latex beads – commonly used in agglutination tests. Colloidal gold nanoparticles – used for visualisation in electron microscopy, Immunoliposomes – antibody-targeted liposomes.	[52–54]
Electro-chemiluminophore	Ruthenium tris(bipyridyl)	[55]

Table 1.3 Commonly used colourimetric, fluorescent and chemiluminescent signalling reagents

	Antibody conjugate enzyme	Substrate	Signalling properties	Read-out
Enzyme-linked immunosorbent (ELISA) - colourimetric	Alkaline phosphatase (AP)	*p*-nitrophenyl phosphate disodium salt (*p*-NPP)	Hydrolysis of *p*-NPP to chromogenic *p*-nitrophenol	Absorbs at 405 nm; yellow coloured product.
	Horse radish peroxidase (HRP)	H_2O_2 coupled to 3,3′,5,5′-Tetramethylbenzidine (TMB)	Very sensitive; fast colour development; may have high background if too much analyte used.	Absorbs at 650 nm; Blue coloured product.
		H_2O_2 coupled to 2,2′-azino-bis(3-ethylbenzothiazoline-6-sulphonic acid (ABTS)	Slow colour development.	Absorbs at 410 nm and 650 nm; green coloured product.
		H_2O_2 coupled to o-phenylenediamine (OPD)	Slightly less sensitive than TMB	Absorbs at 492 nm; yellow-orange coloured product.
Fluorescence-linked immunosorbent assay (FLISA) - fluorescent	Alkaline phosphatase (AP)	4-MUP, dissolved in 0.1 to 0.2 mg ml^{-1} in 100 mM diethanolamine, 1 mM $MgCl_2$, pH 9.6 (Corning) AttoPhos® (Promega)	Fluorescence-based assays are only slightly more sensitive than colourimetric assays; however, fluorescence-based read-outs can give a wider dynamic range.	Excitation 360 nm, emission 440 nm
	β-galactosidase	4-MUG, (Corning)		Excitation 360 nm Emission 440 nm
	Peroxidase (e.g. horse radish peroxidase (HRP))	HPA and HPPA, addition of H_2O_2 is necessary (Corning)		Excitation 320 nm Emission 404 nm
		Quantiblue (Pierce)		Excitation 325 nm Emission 420 nm
		QuantaRed (Pierce)		Excitation 570 nm Emission 585 nm

(*Contd.*)

	Antibody conjugate enzyme	Substrate	Signalling properties	Read-out
Chemiluminescent ELISA	HRP	Supersignal ELISA Pico Chemiluminescent substrate (Pierce)	Full compatibility with all formats of immunoassay.	Light output should be measured
		Supersignal ELISA Femto Maximum sensitivity from Pierce		
	AP, HRP	Lumigen® from Beckman Coulter	Range of different products that will generate chemiluminescence in the presence of AP or HRP	

peroxidases in industrial settings, an interesting study was carried out by Loughran et al. The authors resurrected a 110 million year old active ancestral plant peroxidase gene called 'Grandparent' (GP). It was thought that in 110 million years of evolution, some enzymatic properties may have been lost. Loughran et al. compared the properties of GP to the existing peroxidases, HRP isoenzyme A2, HRP isoenzyme C and SBP. The results found that GP displays moderate thermal stability but exceeded the extant peroxidases in increased tolerance to H_2O_2, a desirable attribute in the biotechnological industries [56]. An advantage of using peroxidase as an enzymatic label is its small size, which rarely causes steric hindrance when conjugated to antibodies (usually at a 4:1 ratio). Its limitation lies in the fact that the peroxidase reaction requires a substrate for H_2O_2 and is incompatible with buffers that contain sodium azide or metals, as they inactivate peroxidase.

The enzyme, alkaline phosphatase (AP), is an alternative signal-producing enzymatic label. It has an approximate molecular weight of 86 kDa. Due to its larger size, care must be taken when labelling antibodies with AP, to ensure that the conjugation level does not hinder access for antigen binding. AP is more expensive than peroxidase but it is more stable. A disadvantage associated with using AP is that it is rendered inactive in acidic conditions (pH < 4.5), in chelating agents or in inorganic buffers. However, these attributes may be advantageously used as reaction stopping mechanisms. The substrates of AP are non-toxic and relatively stable, for example *p*-nitrophenyl phosphate (PNPP) is stable for months at 4°C (Table 1.3).

1.4.1.2 Luminescence as a method of immuno-detection

Luminescence refers to the release of energy from an electronically excited molecule in the form of visible light. When the excited molecule returns to the ground state it releases a photon of light. The 'catch-all' title of luminescence covers a range of detection systems, including chemiluminescence, phosphorescence, bioluminescence and fluorescence.

1.4.1.2.1 *Chemiluminescence*

Chemiluminescence refers to the release of energy from chemical reactions in the form of light and does not require a light source for excitation (unlike fluorescence) [44]. The photons generated from luminescent compounds can be triggered in a very short period of time and the sensitivity reached can be higher than that achieved with conventional labelling [37, 57]. Examples of chemical labels were previously given in Table 1.3 [37, 58].

Two methods can be chosen: (i) using a chemically labelled substrate which converts to a chemiluminescent product, (ii) using a chemiluminescent molecule directly attached to the antibody. The labelling of a ligand (e.g. an antibody) with an enzyme that generates chemiluminescence is frequently used as it can initiate multiple chemiluminescent reactions making the reaction highly sensitive. Alternatively, the chemiluminescent compound can be covalently labelled to one of the complementary binding partners. This is a straightforward approach, however, not many chemiluminescent tags exist and there is usually limited surface space on the antibody to fit multiple tags.

Advantages of chemiluminescent detections systems include, fast emission of light, wide dynamic range, high stability of reagents and low consumption of expensive reagents, short incubation times, high sensitivity, elimination of background effects and low toxicity [58, 59].

1.4.1.2.2 *Bioluminescence, a natural form of signal generation*

Bioluminescence refers to the phenomena whereby biological reactions produce light [42]. Bioluminescence has often proven advantageous when used in immunoassays due to its unique properties, since unlike fluorescence, there is virtually no associated background, and it has a high quantum yield and rapid kinetics of reaction [44].

Many bright photoproteins have been discovered in the darkest places. Aqueorin was originally found in the jellyfish *Aequoria victoria* [43] and is a stable complex composed of an apoprotein (apoaequorin), a chromophore (coelenterazine) and molecular oxygen [60]. Recombinant aequorin has successfully been used in immunoassays to detect the hormone cortisol [61]. Recombinant aequorin is chemically conjugated to cortisol at different molar ratios, and the resulting conjugates are assessed for the highest level of bioluminescence [61]. The development of a chimeric antibody incorporating aequorin has also been shown to be useful. The apoaequorin gene was sub-cloned into a mammalian expression vector and the constant domain of the antibody replaced by the photoprotein. This method is more reliable than chemically linking the photoprotein to the antibody as chemical modifications can often lead to 'batch-to-batch' variations or loss of antibody binding activity [45]. When aequorin was first discovered in 1962, Shimomura et al. simultaneously discovered a second protein that has also become a fundamental bioimaging tool [43]. Green fluorescence protein (GFP) has been frequently used as a genetically encoded fluorescence marker. The fluorescence protein (FP) family has expanded to over 1000 variant forms, each exhibiting different excitation and emission wavelengths, thus, all displaying different colours (e.g. monomeric Orange (mOrange) (excitation 548 nm/emission 562 nm) to mRuby (ex. 558 nm/em. 605 nm)). A review by Nienhaus and colleagues contains a selection of some of the most widely used FPs [62].

1.4.1.2.3 *Fluorescence, a widely used method of immunoassay signal generation*

Fluorescence is a phenomenon that occurs when electromagnetic energy (a photon of light) is absorbed by a substance, thus activating its electrons and elevating them into higher energy states. The return to ground state energy causes the release of energy in the form of light, called fluorescence. Fluorescence only occurs for as long as the substance is absorbing light, however, the fluorescent molecule can be excited again, thus continuing the cycle. Emitted fluorescence occurs at a longer wavelength than the wavelength for excitation and the change in wavelength is referred to as the 'Stokes shift'. This change in wavelength occurs due to a loss of energy between the excitation of the electron and the release of the energy as fluorescence. The degree of 'Stokes shift' depends on the inherent electronic structure of the fluorophore.

A fluorophore is excited over a range of wavelengths. The wavelength at which the molecule is excited most optimally is called the excitation maximum. Likewise, the fluorophore emits fluorescence over a range of wavelengths. The emission maximum is the wavelength at which the fluorophore emits light (fluorescence) most intensely. Since the fluorophores absorb and emit over a range of wavelengths, it is important to choose two fluorophores with distinct excitation and emission peaks, so that they do not overlap and can be detected individually.

Fluorescent molecules can be used in fluorescence immunoassays as an alternative to colourimetric readouts. Fluorescent substrates can be utilised in place of TMB or PNPP as substrates for AP, β-galactosidase and HRP detection enzymes (previously listed in Table 1.3). The production of a fluorescent signal is influenced by many different parameters including pH, temperature, ion concentration, drying, light scattering, quenching and bleaching, and all must be accounted for during experimentation [63, 64].

1.4.2 Nanomaterials, for Signal Generation and Immobilisation

Nano-sized entities (between 1–100 nanometers) are becoming increasingly prevalent in immunoassays for use in both detection and immobilisation. They permit very low levels of detection, and are increasingly being utilised in 'point-of-care' diagnostics.

Quantum dots (QDs) are fluorescent nanostructures composed of semiconducting materials that are now being used in a wide range of biological imaging techniques [65–67]. They were first discovered in 1980 by Ekimov and Onushchenko who found that QDs could produce a range of fluorescence signals based on their size [68]. Currently, QDs can be classified into three different categories based on their composition. The first, 'core-type' QDs are composed of a single material e.g. cadmium selenide (CdSe) or cadmium sulphide (CdS) [69]. Secondly, 'core-shell' QDs are composed of two semiconducting materials, one 'core' material embedded within a 'shell' material (Fig. 1.10). These 'core-shell' QDs display improved brightness and quantum-yields over 'core-type'

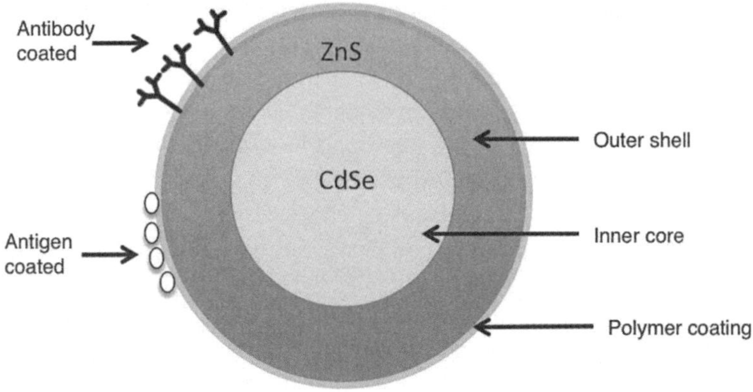

Figure 1.10 Quantum dot (QD) structure displaying inner core and outer shell. Inner core materials that can be used in QDs include zinc sulphide (ZnS), cadmium sulphide (CdS), zinc selenide (ZnSe), cadmium telluride (CdTe), lead sulphide (PbS), PbSe/Te and CdSe/Te and cadmium mercury/tellurium (CdHg/Te) alloys. The outer core is usually ZnS. The QD is surrounded by a polymer coating which increases water solubility and facilitates binding of antibody/antigen.

QDs. Finally, the third type of QD is the 'alloy' QD, composed of zinc selenium-cadmium selenide (ZnSe-CdSe). Alloy QDs are unique, as their fluorescence properties can be altered without changing the size of the QD. The change in the ratio of alloy components facilitates the change in colour [69]. QDs have become a new resource in the field of disease detection and diagnosis and have been used in many biological assays such as fluorescence resonance energy transfer (FRET)-based sensing, cellular imaging and immunoassays [66, 70–72].

Numerous QD attributes have been identified to differentiate them from fluorescent organic dyes or protein fluorophores [73]. These include:

- wide excitation spectra
- narrow-size-tunable photo-luminescent emission spectra
- large Stokes shifts
- high quantum yields
- increased photostability (over fluorescent dyes)
- highly suitable to multicolour applications

- distinct populations of QDs can be excited by a single excitation wavelength
- higher resistance to **photobleaching** under continuous illumination

Gold nanoparticles (AuNPs or GNPs), have increased in popularity due to their stability over long periods of time. Their inherently high electron densities renders them easily detectable by a wide range analytical technologies, e.g. atomic force microscopy (ATM), Fourier transform infrared spectroscopy (FT-IR) and scanning electron microscopy (SEM). Depending on their size, AuNPs produce different colours; if less than 100 nm, AuNPs are red, while greater than 100 nm, AuNPs are yellowish in colour [74]. AuNPs non-covalently linked to antibodies, have been successfully integrated into lateral flow immunoassays, due to their robust nature, stability and ability to produce an intense colour [74].

Carbon nanotubes (CNTs) are cylinders of carbon composed of one (single walled nanotubes (SWNT)) or more layers of graphene (multiwall nanotubes (MWNT)) [75]. Increasingly, CNTs are being used for industrial applications displaying up to 10-fold greater tensile strength than typical industrial fibres. CNTs can be metallic or semiconducting in nature [76] and can act as antibody supports. Wan and colleagues have exploited their potential use as immunosensing labels as well as availing of their signal transducing capabilities [77]. A universal MWNT, covalently coated in HRP and goat anti-rabbit, was used as a universal electrochemical-based detector for the presence of cancer markers, prostate specific antigen (PSA) and interleukin-8 (IL-8). The system provided the detection of very low levels of PSA and IL-8 (5 pg mL^{-1} and 8 pg mL^{-1}, respectively). However, the numerous steps involved rendered it quite labour intensive.

1.5 Next Generation Signal Transduction Systems

In a concerted effort to simplify detection mechanisms, shorten assay times, reduce the number of assay steps and to facilitate multiplexing of immunoassays, signal transduction methods employing electrochemical, mechanical and optical mechanisms have increased in popularity. The following section will investigate these signal transduction mechanisms in more detail.

1.5.1 Electrochemical Transducers for Immunoassay Applications

Electrochemical transducers are an integral part of immunoassay signalling, hence, Chapter 10 of this book is dedicated solely to this important area. In short, electrochemistry relates to the production of an electric current during a chemical reaction. The most common type of electrochemical reaction used in biotechnology is the reduction/oxidation reaction or redox reaction, during which electrons are transferred between two interacting species. Electrochemical techniques are often employed for use in coloured and turbid media [78, 79]. Additional advantages that apply to electrochemical immunoassay transducers are the high sensitivities that can be achieved and the instruments used for measurement are relatively inexpensive. Electrochemical immunosensors generally have low power requirements and are capable of being incorporated into automated detection platforms [78]. Examples of **amperometric**, **potentiometric**, electrochemical impedance spectroscopy (EIS) and **magnetoresistance** sensing technologies and are discussed further in Chapter 10 of this book.

1.5.2 Nanomechanical Sensors/Piezoelectric Mass Sensors

Nanomechanical transducers detect changes in mass, pressure or resonance frequency. Nanomechanical immunosensors differ from traditional fluorescence-based immuno-detection systems in that they do not require labelling of analytes or antibodies [80]. These sensors have been used to measure a range of analytes such as bacteria, viruses, oligonucleotides, disease markers and inflammatory mediators such as prostate specific antigen (PSA) and interleukins [81, 82].

The piezoelectric effect was first described by Jacques and Pierre Curie in 1880. The term is derived from the Greek word *piezein* meaning to press [83]. When a voltage is applied across a piezoelectric quartz crystal (SiO_2), it induces stress in the material and the quartz undergoes a change in volume, conversely, when the quartz undergoes a change in volume it generates a voltage [83, 84]. Piezoelectricity facilitates the 'label-free' detection of analytes at a surface by measuring a change in mass, and, in the case of immuno-sensing, a change in mass is observed when an analyte binds to an antibody or an antibody binds to immobilised antigen [85]. Two different types of acoustic sensor have been developed, a bulk acoustic wave (BAW) device and a surface acoustic wave (SAW) device and these will be discussed further in the next two sections.

Bulk acoustic wave (BAW) devices or quartz crystal microbalances (QCMs) can be used for the 'label-free' detection of analytes. A BAW device consists of a thin layer of quartz crystal embedded between two electrodes. The quartz crystal produces a characteristic resonant frequency when an alternating current (AC) is applied; this frequency is based on the total oscillating mass of the quartz crystal, and changes when a biomolecule attaches. Comprehensive reviews of the fundamental principles of quartz crystal microbalances and their uses in biological detection have been published by Ferreria et al. and more recently by Ferrier et al. [84, 85]; in addition, the applications of quartz microbalances have been extensively described [86–88]. A study by Seo and colleagues described the use of a novel QCM immunosensor for the detection of alpha-fetoprotein (AFP) developed using TiO_2 nanoparticle-based immunoassay incorporating a silver enhancement reaction [80]. Their system used a sandwich-immunoassay format. The quartz crystal was immobilised with anti-AFP antibody, AFP was added and bound to the antibody, a second anti-AFP antibody conjugated to TiO_2 was then added and bound. A silver enhancement reaction was subsequently carried out; the complex was photo-irradiated (exposed to UV light) in the presence of silver nitrate ($AgNO_3$). Silver (Ag) molecules bound to titanium oxide (TiO_2), and enhanced the mass of the complex by three orders of magnitude, thus making the variations in the resonant frequency of the quartz crystals easier to observe (measured using a QCM200, Stanford Research Systems Sunnyvale CA, USA) [80].

Surface acoustic waves sensors (SAWS) exploit the piezoelectric properties of certain crystalline materials e.g. quartz (SiO_2), lithium niobate ($LiNbO_3$) or lithium tantalate ($LiTaO_3$). SAWS detect changes in mass along the surface of the crystal. Interdigitated electrodes (IDEs) on the surface of the crystal generate acoustic waves, which travel parallel to the surface and are sensitive to changing mass. SAWS have been easily incorporated into **'point-of-care'** (POC) or **microfluidic** devices. Lee and colleagues developed a microfluidic CD device encasing whole blood, wash buffer and assay reagents in a microfluidic compact disc (CD) [89].

The main advantages of acoustic wave sensors is their 'label-free' capabilities, fast assay times ($<$10 min), high sensitivities and the ability to perform assays in turbid and coloured solutions with little pre-assay clean-up required, making them highly applicable to 'real-time', POC in-vitro diagnostics [90]. Lee and colleagues also developed a POC device that uses SAWS to detect the presence of cardiac disease markers cardiac troponin I (cTnI), creatine kinase-MB and myoglobin [89] below the clinical 'cut-off' level required. The SAW relied on changes in mass to generate its signal, however, this rendered it susceptible to changes in density and viscosity of the sample medium. Another limitation to SAW sensing is sensitivity to temperature and mechanical stress, which need to be controlled during experiments [84].

Cantilevers can be manufactured at micro- or nano-scale depending on the requirements of the detection system [91]. The first cantilevers were 'deflection' or 'static' mode cantilevers. They operate on the basis that the cantilever physically bends upon the binding of an analyte to an antibody [92–95]. These were followed by the introduction of 'resonant' or 'dynamic' mode cantilevers, which operate by generating an oscillating signal [96–98]. Both are efficient at measuring the presence of molecules in solution and in air, thus, making them applicable to both biological (e.g. proteins, viruses, bacteria, small molecules and gases) and environmental sensing (e.g. temperature and pH) [84]. Micro-cantilevers are usually made of 1 μm thick rectangular silicon sheets that are anchored at one end. Upon binding of specific sample analyte to an immobilised antibody (or similar binding molecule e.g. cDNA for oligonucleotide detection), a surface stress is imposed on the micro-cantilever, causing it to bend. Deflection of a laser beam detects the bending cantilever. Advantages of micro-cantilevers include their 'label-free' configurations, 'ease-of-functionalisation', 'low-cost', 'ease-of-detection', their potential for miniaturisation and multiplexing. Some drawbacks that arise during the use of cantilever-based sensors include their sensitivity to temperature and changes in refractive index as well as sensitivity to the flow of fluid in the sample medium [99]. Micro-cantilevers have been successfully applied to the detection of tumour markers e.g. angiopoietin-1, a potential marker for tumour progression and to detect small molecules such as mycotoxins [100, 101].

1.5.3 Optical Signal Transduction

Optical biosensors utilise light properties such as **refraction**, production of **evanescent waves** and **reflection**, and measure changes in these properties during biomolecular interactions.

Optical signalling methodologies including a focus on surface plasmon resonance are discussed in Chapter 11 of this book.

1.6 Conclusions and Key Issues

The myriad of immunosensing possibilities presented in this chapter are just a taste of the sensing capabilities that are on offer today. Firstly, the type of antibody for a particular application must be taken into account, and, due to their 'ease-of-manipulation' and capacity for sensitivity improvement, renders recombinant antibodies increasingly attractive.

The strategy used for the immobilisation of antibodies is crucial to maximise stability, enhance sensitivity by ensuring antibodies are correctly orientated and available for binding and to maximise reproducibility. This will be investigated in greater detail in Chapter 3 of this book.

It is also clear that 'label-free' immunosensing has become an important element in analyte monitoring. Despite the technologies available, there are still the fundamental issues of sensitivity, 'signal-to-noise' ratios and aggregation that afflict solid surfaces in use today. The elimination of non-specific binding is key to optimum performance and must be carefully controlled in complex matrices.

Ultimately, a system that requires little pre-assay preparation, is fully integrated, with the ability to multiplex, can be carried out in situ with minimum user intervention, and is affordable will always be the gold standard in immunosensing. 'Lab-on-a-chip' immunoassay systems are currently revolutionising diagnostics with both fluorescence and colourimetric-based detection systems but also with cantilever-based approaches. They facilitate the combination and reduction of assay steps, reagents are encased within the system (which addresses safety issues) and the microfluidics allows the reduction of assay reagent volumes required to complete a test. 'Lab-on-a-chip' can permit the analysis of a number of different analytes in parallel. More information on 'lab-on-a-chip' technology will be addressed in greater detail in Chapter 5 of this book.

Immunoassays should not solely be chosen based on analytical sensitivity, but must address the detection requirements for each situation. For example, an immunoassay may need to generate quantitative data or generate a simple yes/no read-out. The question should also be asked, can multi-component analysis be integrated into the system, as this will greatly increase the value of the immunoassay.

Finally, the translation from laboratory to commercially available systems is an important step and must be pursued so that detection systems can be distributed and used to address global monitoring issues e.g. in remote and resource-limited locations.

Acknowledgments

The authors would like to acknowledge the support of Dublin City University and the Biomedical Diagnostics Institute, Science Foundation Ireland (through grants 08/US/I1512, 10/CE/B1821 and 14/IA/2646), and The Irish Cancer Society Programme grant (PCI11WAT) as part of the Prostate Cancer Research Consortium, Dublin, Ireland.

References

1. Finlay, W.J.J., and J.C. Almagro, Natural and man-made V-gene repertoires for antibody discovery. *Front Immunol*, 2012. **3**.
2. Conroy, P.J., et al., Reconciling the structural attributes of avian antibodies. *J Biol Chem*, 2014. **289**(22):15384–15392.
3. Leenaars, M., and C.F. Hendriksen, Critical steps in the production of polyclonal and monoclonal antibodies: evaluation and recommendations. *ILAR J*, 2005. **46**(3):269–279.
4. Zhu, K., et al., Recent developments in antibody-based assays for the detection of bacterial toxins. *Toxins (Basel)*, 2014. **6**(4):1325–1348.
5. Howard, G.C., and M.R. Kaser, eds. *Making and Using Antibodies: A Practical Handbook*. 2nd. 2013, CRC Press: Florida.
6. Andris-Widhopf, J., et al., Methods for the generation of chicken monoclonal antibody fragments by phage display. *J Immunol Methods*, 2000. **242**:159–181.
7. International Chicken Genome Sequencing Consortium, Sequence and comparative analysis of the chicken genome provide unique perspectives on vertebrate evolution. *Nature*, 2004. **432**(7018):695–716.
8. Narat, M., Production of antibodies in chickens. *Food Technol Biotechnol*, 2003. **41**(3):259–267.
9. Kohler, G., and C. Milstein, Continuous cultures of fused cells secreting antibody of predefined specificity. *Nature*, 1975. **256**(5517): 495–497.
10. Conroy, P.J., et al., Antibody production, design and use for biosensor-based applications. *Semin Cell Dev Biol*, 2009. **20**(1):10–26.
11. Hayes, C.J., P. Leonard, and R. O'Kennedy, Overcoming antibody expression and screening limitations by smart design: applications to PSA immunoassay development. *Protein Expr Purif*, 2012. **83**(1):84–91.
12. Hudson, P.J., Recombinant antibody fragments. *Curr Opin Biotechnol*, 1998. **9**(4):395–402.
13. Holliger, P., and P.J. Hudson, Engineered antibody fragments and the rise of single domains. *Nat Biotechnol*, 2005. **23**(9):1126–1136.
14. Barbas, C.F., et al., *Phage Display: A Laboratory Manual*. 2001, Cold Spring Harbour, New York: Cold Spring Harbour Press.

15. Joosten, V., et al., The production of antibody fragments and antibody fusion proteins by yeasts and filamentous fungi. *Microb Cell Fact*, 2003. **2**:1–15.
16. Hayhurst, A., et al., Isolation and expression of recombinant antibody fragments to the biological warfare pathogen *Brucella melitensis*. *J Immunol Methods*, 2003. **276**(1–2):185–196.
17. Birtalan, S., et al., The intrinsic contributions of tyrosine, serine, glycine and arginine to the affinity and specificity of antibodies. *J Mol Biol*, 2008. **377**(5):1518–1528.
18. Muller, B.H., et al., In vitro affinity maturation of an anti-PSA antibody for prostate cancer diagnostic assay. *J Mol Biol*, 2011. **414**(4):545–562.
19. Smith, G.P., Filamentous fusion phage: novel expression vectors that display cloned antigens on the virion surface. *Science*, 1985. **228**(4705):1315–1317.
20. McCafferty, J., et al., Phage antibodies: filamentous phage displaying antibody variable domains. *Nature*, 1990. **348**(6301):552–554.
21. Hoogenboom, H.R., Selecting and screening recombinant antibody libraries. *Nat Biotech*, 2005. **23**(9):1105–1116.
22. Bradbury, A.R.M., et al., Beyond natural antibodies: the power of in vitro display technologies. *Nat Biotech*, 2011. **29**(3):245–254.
23. Bradbury, A.R., and J.D. Marks, Antibodies from phage antibody libraries. *J Immunol Methods*, 2004. **290**(1–2):29–49.
24. Nuwayhid, N.F., Laboratory tests for detection of human immunodeficiency virus type 1 infection. *Clin Diagn Lab Immunol*, 1995. **2**(6):637–645.
25. Jeong, M.S., and D.R. Ahn, A microwell plate-based multiplex immunoassay for simultaneous quantitation of antibodies to infectious viruses. *Analyst*, 2015. **140**(6):1995–2000.
26. Abcam. Available from: http://www.abcam.com.
27. Byrne, B., et al., Antibody-based sensors: principles, problems and potential for detection of pathogens and associated toxins. *Sensors (Basel)*, 2009. **9**(6):4407–4445.
28. Uraipong, C., V. Wong, and N.A. Lee, A testosterone-specific competitive enzyme immunoassay for monitoring water quality. *Bull Environ Contam Toxicol*, 2013. **90**(5):585–590.
29. Czeh, A., et al., A flow cytometry-based competitive fluorescent microsphere immunoassay (CFIA) system for detecting up to six mycotoxins. *J Immunol Methods*, 2012. **384**(1–2):71–80.

30. Murphy, C., et al., Detection of the cyanobacterial toxin, microcystin-LR, using a novel recombinant antibody-based optical-planar waveguide platform. *Biosens Bioelectron*, 2015. **67**:708–714.
31. Gan, S.D., and K.R. Patel, Enzyme immunoassay and enzyme-linked immunosorbent assay. *J Invest Dermatol*, 2013. **133**(9):e12.
32. Yalow, R.S., and S.A. Berson, Assay of plasma insulin in human subjects by immunological methods. *Nature*, 1959. **184**(Suppl 21):1648–1649.
33. Yalow, R.S., and S.A. Berson, Immunoassay of endogenous plasma insulin in man. *J Clin Invest*, 1960. **39**:1157–1175.
34. Kuznetsov, et al., On applicability of laccase as label in the mediated and mediatorless electroimmunoassay: effect of distance on the direct electron transfer between laccase and electrode. *Biosens Bioelectron*, 2001. **16**(1–2):73–84.
35. Du, D., et al., Immunological assay for carbohydrate antigen 19-9 using an electrochemical immunosensor and antigen immobilization in titania sol-gel matrix. *J Immunol Methods*, 2003. **283**(1–2):67–75.
36. Liu, Y., and Y. Li, An antibody-immobilized capillary column as a bioseparator/bioreactor for detection of *Escherichia coil* O157:H7 with absorbance measurement. *Anal Chem*, 2001. **73**(21):5180–5183.
37. Dodeigne, C., L. Thunus, and R. Lejeune, Chemiluminescence as a diagnostic tool. A review. *Talanta*, 2000. **51**(3):415–439.
38. Kricka, L.J., G.H.G. Thorpe, and R.A.W. Stott, Enhanced Chemiluminescence Enzyme-Immunoassay. *Pure Appl Chem*, 1987. **59**(5):651–654.
39. Alegria-Schaffer, A., A. Lodge, and K. Vattem, Performing and optimizing Western blots with an emphasis on chemiluminescent detection. *Methods Enzymol*, 2009. **463**:573–599.
40. Kamidate, T., et al., Application of 4-iodophenol-enhanced luminol chemiluminescence to direct detection of horseradish peroxidase encapsulated in liposomes. *Anal Sci*, 2009. **25**(9):1163–1166.
41. Hicks, J.M., Fluorescence immunoassay. *Hum Pathol*, 1984. **15**(2):112–116.
42. Shim, Y.N., and I.R. Paeng, Development of bioluminescence immunoassay using photoprotein, aequorin and site-directed immobilization. *Bull Korean Chem Soc*, 2003. **24**(1):70–74.
43. Shimomura, O., F.H. Johnson, and Y. Saiga, Extraction, purification and properties of aequorin, a bioluminescent protein from the luminous hydromedusan, Aequorea. *J Cell Comp Physiol*, 1962. **59**(3):223–239.

44. Roda, A., et al., Biotechnological applications of bioluminescence and chemiluminescence. *Trends Biotechnol*, 2004. **22**(6):295–303.
45. Casadei, J., M.J. Powell, and J.H. Kenten, Expression and secretion of aequorin as a chimeric antibody by means of a mammalian expression vector. *Proc Natl Acad Sci USA*, 1990. **87**(6):2047–2051.
46. Naylor, L.H., Reporter gene technology: The future looks bright. *Biochem Pharmacol*, 1999. **58**(5):749–757.
47. Alam, J., and J.L. Cook, Reporter genes: Application to the study of mammalian gene transcription. *Anal Biochem*, 1990. **188**(2):245–254.
48. Jia-Ming, L., et al., Determination of human IgG by solid substrate room temperature phosphorescence immunoassay based on an antibody labeled with nanoparticles containing Rhodamine 6G luminescent molecules. *Spectrochim Acta A Mol Biol Spectrosc*, 2005. **61**(5):923–927.
49. Goldman, E.R., et al., Conjugation of luminescent quantum dots with antibodies using an engineered adaptor protein to provide new reagents for fluoroimmunoassays. *Anal Chem*, 2002. **74**(4):841–847.
50. Maple, P.A., et al., Performance of a time-resolved fluorescence immunoassay for measuring varicella-zoster virus immunoglobulin G levels in adults and comparison with commercial enzyme immunoassays and Merck glycoprotein enzyme immunoassay. *Clin Vaccine Immunol*, 2006. **13**(2):214–218.
51. Maple, P.A.C., C.S. Jones, and N.J. Andrews, Time resolved fluorometric immunoassay, using Europium labelled antihuman IgG, for the detection of human tetanus antitoxin in serum. *J Clin Pathol*, 2001. **54**(10):812–815.
52. Tully, E., et al., The development of rapid fluorescence-based immunoassays, using quantum dot-labelled antibodies for the detection of *Listeria monocytogenes* cell surface proteins. *Int J Biol Macromol*, 2006. **39**(1–3):127–134.
53. Kozlowska, D., et al., Molecular and magnetic resonance imaging: The value of immunoliposomes. *Adv Drug Deliv Rev*, 2009. **61**(15):1402–1411.
54. Xing, Y., et al., Bioconjugated quantum dots for multiplexed and quantitative immunohistochemistry. *Nat Protoc*, 2007. **2**(5):1152–1165.

55. Doeven, E.H., et al., Selective excitation of concomitant electrochemiluminophores: tuning emission color by electrode potential. *Angew Chem Int Ed Engl*, 2012. **51**(18):4354–4357.
56. Loughran, N.B., et al., Stability properties of an ancient plant peroxidase. *Biochimie*, 2014. **104**:156–159.
57. Girotti, S., et al., Trace analysis of pollutants by use of honeybees, immunoassays, and chemiluminescence detection. *Anal Bioanal Chem*, 2013. **405**(2–3):555–571.
58. Rongen, H.A.H., et al., Chemiluminescence and immunoassays. *J Pharm Biomed Anal*, 1994. **12**(4):433–462.
59. Bi, S., H. Zhou, and S. Zhang, Multilayers enzyme-coated carbon nanotubes as biolabel for ultrasensitive chemiluminescence immunoassay of cancer biomarker. *Biosens Bioelectron*, 2009. **24**(10):2961–2966.
60. Ohmiya, Y., and T. Hirano, Shining the light: The mechanism of the bioluminescence reaction of calcium-binding photoproteins. *Chem Biol*, 1996. **3**(5):337–347.
61. Mirasoli, M., et al., Bioluminescence immunoassay for cortisol using recombinant aequorin as a label. *Anal Biochem*, 2002. **306**(2):204–211.
62. Nienhaus, K., and G.U. Nienhaus, Fluorescent proteins for live-cell imaging with super-resolution. *Chem Soc Rev*, 2014. **43**(4):1088–1106.
63. Brand, L., and M.L. Johnson, eds. Fluorescence spectroscopy. *Methods Enzymol*. Vol. 480. 2008, Academic Press.
64. Albani, J.R., ed. *Principles and Applications of Fluorescence Spectroscopy*. 2007, Wiley-Blackwell.
65. Bruchez, M., Jr., et al., Semiconductor nanocrystals as fluorescent biological labels. *Science*, 1998. **281**(5385):2013–2016.
66. Medintz, I.L., et al., Quantum dot bioconjugates for imaging, labelling and sensing. *Nat Mater*, 2005. **4**(6):435–446.
67. Smith, A.M., and S. Nie, Next-generation quantum dots. *Nat Biotechnol*, 2009. **27**(8):732–733.
68. Ekimov, A.I., and A.A. Onushchenko, Quantum size effect in three-dimensional microscopic semiconductor crystals. *JETP Letters*, 1981. **34**(6):345–349.
69. Groeneveld, E., et al., Tailoring ZnSe-CdSe colloidal quantum dots via cation exchange: from core/shell to alloy nanocrystals. *ACS Nano*, 2013. **7**(9):7913–7930.

70. Michalet, X., et al., Quantum dots for live cells, in vivo imaging, and diagnostics. *Science*, 2005. **307**(5709):538–544.

71. Xing, Y., and J. Rao, Quantum dot bioconjugates for in vitro diagnostics & in vivo imaging. *Cancer Biomark*, 2008. **4**(6):307–319.

72. Jamieson, T., et al., Biological applications of quantum dots. *Biomaterials*, 2007. **28**(31):4717–4732.

73. Goldman, E.R., I.L. Medintz, and H. Mattoussi, Luminescent quantum dots in immunoassays. *Anal Bioanal Chem*, 2006. **384**(3):560–563.

74. Omidfar, K., F. Khorsand, and M. Darziani Azizi, New analytical applications of gold nanoparticles as label in antibody-based sensors. *Biosens Bioelectron*, 2013. **43**:336–347.

75. De Volder, M.F.L., et al., Carbon nanotubes: present and future commercial applications. *Science*, 2013. **339**(6119):535–539.

76. Kurkina, T., and K. Balasubramanian, Towards in vitro molecular diagnostics using nanostructures. *Cell Mol Life Sci*, 2012. **69**(3):373–388.

77. Wan, Y., et al., Carbon nanotube-based ultrasensitive multiplexing electrochemical immunosensor for cancer biomarkers. *Biosens Bioelectron*, 2011. **30**(1):93–99.

78. Ghindilis, A.L., et al., Immunosensors: electrochemical sensing and other engineering approaches. *Biosens Bioelectron*, 1998. **13**(1):113–131.

79. Sharma, M.K., et al., Highly sensitive amperometric immunosensor for detection of *Plasmodium falciparum* histidine-rich protein 2 in serum of humans with malaria: comparison with a commercial kit. *J Clin Microbiol*, 2008. **46**(11):3759–3765.

80. Seo, H., et al., Photocatalytic silver enhancement reaction for gravimetric immunosensors. *Nanotechnology*, 2010. **21**(50):505502.

81. Uludag, Y., and I.E. Tothill, Cancer biomarker detection in serum samples using surface plasmon resonance and quartz crystal microbalance sensors with nanoparticle signal amplification. *Anal Chem*, 2012. **84**(14):5898–5904.

82. Godber, B., et al., Direct quantification of analyte concentration by resonant acoustic profiling. *Clin Chem*, 2005. **51**(10):1962–1972.

83. Ward, M.D., and D.A. Buttry, In situ interfacial mass detection with piezoelectric transducers. *Science*, 1990. **249**(4972):1000–1007.

84. Ferrier, D.C., M.P. Shaver, and P.J. Hands, Micro and nano structure-based oligonucleotide sensors. *Biosens Bioelectron*, 2015. **68**:798–810.

85. Ferreira, G.N., A.C. da-Silva, and B. Tome, Acoustic wave biosensors: physical models and biological applications of quartz crystal microbalance. *Trends Biotechnol*, 2009. **27**(12):689–697.
86. Becker, B., and M.A. Cooper, A survey of the 2006–2009 quartz crystal microbalance biosensor literature. *J Mol Recognit*, 2011. **24**(5):754–787.
87. Cooper, M.A., and V.T. Singleton, A survey of the 2001 to 2005 quartz crystal microbalance biosensor literature: applications of acoustic physics to the analysis of biomolecular interactions. *J Mol Recognit*, 2007. **20**(3):154–184.
88. Speight, R.E., and M.A. Cooper, A survey of the 2010 quartz crystal microbalance literature. *J Mol Recognit*, 2012. **25**(9):451–473.
89. Lee, W., et al., A centrifugally actuated point-of-care testing system for the surface acoustic wave immunosensing of cardiac troponin I. *Analyst*, 2013. **138**(9):2558–2566.
90. Arruda, D.L., et al., Microelectrical sensors as emerging platforms for protein biomarker detection in point-of-care diagnostics. *Expert Rev Mol Diagn*, 2009. **9**(7):749–755.
91. Lang, H.P., M. Hegner, and C. Cerber, Cantilever array sensors. *Mater Today*, 2005. **8**:30–36.
92. Fritz, J., Cantilever biosensors. *Analyst*, 2008. **133**(7):855–863.
93. Hansen, K.M., and T. Thundat, Microcantilever biosensors. *Methods*, 2005. **37**(1):57–64.
94. Hwang, K.S., et al., Micro- and nanocantilever devices and systems for biomolecule detection. *Annu Rev Anal Chem (Palo Alto Calif)*, 2009. **2**:77–98.
95. Ziegler, C., Cantilever-based biosensors. *Anal Bioanal Chem*, 2004. **379**(7–8):946–959.
96. Lange, D., et al., Complementary metal oxide semiconductor cantilever arrays on a single chip: mass-sensitive detection of volatile organic compounds. *Anal Chem*, 2002. **74**(13):3084–3095.
97. Ilic, B., et al., Mechanical resonant immunospecific biological detector. *Appl Phys Lett*, 2000. **77**(3):450–452.
98. Ilic, B., et al., Enumeration of DNA molecules bound to a nanomechanical oscillator. *Nano Lett*, 2005. **5**(5):925–929.
99. Arlett, J.L., E.B. Myers, and M.L. Roukes, Comparative advantages of mechanical biosensors. *Nat Nanotechnol*, 2011. **6**(4):203–215.

100. Ricciardi, C., et al., Development of a microcantilever-based immunosensing method for mycotoxin detection. *Biosens Bioelectron*, 2013. **40**(1):233–239.

101. Ricciardi, C., et al., Development of microcantilever-based biosensor array to detect angiopoietin-1, a marker of tumor angiogenesis. *Biosens Bioelectron*, 2010. **25**(5):1193–1198.

Chapter 2

Recombinant Antibodies for Diagnostic Applications: Design Considerations and Structural Correlates

Stephen Hearty and Richard O'Kennedy

Biomedical Diagnostics Institute, Dublin City University, Collins Avenue, Dublin 9, Ireland

stephen.hearty@gmail.com

The range of analytes that require monitoring in the modern age is ever increasing and can range from very discrete small molecules (haptens) to larger macromolecules and even whole cells. Instrumentation capable of efficiently processing sample material and reporting biophysical metrics is now widely available and this has facilitated automation, miniaturisation and improved throughput of many analytical platforms. Irrespective of the technology platform, the analyte recognition element can often be the most crucial performance differentiator. Antibodies are ubiquitous (bio)recognition molecules that have proven their efficacy repeatedly against a huge variety of challenging analytes. Dependence on antibodies remains a key paradigm in diagnostics and it is important to appreciate just why and how these molecules so effectively meet the diagnostic challenges of today.

Immunoassays: Development, Applications and Future Trends
Edited by Richard O'Kennedy and Caroline Murphy

ISBN 978-981-4669-97-9 (Hardcover), 978-1-315-20654-7 (eBook)
www.panstanford.com

2.1 Diagnostic Antibodies: Co-opting Natural Immunity

One of the best established approaches in the immunoassay toolbox involves the exploitation of the natural immune response of an animal by exposing it to an analyte of interest. Typically, this involved purifying the designated proteinaceous target analyte (e.g. a pathogenicity marker protein from a bacterial cell or a cancer biomarker from serum or tumour cell surface marker) and injecting (usually in the presence of an adjuvant) into the animal. Following this primary immunisation, the animal is boosted intermittently over a period of several weeks to months to take advantage of the in vivo affinity maturation process. Recombinant techniques now enable production of protein **immunogens** by heterologous expression, thereby avoiding the need to culture large amounts of clinical material and the risks associated with handling such material. DNA immunisation is another recombinant enabling technology that bypasses expression and purification steps by co-opting the host animals' translational machinery to produce the target protein in vivo. This initial 'prime' is often performed in conjunction with subsequent 'boosts' with purified antigen. **Haptens** (molecules of low molecular weight such as drugs) generally need to be conjugated to larger carrier proteins [1] such as keyhole limpet hemocyanin (KLH), bovine serum albumin (BSA) or bovine thyroglobulin (BTG) so that they can be effectively 'seen' by the immune system and efficiently engage T-cells. Likewise, peptides can be conjugated to carrier proteins and used to prime immune responses. However, although this strategy can be successful [2], it must be realised that the conjugated peptide is artificial and might not always faithfully represent the native context of the peptide, especially if the peptide represents an epitope within a macromolecule exhibiting hierarchical structural complexities.

2.2 Harnessing Natural Diversity

Traditionally, serum-derived polyclonal antibodies and hybridoma-derived monoclonal antibodies have proved the principal source of such reagents [3]. However, both of these antibody types are limited in their absolute diagnostic utility. For instance, polyclonal antibodies must be serially harvested and isolated from immunised animals and batch heterogeneity is a major problem. Likewise, by virtue of their polyclonality and inherent heterogeneity, there is the very real possibility of cross-reactivity arising, unless secondary purification steps are introduced. Monoclonal antibodies produced using B-cell immortalisation or hybridoma technologies are superior by virtue of their true monospecificity, which can be exploited to detect class-specific or even unique analytes such as pathogenic bacterial cells within a predominantly non-pathogenic genus background [4]. However, as they are predominantly rodent-derived, conserved mammalian proteins often prove refractory to such antibody generation methodologies. Once an adequate antigen-specific serum titre is obtained, the polyclonal population is suitably enriched and the B-cell population is adequately biased and this stacks the immunological dice in favour of isolating and immortalising a stable B-cell candidate. Although a very robust technology, it is important to realise that it really is a numbers game and also that what is returned is essentially a snapshot of the immune repertoire.

It is now possible to capture routinely the entire variable (V) gene repertoire of an immunised animal by specifically amplifying the V genes using PCR and creating a recombinant V gene library. Thus, rather than a snapshot, this strategy documents the entirety of the antigen-driven humoral response. It is then possible to recapitulate the fragment variable (Fv) pairing by synthetically linking the V_H and V_L domains with a flexible linker sequence. At this point it is useful to consider the various antibody domains as modular entities and it can then be appreciated that it is a facile exercise to reformat this minimalist single-chain Fv (scFv) construct into a range of alternative configurations (Fig. 2.1) ranging from dimerised scFv to Fab and even completely retro-engineered IgG. The random nature of the recombinant combinatorial process can lead to scFv's with entirely novel specificities and affinities.

Typically, recombinant scFv libraries from immune animals are of the order of 10^7–10^{10} independent transformants and this is usually more than adequate. Following a final boost, the major

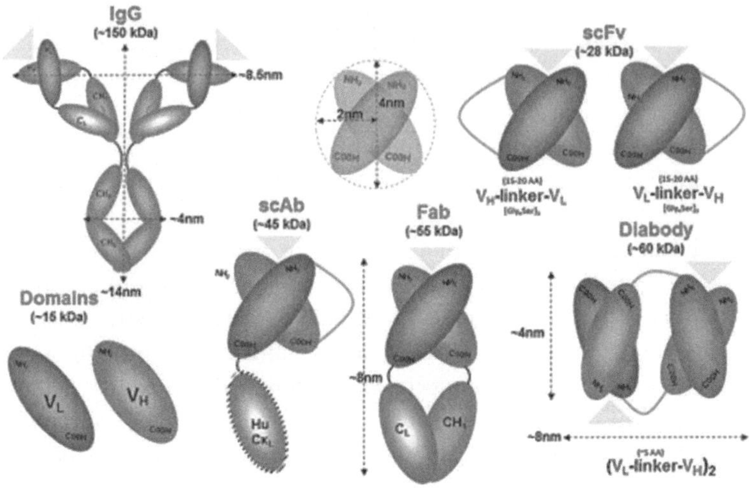

Figure 2.1 Typical IgG and representative iterations of modular recombinant antibody formats. An IgG molecule is approximately 150 kDa and consists of two heavy (H) and two light (L) polypeptide chains (shown) that are linked together by disulphide bonds. The IgG is a 'Y-shaped' molecule. The two arms of the 'Y' are composed of variable heavy (V_H) and variable light (V_L) regions that contain the antigen binding sites and together are known as the Fv portion (shown). The IgG is also composed of the constant (C) region that determines the antibody isotype and is important in signalling to the immune system. The single-chain fragment variable (scFv) is comprised of V_H and V_L regions that are connected at their terminal ends by a flexible glycine-serine $(Gly_4Ser)_3$ linker. A single-chain antibody (scAb) consists of an Fv region, and tethered to the V_L region is a human constant κ light chain. A fragment antigen binding (Fab) (or fragment antigen binding molecule) is composed of one complete light chain connected by a disulphide bond to a V_H and C_{H1} chain. A diabody is a bispecific recombinant antibody molecule, composed of two Fv molecules connected by flexible Gly-Ser linkers.

lymphoid organs (e.g. spleen and bone marrow) are harvested, RNA is extracted and reverse transcribed to yield a cDNA template from which is amplified the V gene repertoire. Peripheral blood lymphocytes can also be used for library construction in cases where it is not practicable to remove lymphoid organs and, indeed, are more often preferentially used for the construction of nonimmune libraries. The latter scenario exploits the naïve immune repertoire, since the animals are not systematically primed with any dedicated immunisation regimens, although the actual degree of naïvety will depend on the age, immunological fitness and extent of exposure to environmental antigens for a given animal. In order to augment diversity it is preferable to prepare a pooled naïve library comprising representative cloned repertoires from multiple animals. The obvious advantage of naïve libraries is that once constructed, they essentially represent a universal shelf library that is ready to screen any target antigen. The time lag between immunisation and library construction is eliminated. Furthermore, highly toxic antigens can be readily screened. The consequence of naïvety, however, is that in vivo affinity maturation events are bypassed, and thus, clones frequently return antibodies with lower affinity constants.

2.3 Affinity

It is salient to note that in vitro antibodies are not subject to the same kinetic binding constraints that prevail in natural B-cell receptor (BCR) evolution [5] and, consequently, it is theoretically possible to isolate very high-**affinity** binders from recombinant antibody libraries using available display technologies. This is dependent on library quality with respect to intrinsic diversity and the selection stringency used.

The on-rate i.e. rate at which an antibody binds its cognate antigen, will always be largely dictated by limiting factors such as antibody size and charge, which impact on diffusion constants in a given matrix and becomes particularly limiting when in vitro selections are performed under static incubation conditions on antigen-coated wells or immunotubes. As a consequence of this, affinity-based selections designed with suitable stringency (decreasing antigen concentrations and increasing washing steps) factored in to encourage higher-affinity binders frequently return 'hits' with greater spread and extremes in k_d than k_a. Surface plasmon resonance (SPR) (described in greater detail in Chapter 11 of this book) has established itself as the technology *de rigeur* for measuring antibody-antigen interactions [6]. It is favoured because it enables binding events to be monitored in real time (Fig. 2.2) and without the need for ancillary labels. Cumulatively, these attributes enable robust analysis and faithful return of kinetic constants. It is often easier to relate the off-rate to the antibody-antigen complex half-life ($t_{1/2}$). This simply reflects the time needed for 50% of the complex to dissociate is independent of concentration and can readily be resolved as $t_{1/2} = \ln 2/k_\text{d}$. For instance, for an off-rate of $10^{-4}(\text{s}^{-1})$, the time to reach 50% dissociation will be 115.5 minutes. Some phage display exponents routinely employ competition with free antigen either as a specific means of elution or to specifically deplete weaker binding clones prior to eluting the more tightly bound clones.

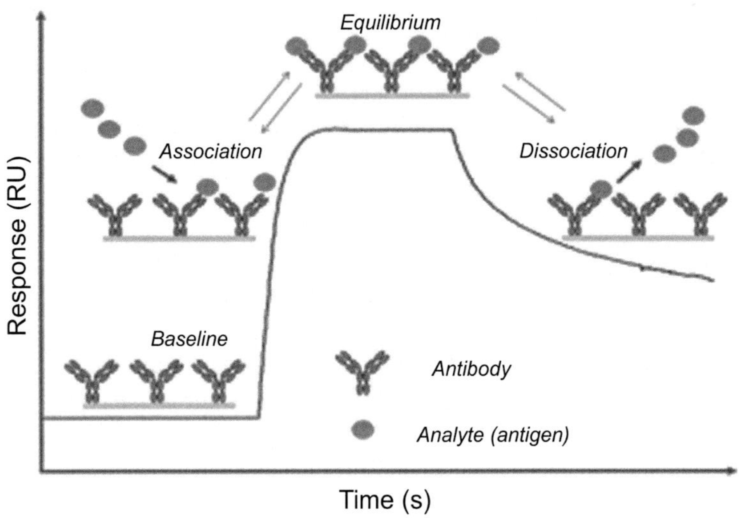

Figure 2.2 A typical SPR sensorgram profile. Binding of target analyte to cognate ligand (antibody) immobilised on the sensor chip surface is monitored in real time and reported in arbitrary response units (RUs). The affinity of the antibody (the equilibrium dissociation constant K_D) is easily resolved from the ratio of the dissociation ('off-rate', k_off or k_d) and association ('on-rate', k_on or k_a) according to $K_\text{D} = k_\text{d}/k_\text{a}$.

2.4 Exploiting Synthetic Diversity in vitro

It is possible to generate artificial diversity entirely ex vivo using synthetic chemistry and molecular biological tools. Like naïve libraries, these also remove the need for immunisation, and even more importantly, they can subvert tolerance and, thus, are increasingly becoming the library type of choice when dealing with difficult-to-isolate antibodies such as those against human biomarkers and therapeutic targets. Similarly, they can be readily screened against toxic target analytes. From a practical perspective, in any antibody selection campaign, the composition of the clonal output population can often be heavily dictated by expression bias. Although expression can be variably influenced by complementarity determining region (CDR) heterogeneity, particularly when harbouring indiscriminate cysteines and stop codons, it is often a more direct reflection of the cumulative framework contributions. This can be at least partly circumvented by carefully designing the synthetic diversity within the context of a well-validated, acquiescent framework. The resultant normalisation of expression, it will be appreciated, has a huge translational impact on the screening campaign and facilitates more seamless assimilation into high-throughput (HT) platforms. Accordingly, due to its marked overrepresentation in the expressed human repertoire [7, 8], the DP47 (VHIII) germline variable heavy domain is considered a particularly suitable generic heavy chain scaffold for human synthetic antibody libraries wherein it confers superior thermodynamic stability profiles [9]. Similarly, a restricted set of overrepresented light chain germline frameworks (e.g. DPK22 (VkIII)) are frequently incorporated. Indeed, the very obvious light chain inactivity reflects a heightened degree of promiscuity of discrete heavy chains and, certainly in the earliest pioneering semi-synthetic libraries, such apparently 'universal light chains' [10] were exploited to demonstrate the feasibility of affinity isolation from a CDRH3-restricted diversity. In a therapeutic setting, due diligence with respect to selection of framework can help ensure that candidate therapeutic antibodies are less likely to impact the patient's immune system, although it is still possible for the CDR region itself to stimulate an adverse immune response. Fortunately, with the exception of some clinical diagnostic applications, the latter scenario is one that poses fewer constraints in the broader diagnostic arena. The vast majority of reported synthetic libraries are designed based on the large and growing repositories of antibody sequence data which allow identification of key residues and a deeper understanding of mutational residues. One cannot help but think that at this stage of the antibody engineering revolution, such foundations are rather conservative and safe, perhaps, particularly focused on therapeutic constraints. The diagnostic field has the opportunity to more fully probe and indeed exploit the totality of the benefits that traditional and more novel library design has to offer.

If the library is suitably designed and constructed, so as to be biased towards target-specific traits (e.g. long loops for cleft-binding or biased hydrophobicity) then it could legitimately be expected that such a synthetic antibody library might confidently return a proportion of potential binding singularities. However, such bespoke in silico design is entirely predicated on comprehensive a priori knowledge of target structure and precise epitope definition. It may be argued that this is in fact a more accurate representation of natural immune repertoires as constructed following potent stimulation and invoking of memory responses. Such designs will undoubtedly benefit from more comprehensive mining of the B-cell bias in response to defined immunogen or immunogen classes, an exercise made possible by increasing accessibility to HT sequencing facilities [11]. This could also involve iterative exploration of tolerable and contributory functional diversity ranging from purely CDR-H3-focused minimalist, and even binary-restricted diversity [12, 13], to more expansive inclusion of non-paratope residues likely to contribute conformational complexities and additive favourable thermodynamic stabilisation and binding energetics.

2.4.1 Introducing Diversity

The simplest and most ubiquitously applied generic strategy for introducing diversity within designated CDR region(s) exploits codon degeneracy within the amino acid code. For instance, by using the NNS codon (where N = A, G, C or T S = G or C) we effectively assign a 32 codon redundancy to address the complete range of 20 amino acids at discrete positions. In practice, NNK (K = G or T) is often preferentially used because of the lower intrinsic GC coverage which may compromise downstream sequencing efforts. Unlike the loosest NNN codon, the NNK and NNS codons only encode for a single, amber (TAG) stop codon. Intuitively then, the greater the sequence space one wishes to randomise, the greater the library size must be. Therein lies one of the key limitations. If, for instance, one were to target a nine residue CDR and 'hard randomise' this using NNK degeneracy, then 20^9 (i.e. 5.1×10^{11}) discrete amino acid combinations would be possible. Such numbers are beyond the current maximal achievable transformation efficiencies in bacteria. Even if transformation efficiencies in the range of 10^9–10^{10} are routinely achieved, it is likely that library quality would be compromised by disparate codon redundancy, spurious amber (TAG) stop codons, arbitrary cysteines and other disadvantageous combinations that would reduce overall expression and particularly, functional expression. Thus, the likelihood for a large disparity between designed saturated sequence diversity and accessible functional diversity can be detrimental to overall output quality. For this reason, it is common to include at least a degree of 'soft randomisation' usually premised on knowledge of the epitope characteristics or inertial residues in the CDR which can be adequately countenanced within an altogether less speculative degeneracy. This might entail restricting diversity at a particular position to a small subset of hydrophobic residues like F, I, L and V which can be coded for using the NTT codon. Cassette mutagenesis (Fig. 2.3) is one of the simplest and most commonly used synthetic library and mutagenesis strategies.

Trimer oligonucleotide synthesis gives much more precise control over the positional codon assignation and thus, allows one to better account for codon usage bias, eliminate spurious stop codons and sequence repeats. It is likely that in the future trimer oligonucleotide technology will become more efficient, affordable and accessible, just like extended length oligonucleotide and chemical gene synthesis have almost displaced traditional gene cloning by PCR of genomic or cDNA. The evolution of the HuCAL® libraries attest just how refined libraries can be when using codon-controlled

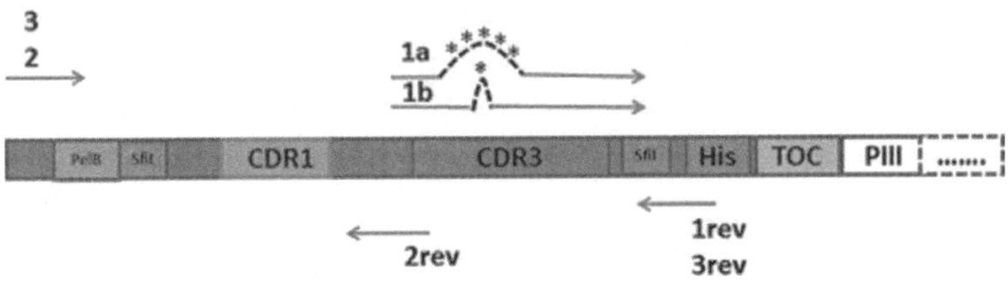

Figure 2.3 Cassette mutagenesis. This is simply a series of sequential PCRs. The first PCR (primers 1a or 1b + 1rev) incorporates the synthetic diversity into CDR3. This diversity can be designed to be more (1a) or less (1b) saturating, with the asterisk '*' indicating targeted mutagenic sites. The second PCR (primer 2 + 2rev) amplifies the N-terminal region comprising the CDR1 and CDR2 regions and incudes a 1a/1b-overlapping sequence encoded on 2rev. Both PCR products are then purified and combined in a standard SOE overlap PCR. This third and final PCR step, yields the complete, mutagenized library and is ready for cloning into the vector of interest. His = Histidine tag (common feature of phagemid and expression vectors to enable purification by immobilised metal affinity chromatography (IMAC). TOC = 'tag of choice', this is an additional tag often incorporated as a detection moiety (e.g. FLAG or HA peptide sequences).

library construction approaches [8, 14, 15]. The acquisition of Slonomics technology by Morposys will no doubt further bolster codon controlled library design as the 'sloning' approach using synthetic double stranded triplet sequences very precisely removes the risk of spurious stop codons, sequence repeats, indiscriminate cysteines, N-linked glycosylation sites and other destabilising motifs are also known to improve library capabilities [16].

2.4.2 Introducing Diversity: Affinity Maturation

In vitro affinity maturation can be achieved by random or site-directed mutation strategies using the same basic principles as used for introduction of diversity into the synthetic CDR libraries, but at a lower degree. The mutational loading can be further increased by using error-prone PCR (EP-PCR), although sometimes this can introduce mutations at key contributing residues positioned outside of the principle CDR-defined paratope. This may invoke antipathy in therapeutic circles, but as long as expression and stability are not compromised, such mutant progeny are generally acceptable for diagnostic applications. Light chain shuffling is often viewed as a conservative means of fine tuning the affinity of clones. Often this strategy is successful in terms of returning improved affinity clones but, especially in the case of immune libraries, it might be argued that if the original library (depending on its size and diversity) was interrogated more comprehensively or stringently then an equally high-affinity clone might be isolated. In certain cases it might well be that the higher affinity clone resulted from more stringent selection conditions being exerted on the shuffled library.

Even with the most optimally constructed libraries, the success of any antibody isolation campaign, particularly from recombinant and synthetic libraries comes down to a simple game of numbers. It is long acknowledged that there is a clear correlation between the accessible clonal diversity and the affinity of antigen-binding clones returned [17]. This is not only a limitation of recombinant antibody libraries as, in fact, the theoretical cumulative (sequence + combinatorial) diversity of the natural repertoire is much too large to be accommodated within the available B-lymphocyte reservoir. This is why the natural in vivo repertoire must be considered a dynamic repertoire relentlessly depleting, enriching and focusing the immune B-cell inventory to deliver the requisite immunity.

Extending this purely arithmetic interpretation, it will be appreciated that the major limitation, whether natural or synthetic libraries are employed, is actually compartmentalising and addressing the available diversity. In contrast to in vivo immunity, with in vitro we have the capacity to use rational and stringent selection techniques to bias or focus the library repertoire. Importantly, we are not subject to the same kinetic binding constraints that prevail in BCR evolution in vivo, and thus, it is theoretically possible to isolate very high-affinity binders from immune combinatorial libraries. In effect, the only constraining factor is how to actually compartmentalise and sample such large diversities.

2.5 Paradigms Challenged

Immunological convention asserts that the H-chain and in particular the CDRH3 domain is the main foci of humoral sequence diversity and by consequence is the de facto principal determinant of paratope functionality. This is substantiated by the plentiful examples of light chain promiscuity arising in antibodies of both natural and recombinant origin. Accordingly, the dogma consigns the L chain and subordinate H chain CDRs (CDRH1 and CDRH2) to ancillary 'bit-player' roles in the theatre of humoral immunity. Rather than dictating specificity, these subordinate elements play auxiliary roles that ostensibly contribute to fine-tuning the affinity. Hence, it is common practice to perform light chain and subordinate CDR shuffling on lead antibody candidates that require affinity enhancements. Indeed, our very existence is predicated on the 'adequacy' of this perceived convention. However, the huge strides forward in refining synthetic antibody library design have begun to challenge this convention. Such libraries can overcome the limitations imposed by the diversity-creating capacity of the humoral system with respect to CDRL3 [18] and when adequate diversity is ascribed to the CDL3 it can indeed assume the dominant role and dictate paratope functionality [19].

Until quite recently [20] antibodies bearing longer CDR3 loops (>14–16 residues) were thought to be immunological anomalies which escaped de-selection in the bone marrow and persisted to potentiate and exacerbate autoimmune events such as rheumatoid arthritis (RA). The amassing portfolio of broadly neutralising antibodies (bnAbs) against HIV [21–26] (VH3-23 and Vk1-33*01) are clear exceptions to this rule and force us to consider extended CDR loop lengths as legitimate and advantageous components of the immunological repertoire. It seems reasonable to speculate that such apparent incongruities of the antibody class are advantageous for viral neutralisation as they can access crevices or areas partly occluded due to membrane proximity, domain folding or glycan shielding and as the antigenic footprint is reduced, there is also a concomitant reduction in the potential for escape mutants to arise. Such paratopic dexterity is easily appreciated by considering the difficulty one might encounter if trying to type on a keyboard while wearing boxing gloves.

There is increasing credence to an alternative natural humoral immunity mediated by germline-encoded antibodies. These are antibodies which are immunologically active despite not having gone through any in vivo somatic maturation events. The strongest evidential basis to date for this so-called SOS antibody response [27] concerns the fascinating case of 3 potent influenza neutralising antibodies, each arising from the same VH1-69 germline gene, isolated independently from patients on three different continents. This is in keeping with the view that the totality of the immune repertoire is so well adapted to its ligand role that defined discrete antibody specificity can justifiably be described based on a manifestation of greater apparent affinity for cognate antigen over the broader antigenic landscape. This SOS component is necessary particularly in cases of viral infection where survival is dependent on an immediate response and the elaborate symphony of the diversity-generating humoral machinery is effectively de-mobbed and rendered redundant in a true example of 'survival of the fittest'. This subset of antibodies is postulated to function by virtue of possessing particularly hydrophobic CDRH2 loops. It is unlikely that stringent affinity-based selections would return such an antibody consensus. Fortunately, for the majority of diagnostic applications it is the specificity, affinity and stability which are the outstanding metrics we strive to maximise.

2.6 Single-Domain Antibodies

The abilities of antibodies such as 'C05' to mediate binding primarily through the V_H domain with the dominant extended CDRH3 and with only a minor contribution from CDRH1 is interesting in light of the burgeoning single-domain antibody field [28].

Given the supradomain complexity of the obligately heterodimerised mammalian immunoglobulin, it is intuitive that if the V_H and V_L domains are expressed independently they would be unstable and prone to aggregation by virtue of having exposed hydrophobic interfacial regions. Accordingly, such aberrancies are extremely rare in humans although there is at least one case of a stable anti-melanoma V_H antibody which was isolated from a vaccinated patient using phage display [29] and the company Domantis (now part of GSK) has positioned itself as a human single-domain antibody (DAb) platform [30] exponent.

Camelids (camels, llamas and alpacas) produce a class of 'heavy chain only' antibodies in which binding is mediated through unpaired variable heavy domains termed 'V_{HH}' [31]. Whereas conventional human and mouse V domains are stabilised by heterodimerisation, V_{HH} domains are characterised by a series of hallmark substitutions [32] which confer increased hydrophilicity in the region corresponding to the site of light chain heterodimerisation in conventional IgG. This translates into improved soluble expression, a feature which renders libraries of V_{HH} domain's a very efficient means of harnessing and mining natural and synthetic camelid antibody diversity.

Much of the excitement around these types of single domain antibodies emanates from their stability and amenability to multiple heterologous expression systems [33] and their impressive ability to refold to recapitulate native biding affinity [34, 35]. However, as with every class of antibody, it is dangerous to make such sweeping generalisations as thermodynamic anomalies can occur [36] and efforts have gone into identifying a more suitable universal V_{HH} candidate framework (e.g. cAbBCII10) to confer improved thermodynamic properties on grafted V_{HH} CDRs [37]. Such improved thermodynamic characteristics will have significant merit in diagnostic settings. It is also interesting that they often have a long CDR3 that correlates well with their proposed cleft-binding propensity [38]. It is tempting to use a bowling ball analogy whereby conventional IgG or scFv/Fab heterodimers are seen to engage their targets in an 'Atlas'-style cupping fashion and while V_{HH} target the cavities. However, in the case of the archetypal lysozyme active site-binding V_{HH} [39], although the CDR3 very patently interrogates the binding site, the antigen interfacial area of the V_{HH} and conventional heterodimeric Fv elements towards lysozyme are actually quite similar [40].

One might reasonably speculate that such a CDR3 prominence would militate against hapten binding. However, there are several cases of reported hapten-binding V_{HH} antibodies such as that against (admittedly, a rather large) Cu-complexed azo dye compound [41, 42] and also the prototypical hapten, methotrexate [43]. It now appears that methotrexate binding could well be mediated by a cryptic binding pocket created by additive contributions from a non-hypervariable loop region [44], in line with the postulated CDR4 element [45]. This co-ordinated interaction mechanism may mean that V_{HH}'s offer a greater potential for hapten binding than was first thought, particularly in light of their apparent ability to perform reproducibly in high levels of solvent [46], which so frequently presents a significant complication following generic sample extraction protocols for haptenic contaminants in environmental and food samples.

In what must be classed as a quintessential example of convergent evolution, the shark new antigen receptor immunoglobulin (IgNAR) comprises a dimeric, non-heterodimerised variable domain component (VNAR). Whereas V_{HH} is a bona fide descendent of the mammalian IgG, IgNAR arose independently, as a distinct isotype in its own right. At approximately 12kDa in size, VNARS are the smallest single domain antibodies capable of independent antigen binding.

It is plausible that as result of their small size, paucity of light chain permutations and concomitant limited diversity, they more frequently adopt long CDR3 loops that are very heavily diversified, even at the primary repertoire level, by 4 rearrangement events as distinct from higher order mammalian translocon-mediated diversity. Similar to V_{HH}, they retain invariant hallmark canonical cysteine residues, often in conjunction with additional CDR1 and/or CDR3 bridging cysteine residues (Fig. 2.4). These confer an additional level of structural diversity and also contribute to the pronounced stability of VNAR domains. Although conventional mAbs have been shown to bind comparable cleft regions [47] it would appear that VNARs and V_{HH}s share a remarkable preference for cleft binding. This is elegantly demonstrated by crystal structure determinations of VNARs in complex with cognate antigen [48, 49] and also tentatively suggests that an induced fit binding mechanism might be involved.

From a diagnostic perspective there are obvious advantages to using VNARs. The phylogenetic distance of sharks from mammals has proven value in targeting intractable mammalian antigens [50] is another key inherent advantage. The stability inherent in a disulphide-stabilised domain designed to circulate and persist in the high osmolar and 350 mM urea-loaded environs of shark

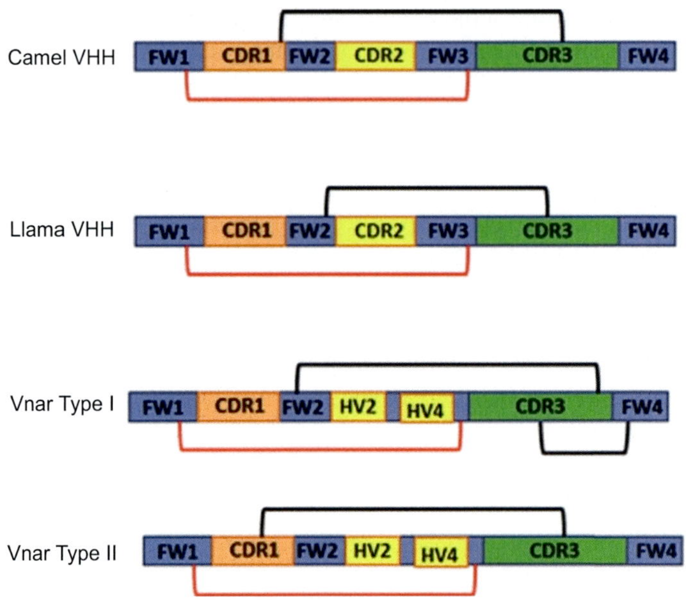

Figure 2.4 Diagrammatic representation of the structural blueprint of rearranged camelid and shark variable heavy domains. Antigen binding regions are composed of hypervariable regions (HV) where the propensity to insert amino acids at a given position is highly diverse, these HV regions are flanked by regions of reduced amino acid diversity and these are known as framework (FW) regions. In addition to a classical canonical cysteines bridge (red line), both shark and camelid variable heavy chains exhibit non-canonical intra-molecular disulphide-linked cysteine residues.

serum could be extremely beneficial in field applications and would also have likely advantageous implications for reagent shelf-life and point-of-care integrity, particularly in low resource environments. The ability of VNARs to retain binding functionality when covalently immobilised onto biosensor surfaces as important implications for ease of characterisation, development of biosensor-based diagnostic assays and chemical conjugation of labels. Conversely, scFv molecules often fail to tolerate such adulterations and chemical conjugation or immobilisation frequently leads to ablation of functionality (personnel observation). Coupled with facile heterologous expression, it is understandable that VNARs are seen as legitimate reagents to target diagnostically relevant analytes [51]. Both shark and llama single domain antibodies were recently evaluated for Ebola virus detection [52, 53] and it is likely that development of portable biosensors for field applications such as this could benefit immensely from this currently under-exploited class of thermodynamically robust single domain antibodies.

2.7 Conclusion

The ability to readily modularise, affinity mature, format and easily express in heterologous expression systems make recombinant antibodies a rich resource for the very wide array of modern diagnostic challenges. At a time when high affinity and specificity are almost taken for granted, recombinant antibodies offer many additional inherent advantages. Their small size can be exploited for imaging applications where shorter half-life and tissue penetration are requisite characteristics. It is possible to readily engineer and interchange fusion tags or labels to facilitate detection or site-specific conjugation for chemical modification or directed immobilisation. The minimal molecular footprint they present compared to whole IgG can reduce assay interference arising from heterophile antibodies, complement engagement or other spurious Fc interactions that can compromise analysis of clinical samples.

Using a holistic approach, it is possible to make an antibody against almost any target analyte. The key is to know exactly what one requires in the endpoint assay and to base the generation strategy (e.g. immune or synthetic, mouse or chicken) and selection (e.g. biased for high affinity, class cross-reactivity, slow off-rate or improved thermodynamic stability at low pH/high temperature) criteria on this comprehensive appreciation of the target analyte and the envisaged endpoint. A useful mantra is to know what the analyte is, know how much of it one needs to be able to detect and in what setting one needs to detect it. The approaches are now well established to successfully deliver these powerful reagents.

References

1. Fitzpatrick, B., and R. O'Kennedy, The development and application of a surface plasmon resonance-based inhibition immunoassay for the determination of warfarin in plasma ultrafiltrate. *J Immunol Methods*, 2004. **291**(1–2):11–25.
2. Conroy, P.J., R.J. O'Kennedy, and S. Hearty, Cardiac troponin I: a case study in rational antibody design for human diagnostics. *Protein Eng Des Sel*, 2012. **25**(6):295–305.
3. Kohler, G., and C. Milstein, Continuous cultures of fused cells secreting antibody of predefined specificity. *Nature*, 1975. **256**(5517):495–497.
4. Hearty, S., et al., Production, characterisation and potential application of a novel monoclonal antibody for rapid identification of virulent *Listeria monocytogenes*. *J Microbiol Methods*, 2006. **66**(2):294–312.
5. Hearty, S., and R. O'Kennedy, Exploiting recombinant antibodies in point-of-care (POC) diagnostics: the combinatorial advantage. *Bioeng Bugs*, 2011. **2**(3):182–186.
6. Hearty, S., P. Leonard, and R. O'Kennedy, Measuring antibody-antigen binding kinetics using surface plasmon resonance. *Methods Mol Biol*, 2012. **907**:411–442.
7. de Wildt, R.M.T., et al., Analysis of heavy and light chain pairings indicates that receptor editing shapes the human antibody repertoire. *J Mol Biol*, 1999. **285**(3):895–901.
8. Knappik, A., et al., Fully synthetic human combinatorial antibody libraries (HuCAL) based on modular consensus frameworks and CDRs randomized with trinucleotides. *J Mol Biol*, 2000. **296**(1):57–86.
9. Ewert, S., et al., Biophysical properties of human antibody variable domains. *J Mol Biol*, 2003. **325**(3):531–553.
10. Burton, D.R., and C.F. Barbas, 3rd, Human antibodies from combinatorial libraries. *Advances in Immunology*, 1994. **57**:191–280.
11. Glanville, J., et al., Precise determination of the diversity of a combinatorial antibody library gives insight into the human immunoglobulin repertoire. *Proc Natl Acad Sci USA*, 2009. **106**(48):20216–20221.
12. Fellouse, F.A., et al., Molecular recognition by a binary code. *J Mol Biol*, 2005. **348**(5):1153–1162.
13. Fellouse, F.A., et al., High-throughput generation of synthetic antibodies from highly functional minimalist phage-displayed libraries. *J Mol Biol*, 2007. **373**(4):924–940.

14. Rothe, C., et al., The human combinatorial antibody library HuCAL GOLD combines diversification of all six CDRs according to the natural immune system with a novel display method for efficient selection of high-affinity antibodies. *J Mol Biol*, 2008. **376**(4):1182–1200.
15. Prassler, J., et al., HuCAL PLATINUM, a synthetic Fab library optimized for sequence diversity and superior performance in mammalian expression systems. *J Mol Biol*, 2011. **413**(1):261–278.
16. Kronqvist, N., et al., Combining phage and staphylococcal surface display for generation of ErbB3-specific Affibody molecules. *Protein Eng Des Sel*, 2011. **24**(4):385–396.
17. Perelson, A.S., and G.F. Oster, Theoretical studies of clonal selection: minimal antibody repertoire size and reliability of self-non-self discrimination. *J Theor Biol*, 1979. **81**(4):645–670.
18. Nemazee, D., Receptor editing in lymphocyte development and central tolerance. *Nat Rev Immunol*, 2006. **6**(10):728–740.
19. Persson, H., et al., CDR-H3 diversity is not required for antigen recognition by synthetic antibodies. *J Mol Biol*, 2013. **425**(4):803–811.
20. Briney, B.S., J.R. Willis, and J.E. Crowe, Jr., Human peripheral blood antibodies with long HCDR3s are established primarily at original recombination using a limited subset of germline genes. *PLoS One*, 2012. **7**(5):e36750.
21. Pancera, M., et al., Crystal structure of PG16 and chimeric dissection with somatically related PG9: structure-function analysis of two quaternary-specific antibodies that effectively neutralize HIV-1. *J Virol*, 2010. **84**(16):8098–8110.
22. Hearty, S., et al., Surface plasmon resonance for vaccine design and efficacy studies: recent applications and future trends. *Expert Rev Vaccines*, 2010. **9**(6):645–664.
23. McLellan, J.S., et al., Structure of HIV-1 gp120 V1/V2 domain with broadly neutralizing antibody PG9. *Nature*, 2011. **480**(7377):336–343.
24. Walker, L.M., et al., Broad neutralization coverage of HIV by multiple highly potent antibodies. *Nature*, 2011. **477**(7365):466–470.
25. Pancera, M., et al., N332-Directed broadly neutralizing antibodies use diverse modes of HIV-1 recognition: inferences from heavy-light chain complementation of function. *PLoS One*, 2013. **8**(2):e55701.
26. Zwick, M.B., E.O. Saphire, and D.R. Burton, gp41: HIV's shy protein. *Nat Med*, 2004. **10**(2):133–134.

27. Lerner, R.A., Rare antibodies from combinatorial libraries suggests an S.O.S. component of the human immunological repertoire. *Mol Biosyst*, 2011. **7**(4):1004–1012.
28. Ekiert, D.C., et al., Cross-neutralization of influenza A viruses mediated by a single antibody loop. *Nature*, 2012. **489**(7417):526–532.
29. Cai, X., and A. Garen, A melanoma-specific VH antibody cloned from a fusion phage library of a vaccinated melanoma patient. *Proc Natl Acad Sci USA*, 1996. **93**(13):6280–6285.
30. Holt, L.J., et al., Domain antibodies: proteins for therapy. *Trends Biotechnol*, 2003. **21**(11):484–490.
31. Hamers-Casterman, C., et al., Naturally occurring antibodies devoid of light chains. *Nature*, 1993. **363**(6428):446–448.
32. Muyldermans, S., et al., Sequence and structure of VH domain from naturally occurring camel heavy chain immunoglobulins lacking light chains. *Protein Eng*, 1994. **7**(9):1129–1135.
33. Wesolowski, J., et al., Single domain antibodies: promising experimental and therapeutic tools in infection and immunity. *Med Microbiol Immunol*, 2009. **198**(3):157–174.
34. van der Linden, R.H., et al., Comparison of physical chemical properties of llama VHH antibody fragments and mouse monoclonal antibodies. *Biochim Biophys Acta*, 1999. **1431**(1):37–46.
35. Dumoulin, M., et al., Single-domain antibody fragments with high conformational stability. *Protein Sci*, 2002. **11**(3):500–515.
36. Conway, J.O., et al., Llama single domain antibodies specific for the 7 botulinum neurotoxin serotypes as heptaplex immunoreagents. *PLoS One*, 2010. **5**(1):e8818.
37. Saerens, D., et al., Identification of a universal VHH framework to graft non-canonical antigen-binding loops of camel single-domain antibodies. *J Mol Biol*, 2005. **352**(3):597–607.
38. Lauwereys, M., et al., Potent enzyme inhibitors derived from dromedary heavy-chain antibodies. *EMBO J*, 1998. **17**(13):3512–3520.
39. Streltsov, V.A., et al., Structural evidence for evolution of shark Ig new antigen receptor variable domain antibodies from a cell-surface receptor. *Proc Natl Acad Sci USA*, 2004. **101**(34):12444–12449.
40. De Genst, E., et al., Molecular basis for the preferential cleft recognition by dromedary heavy-chain antibodies. *Proc Natl Acad Sci USA*, 2006. **103**(12):4586–4591.

41. Spinelli, S., et al., Camelid heavy-chain variable domains provide efficient combining sites to haptens. *Biochemistry*, 2000. **39**(6):1217–1222.
42. Spinelli, S., et al., Lateral recognition of a dye hapten by a llama VHH domain. *J Mol Biol*, 2001. **311**(1):123–129.
43. Alvarez-Rueda, N., et al., Generation of llama single-domain antibodies against methotrexate, a prototypical hapten. *Mol Immunol*, 2007. **44**(7):1680–1690.
44. Fanning, S.W., and J.R. Horn, An anti-hapten camelid antibody reveals a cryptic binding site with significant energetic contributions from a nonhypervariable loop. *Protein Sci*, 2011. **20**(7):1196–1207.
45. Sircar, A., et al., Analysis and modeling of the variable region of camelid single-domain antibodies. *J Immunol*, 2011. **186**(11):6357–6367.
46. Kim, H.J., et al., Isolation of alpaca anti-hapten heavy chain single domain antibodies for development of sensitive immunoassay. *Anal Chem*, 2012. **84**(2):1165–1171.
47. Coley, A.M., et al., Structure of the malaria antigen AMA1 in complex with a growth-inhibitory antibody. *PLoS Pathog*, 2007. **3**(9):1308–1319.
48. Stanfield, R.L., et al., Maturation of shark single-domain (IgNAR) antibodies: evidence for induced-fit binding. *J Mol Biol*, 2007. **367**(2):358–372.
49. Henderson, K.A., et al., Structure of an IgNAR-AMA1 complex: targeting a conserved hydrophobic cleft broadens malarial strain recognition. *Structure*, 2007. **15**(11):1452–1466.
50. Nuttall, S.D., et al., Isolation and characterization of an IgNAR variable domain specific for the human mitochondrial translocase receptor Tom70. *Eur J Biochem*, 2003. **270**(17):3543–3554.
51. Griffiths, K., et al., Shark variable new antigen receptor (VNAR) single domain antibody fragments: stability and diagnostic applications. *Antibodies*, 2013. **2**(1):68–81.
52. Sherwood, L.J., and A. Hayhurst, Ebolavirus nucleoprotein C-termini potently attract single domain antibodies enabling monoclonal affinity reagent sandwich assay (MARSA) formulation. *PLoS One*, 2013. **8**(4):e61232.
53. Goodchild, S.A., et al., Isolation and characterisation of Ebolavirus-specific recombinant antibody fragments from murine and shark immune libraries. *Mol Immunol*, 2011. **48**(15–16):2027–2037.

Chapter 3

Surfaces and Immobilisation Strategies for Use in Immunoassay Development

Chandra K. Dixit[a,*] **and Paul Conroy**[b,*]

[a]*Department of Chemistry, University of Connecticut, Storrs, CT 06269, USA*
[b]*Department of Biochemistry and Molecular Biology, Faculty of Medicine, Nursing and Health Science, Monash University, Melbourne, VIC3800, Australia*
chandra.kumar_dixit@uconn.edu, paul.conroy@monash.edu

Proteins can easily lose their structure and hence their activity upon modification and immobilisation. The detection of proteins using antibodies is inherently reliant on retention of binding affinity, and therefore sophisticated strategies are required to preserve the bio-recognition element [1]. The immobilisation of antibodies (or their fragments) on solid supports has undergone extensive examination and is widely applied in the life science domain. Key parameters exist for the successful exploitation of antibodies in immunoassay-based applications. These parameters are antibody size (covered in Chapter 2), immobilisation, orientation, labelling (covered in this chapter), sensitivity, selectivity and stability. However, the labelling and immobilisation of antibodies is the most crucial factor for immunoassay development, and the approaches adopted may have far-reaching effects on the assay. Recombinant antibodies are

*Both authors contributed equally.

Immunoassays: Development, Applications and Future Trends
Edited by Richard O'Kennedy and Caroline Murphy

ISBN 978-981-4669-97-9 (Hardcover), 978-1-315-20654-7 (eBook)
www.panstanford.com

an attractive technology to optimise these factors, but chemical modification of fragments, such as the single chain fragment variable (scFv) can limit their broader utilisation. Genetic modification facilitates improvement of several of these parameters and such novel antibody fragments are more amenable to immobilisation. The ability to develop more sensitive and robust systems is reliant on the modification of superior assay-specific antibodies to improve these cumulative performance characteristics. The capacity to enhance antibodies with respect to their modification and suitability for subsequent applications is of strategic importance to robust biosensor development. Likewise, knowledge-driven approaches to optimise surface chemistry, immobilisation and conjugation are crucial to develop the next generation of immunoassay systems for incorporation into high-throughput or multiplex platforms for point-of-care and other analytical applications.

3.1 Introduction

Studies on immobilisation have helped many important techniques to evolve, facilitating the development of rapid basic research tools and systems for advanced analysis, for example, affinity chromatography, biosensors, immunoassays and protein arrays [2, 3]. Antibody-based immunoassay platforms, such as biosensors, provide a rapid and convenient alternative to traditional analytical methods. In an ideal scenario, proteins are deposited homogenously on a substrate in high concentrations and with appropriate orientations such that they retain their activity, in addition to prevention of non-specific interactions. Key to the sensitivity of any assay is the deposition of active antibody onto the assay surface (e.g. transducer surface or plate surface) and the efficient coupling of the reporter molecule to the secondary antibody.

The mode of antibody immobilisation dictates the orientation and the activity of the antibody on the immunoassay surface. The amount and activity of the deposited antibody thus have an impact on the sensitivity of the immunoassay [4]. There are two main modes of antibody immobilisation, passive and covalent attachment. They are reliant on both the antibody and the chemical characteristics of the surface on which covalent attachment is desirable [5]. Adsorption of proteins on solid surfaces is by far the most simplistic approach to immobilise antibodies but random orientation and denaturation are significant factors when this approach is adopted. For chemically crosslinking antibodies to the surface the availability of functional groups on both the partners is required. Numerous chemistries have been investigated for linking biomolecules to immunoassay surfaces (Fig. 3.1), including lipid layers, silane layers, polymer layers and self-assembling monolayers (SAM). These approaches generate pendent functional groups on the surface of choice that can be used to perform immobilisation.

Antibodies also possess several functional groups that have been exploited for immobilisation. Pendent carboxyls and amines along with reduced sulphurs (as sulphydryls), and oxidised carbohydrates (as aldehydes) are the native functional groups on an antibody that are most commonly used. In order to capture antibodies on a functionalised surface, primary amines are the most commonly targeted groups. However, lysine residues, which are the major source of primary amines, are stochastically distributed across the antibody; this mode of non-specific attachment can lead to inactivation of the antibody, and un-ordered surfaces (Fig. 3.1). Such random approaches are shown to have two- to threefold lower antigen-binding activities [6]. Digestion and/or reduction of the antibody molecule can permit covalent attachment via the sulfhydryl groups in a slightly more site specific fashion via cysteine resides which form disulphide bonds (oxidised). Finally, targeting the carbohydrate moieties, to generate reactive aldehydes (by oxidation), facilitates coupling to amines (via reductive amination) or hydrazine activated groups on the surface. On the basis of these native functional groups, several other approaches for antibody functionalisation have also been reported. Additionally, tags are employed for immobilising antibody on surfaces. A tag is usually a molecule that is covalently attached to or genetically integrated into the antibody. Each tag has a highly specific binding partner which is grafted on the surface of interest and, thus, facilitates the immobilisation of antibody via the interaction between tag and its partner. A few commonly used tag systems are summarised in

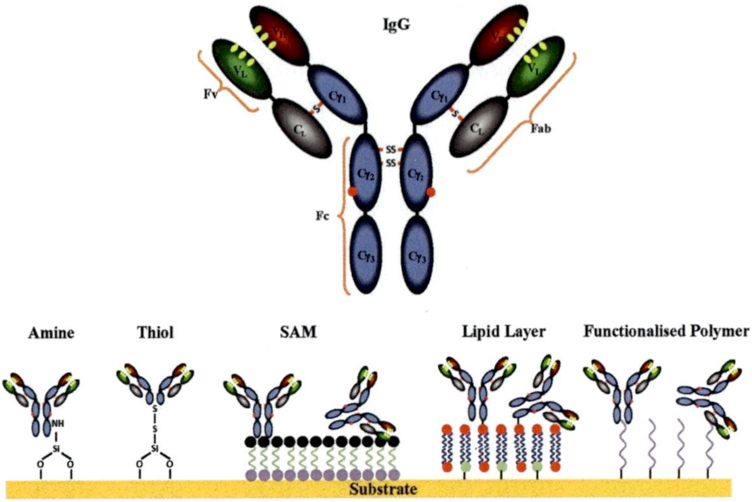

Figure 3.1 Coupling approaches for linking antibodies to surfaces. The classical IgG structure is composed of two heavy and light chains. Critically, the complementarity determining regions (CDRs in yellow) that are housed in the variable heavy (red) and light (green) domains must be preserved for functional binding of antibody with the antigen. In its natural state an antibody possesses primary amines, carboxyls and hydroxyls as target groups for antibody immobilisation. Amine groups are the most abundant of all native pendent groups (approximately 86 amines across the antibody as described on the PDB database) on an antibody and are distributed across the antibody. Therefore, these are the most commonly used for immobilisation applications. In addition, the carboxyl group is another viable group for antibody functionalisation. There are other functional groups that can be utilised following appropriate treatment. The most utilised of such groups are sulfhydryls, which are generated by reduction of the disulphide bonds of an antibody in a controlled fashion with either DTT or mercaptoethanol. Excessive reduction may cause complete release of all the four domains of an antibody leading to loss of activity. The antibody glycosylation sites (red dots) offer an alternative site that can be oxidised with sodium borohydrate to generate pendent aldehydes, which can later bind to amine-functionalised surfaces. Surfaces grafted with polymers having reactive ends, such as epoxy or tosyl groups, can be directly linked to an antibody via amines or hydroxyls. There are other strategies that are crucial for immobilisation of antibodies, e.g. self-assembled monolayers (SAMs) and layer-by-layer assembly of polyelectrolytes, which are also used to capture antibodies on the surface via electrostatic interactions and/or chemisorption.

Table 3.1, which illustrates some approaches to achieve orientated immobilisation of antibodies on surfaces.

Table 3.1 Commonly used antibody conjugates for immobilisation

Conjugate attached to antibody	Complementary biomolecule	Type of interaction	Ref.
Biotin tag	Avidin	Affinity	[7]
SNAP tag	Benzyl (guanine/cytosine)	Affinity	[8]
Polyhistidine tag	Divalent metal ions	Affinity	[9]
Substrate-specific enzyme domains	Enzyme-specific substrate	Affinity	[10–12]
Protein nucleic acid	Nucleotide bases	Hydrogen bonding	[13]

3.2 Tailoring Immunoassay Surfaces

Two crucial points in immunoassays are the efficiency of the capture of an antibody on a given surface and the need to ensure minimum interference of the capture surface and chemistries with the colourimetric/fluorometric signal measurement [1]. Therefore, the selection of a solid support is vital in terms of its potential contribution toward immunoassay sensitivity. A variety of such supports are available. These differ from each other in terms of their chemical, physical and optical properties. On the basis of their chemical properties, they can be characterised into metallic and polymeric (Table 3.2). Polymeric solid supports are employed for microtitre plates, microarray chips or, more recently, fluorocaps, that are widely used to perform immunoassays [1, 14, 15]. Metallic supports are restricted somewhat and are widely applied for use in biosensor-based research and development. However, there are reports from Dixit and colleagues (2012), who have employed nanosphere lithography for generating highly ordered gold surfaces on various solid supports and have demonstrated its potential use in immunoassay development on integrated microfluidic platforms and microarrays [16].

Table 3.2 Various solid supports employed for immunoassay development [15, 17–19]

Support type	Chemical nature	Name	Immunoassay platform
Polymer	Hydrophobic	Polystyrene	Microtitre plate Polymeric sheets
		Polypropylene	Microtitre plate and polymeric sheets
		Polyvinyl chloride	Polymeric sheets
		Polycycloolefin	Microtitre plate
		(Zeonor™ and Zeonex™)	Polymeric sheets and discs
	Hydrophilic	Cellulose acetate	Polymeric sheets
		Polycarbonate	Microtitre plate and Polymeric sheets
		Polymethylmethacrylate	Polymeric sheets
		Polysulphonates	Polymeric sheets
Metallic	Hydrophobic	Gold	Gold-coated surfaces on various supports, e.g. gold on glass
		Silicon	Wafers

3.2.1 Surface Designing/Modulation and Customisation for Antibody Immobilisation and Immunoassay Development

3.2.1.1 Precursor modulation and post-manufacture treatments for controlling the surface properties

The polymeric solid supports employed for performing immunoassays are either hydrophilic or hydrophobic, which is mainly based upon the nature of the monomeric units of these polymers. Hydrophilic polymers are usually composed of monomers that have electronegative functional groups. Conversely, hydrophobic monomers either lack any electronegative functionality or possess resonating structures where electrons are metastabilised due to efficient sharing [20]. Various functional groups are represented and can be ordered according to their hydrophilicity, i.e. hydroxyl >sulphonate >carboxyl >amino >phosphate >alkyl >allyl >aryl.

In terms of its chemical behaviour, an antibody is rich in hydrophobic pockets, which on solvation are exposed towards its surface. These hydrophobic patches are crucial for adsorbing an antibody on solid supports because such hydrophobic interactions between antibody molecules and surface are the key stabilising force involved. An antibody also favours ionic-, covalent- and dative-type interactions [21]. We will first discuss these surfaces for antibody-holding capacity with respect to their chemical nature and then describe various methodologies that are used for improving their protein-holding capacity. Also, a detailed understanding of the chemical nature of an antibody is equally important because this will be decisive in designing and optimising the procedure for antibody capture and for the subsequent selection of the appropriate surfaces and associated reagents.

Based on the classification of surfaces, described in Table 3.1, antibody-holding capacities can be predicted. A hydrophobic surface has a strong tendency to create hydrophobic interactions. However, selection of an appropriate surface is also dependent on the nature of the application for which it is to be employed. For example, microtitre plates are usually made up of polystyrene, which is a hydrophobic polymer, but it comes in various forms with each providing different levels of hydrophobicity and possess different antibody-binding and -holding tendencies [17]. It is evident that the chemical properties of polymeric solid supports can be drastically changed by small adjustments in manufacturing conditions. Manufacturing techniques include the use of pre-functionalised monomer units, which after polymerisation will result in a functionalised surface [20]. Using this approach, surfaces with different functionalities can be generated, given that the required functionality is available in a monomer unit. Classic examples of these are the surfaces from Nunc. These surfaces come with amine functionality and are generated by using an amine-modified monomeric styrene. Relevant commercially available products for this category are summarised in Table 3.3.

In addition, functionalities can be grafted to the solid support after the manufacturing process. There is an array of post-manufacture surface modification methods that are used to confer a specific chemical nature on a given surface for improving its

Table 3.3 Commercially available pre-functionalised surfaces for immunoassay development

Solid support	Functionality	Manufacturer
Polystyrene microplates	Amine (Covalink^{TM}) and carboxy-grafted (Nuclolink^{TM}) surface	Thermo Fisher Nunc
Polystyrene microplates	Maleic anhydride (amine-binding), maleimide-activated (sulfhydryl-binding) and nickel-grafted surface	Thermo Fisher Pierce
Polystyrene microplates	Amine-coated (CarboBind^{R} and DNABind^{R}), and membrane-grafted (FiltrEx^{R})	Corning
Polypropylene microplates	Amine-grafted	Eppendorf

antibody-holding capacity. The most important strategy involves grafting of either small hydrophobic molecules or molecules that terminate in highly hydrophobic functional groups on the surface. The hydrophobicity introduced after the manufacture of polymer substrate by graft method enhances the passivation of the antibodies on it. Several desired functionalities, such as amines, carboxyls, sulphydryls etc., can be incorporated after the solid support manufacturing. A list of such products are summarised in Table 3.4.

Unlike hydrophobic polymers, hydrophilic surfaces have electronegative functionality that significantly increases their affinity towards water (measured by the water droplet flattening using contact angle measurements). These surfaces can also be created following the same manufacturing practices as described for hydrophobic surfaces. However, the nature of the monomer unit or the functionality it bears will change according to the nature of the functional groups required.

Initially it was considered that high-density immobilisation of antibodies can only be achieved on hydrophobic surfaces. However, reports have suggested that hydrophilic surfaces can accommodate significantly larger amounts of antibodies in comparison

Table 3.4 Various methods for improving hydrophilicity and hydrophobicity of the surface

Functionalisation	Strategy/chemical nature of graft	Method of grafting	Ref.
Hydrophilic	Hydroxyl (-OH)	Plasma polymerization in presence of suitable alcohol Adsorbing polysaccharides Grafting hydroxyl-functionalized telechelic polybutadienes (HTPBD)	[22, 23]
	Carboxyl (CO_2H) and amine (NH_2)	Plasma enhanced chemical vapor deposition (PECVD) in the presence of a suitable carboxy or amine precursor, e.g. silanes and non-silane starting molecules. Chemical adsorption using wet method approach for specific amino acids and other related groups.	[24, 25]
Hydrophobic	Aromatic groups (benzene ring-containing amino acids such as phenylalanine), alkyl groups (e.g. methyl, ethyl)	Simple adsorption on a plasma and/or chemically-treated solid support	[26, 27]
	Carbohydrates (e.g. complex polysaccharides such as cellulose and chitin, and glycols such as polyethylene glycol)	PECVD method	

to hydrophobic surfaces [28]. The structural and functional behaviour of antibodies was extensively studied by Vermeer and colleagues [29–32] and their findings laid the foundation for many subsequent reports. An important outcome from their work was that hydrophobic surfaces tend to induce higher degrees of conformational changes in an antibody in comparison to hydrophilic surfaces. This could be explained as follows. Hydrophobic pockets in a protein are buried deep in the three-dimensional structure, and therefore, a significant degree of structural reshuffling is expected when a protein is passivated on a hydrophobic surface. However, higher numbers of electronically-active (polar, charged etc.) functional groups are present on the surface of a protein, hence, when passivated on a hydrophilic surface no significant structural reshuffling is required. In addition, there could possibly be associated factors such as molecular flattening of the antibody after adsorption on the surface. This was demonstrated using a Fourier transform infrared spectroscopy (FTIR) spectrum [33]. Another interesting finding of Vermeer's work was that the heat generated during the release of water of hydration induces significant antibody denaturation which is considerably more than that caused by structural reshuffling. These findings indicate that hydrophilic surfaces are superior in terms of antibody-holding capacity and preservation of antibody activity. However, most of the commercially available solid supports (Table 3.2) such as polystyrene, polymethylmethacrylate, cycloolefin polymers (Zeonor™, Zeonex™) are hydrophobic in nature.

In addition, there are various metallic surfaces employed for developing immunoassays; however, these are mainly restricted to biosensor-based applications. Silicon and gold are widely used metallic surfaces with their applications extending from surface-plasmon resonance to impedance-based immunoassays [34]. Most of these metallic surfaces are not used in their native forms, due to the formation oxide layers on their surface, and require activation. There are various strategies available for activating these surfaces. The most common method is exposing these surfaces to piranha etch [35], which is a solution of sulphuric acid with hydrogen peroxide (acid piranha) or ammonium hydroxide (base piranha) which varies in ratio (3:1, 7:1 and 12:1) according to the requirements. This treatment removes oxides from the surface rendering it hydrophilic.

Activated gold may be employed directly for antibody capture but silicon surfaces require further treatment. These activated surfaces can be grafted with various functional groups such that the hydrophilicity can be precisely governed by the nature of the functional group employed. Gold surfaces are usually functionalised with reagents that have a thiol/sulfhydryl group at one terminal and a desired functional group at the other. Thiol groups are preferred because of their one-step binding to gold. Amino groups also have a tendency to interact with gold surfaces due to coordinate bond formation tendencies with gold. Hence, amine functionalities could also be employed capturing antibodies on gold surfaces. Pakiari and Jamshidi (2007) have suggested that amino, oxygen and thiol groups interact with gold via coordinate-anchoring of the nitrogen atom in the amine, the oxygen (of carbonyl-group) and the sulphur atom of the thiol and non-conventional hydrogen bonding between hydrogen atoms of these functional groups with gold. Dixit and colleagues have employed amino and thiol silane-based functionalities for developing surface plasmon resonance-based immunoassays [36, 37].

This latter method is quick and easy for grafting different functional groups to gold surfaces. Many commercially functionalised gold surfaces, viz. amine, carboxy, nitroloacetic acid and streptavidin, are available from manufacturers, particularly from GE Healthcare. Silicon surfaces are routinely functionalised with silane molecules, which create monolayers on its surface with a specific functionality [37]. Silanes mainly possess amine, carboxy, sulphydryl or epoxy functional groups. Therefore, silicon surfaces can first be functionalised followed by customisation of the surface according to immunoassay-specific requirements.

3.2.1.2 Grafting functional groups by physical and chemical methods

A desired scale of hydrophilicity/phobicity can also be achieved by employing specific surface functionalisation strategies. These strategies are highly robust and relatively easy to perform. The most important of these strategies is layer-by-layer (LBL) assembly of polyelectrolytes. An electrolyte is a substance that possesses free ions, but polyelectrolytes are those substances that have functional groups that are capable of generating free ions in solution or in gel phases. When surfaces of solid supports (metallic or polymeric) are coated with these polyelectrolytes their surface properties change significantly. The most common example of a polyelectrolyte-mediated functionalisation is LBL assembly using polyglutamic acid and poly-L-lysine. Various polyelectrolyte systems used for LBL assemblies with their potential applications in the field of immunoassay development are listed in Table 3.5. The summarised LBL methods were employed for the development of various immunoassays In addition, simple grafting of polyglutamic acid or poly-L-lysine can also improve surface wettability for immunoassay-based applications. In general, wettability increases the more hydrophilic the surface, and hence, better ionic interaction mediated immobilisation could be achieved on such surfaces [38–40].

Table 3.5 Commercially available polyelectrolytes used in surface functionalisation [38–40]

Polyelectrolyte (PE)	Monomeric constituents
Cationic	
Cationic polyacrylamides (co-polymer)	Acrylamide and acrylamide-propyl-trimethyl-ammonium chloride
Cationic dextran	Dextran and 2,3-epoxypropyl-trimethyl-ammonium chloride
Poly(diallyl-dimethyl ammonium chloride)	Diallyl-dimethyl ammonium chloride and acrylamide
Polyamideamine epichlorohydrine	Epichlorohydrine
Anionic	
Carboxymethyl-cellulose	Carboxymethyl-cellulose
Polystyrene sulfonate	Styrene sulphonate
Poly(methacrylic acid)	Methacrylic acid
Polyacrylic acid	Acrylic acid
Polystyrene sulfonic acid	Styrene sulfonic acid
Polyethylene glycol	Ethylene glycol
Polyamino acids	Single or multiple amino acid polymers

Physical and chemical methods for efficient functionalisation of surfaces for immunoassay development include surface activation with silanes that are available with important functionalities such as amino (3-aminopropyltriethoxy silane (APTES)), carboxy (sodium salt of carboxy silane) and epoxy silane. However, there are many associated advantages and drawbacks for using silanes. Silanes are easy to use for surface modifications, but the surfaces require prior treatment such as oxidation for generating 'electron-rich' oxygen-containing functional groups that could facilitate siloxane bonds. High water-mediated degradability of these silanes restrict the exposure time of such surfaces with water-containing buffers and reagents. However, there are various methods developed that improve surface wettability by reducing water-associated degradability of silanes. The most common approach for stabilising silane-mediated functionalities is high temperature baking of the surfaces during or after silane functionalisation [41].

Plasma-enhanced chemical vapour deposition (PECVD) is a major technique that grafts a user-defined thickness of a desired functionality on a surface. This technique enables deposition of a homogeneous layer of functional groups on any type of surface, irrespective of whether the surface is metallic or polymeric [42]. Given the preciseness of surface modification with PECVD this approach is widely employed for preparing surfaces with different levels of wettability used for antibody and protein immobilisation and immunoassay development. PECVD is superior than other conventional spin- or drop-coating approaches because of the high degree of homogeneity and stability of the grafted functionalities [43].

3.3 Antibody Immobilisation

The mode of antibody immobilisation dictates the orientation on the surface which ultimately impacts on the antibodies' activity. Hence, efficient immobilisation of antibodies for immunoassay-based applications, be it 'point-of-care' or otherwise, requires novel and well-designed approaches for ensuring maximisation of assay sensitivity. Table 3.6 illustrates some examples of strategies for antibody immobilisation [44].

Table 3.6 Antibody immobilisation strategies

Method	Mechanism	Surface/coupling strategy
Adsorption	Electrostatic; hydrophobic interactions	Polystyrene/nitrocellulose
Covalent (Random)	Random: Primary amines (lysine)	EDC-NHS, aldehyde
Covalent (Ordered)	Cysteine residues Carbohydrate residues	Maleimide Hydrazine
Capture proteins	Affinity	Protein A, G or A/G derivatised
Functional tags	Affinity	Streptavidin-biotin SNAP-tag

The choice of approach for immobilisation relies on novel chemistries to link the surface functional end groups with the various free sites on the antibody. The use of bi-functional linkers targeting specific amino acid residues on the antibody have utility in ordering the antibody orientation on novel surface chemistries [45]. Preparation of fragments from the IgG molecule also facilitates the use of such linker approaches. Figure 3.2 illustrates common approaches for the generation of fragments using enzymatic and recombinant approaches and Table 3.7 highlights some approaches undertaken for the immobilisation of antibodies on multiple surfaces. In general, the non-specific approaches yield greater surface density. However, it is the ordered approaches that result in higher levels of active antigen-binding capacity.

Shmanai and co-workers highlighted the fact that the ability to specifically orientate antibodies can be masked by the 'non-specific' interaction of other low molecular weight functionalities on the antibodies with the surface. Therefore, a balance between site-specific capture and non-specific interactions must be sought, particularly in hydrophobic macro-supports [46]. Vikholm-Lundin addressed this non-specificity issue by using disulphide bearing polymers that can repel proteins and, hence, block any non-specific interactions for SPR-based applications [47].

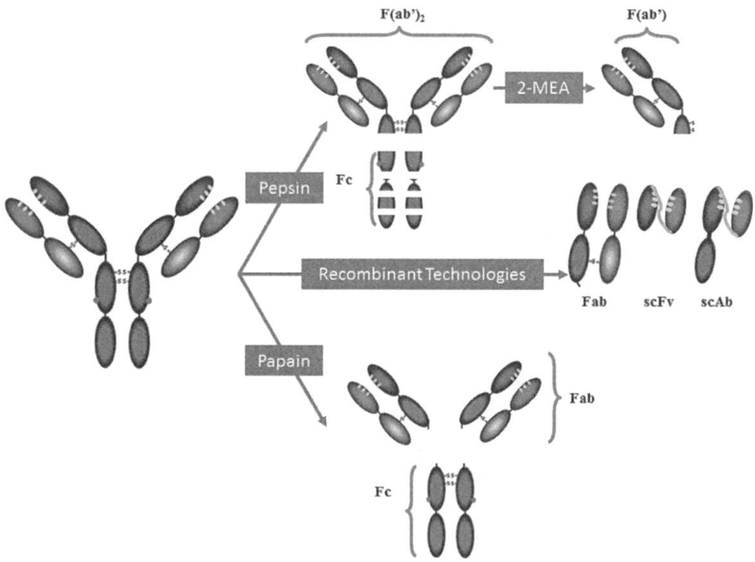

Figure 3.2 Approaches for preparation of IgG fragments. Treatment of the IgG molecule with pepsin generates F(ab')$_2$ and subsequent treatment with 2 mercaptoethylamine (2-MEA) results in the F(ab') fragment. Papain treatment gives rise to Fab fragments, which can be separated from the Fc portion. Recombinant antibodies are an attractive approach for generating superior recognition elements with inclusion of reactive sites to facilitate immobilisation on various fragments. These include the single-chain fragment variable (scFv), fragment antigen binding (Fab) and single-chain antibody (scAb), which facilitates ordered immobilisation. Adapted with permission from Brogan et al. [44].

Table 3.7 highlights the disadvantage of directly attaching antibody fragments (or indeed antibodies in general) to planar surfaces. Brogan and co-workers demonstrated that for a large antigen (alkaline phosphatase, 150 kDa) steric hindrance resulted in lower antigen-binding ability with a planar immobilisation strategy. This could be due to the constrained nature of immobilising antibodies directly on the gold surface, causing denaturation, but it might also be due to inaccessibility of the surface-grafted antibody-binding domains for binding to the epitopes on the antigen. In such a case, increasing the surface density may not increase antigen-binding capacity, as the immobilised fragment may not come into

Table 3.7 Antibody covalent immobilisation approaches

Antibody	Surface chemistry	Detection	Ref.
F(ab') F(ab)	Gold-thiol	QCM	[48]
F(ab') F(ab)	(GOPS)-dextran-amine (GOPS)-thiol	TIRF	[50]
IgG	MOF heterobifunctional Thiol-amine	Fluorescence	[51]
IgG F(ab')	Biotin–hydrazide Biotin–maleimide	Microarray (streptavidin)	[52]
F(ab')	Gold-thiol	SPR	[53]
IgG	DNA-guided protein G	Gold chip (SPR) Gold nanoparticles	[54]
IgG	Antibody-binding peptide-PEG	SPR	[55]
IgG	Thiocyanate - protein A	SPR	[56]
IgG	DDI – Streptavidin Direct immobilisation Affinity ligand	Antibody microarray (3D protein slides)	[57]
IgG	SAM (ssDNA)	SPR	[58]
IgG	Organosilanes Acrylic acid Diethylene glycol Dimethylether	SAF	[42]
IgG	(random IgG/protein G) Sulpho-GMBS Biotin-streptavidin	DPI SPR	[59]
IgG 2-MEA Fragment	Random SAM Orientated SAM Planar gold	SPR	[60]

QCM, quartz crystal microbalance; GOPS, glycidyloxypropyl-trimethoxysilane; TIRF, total internal reflection fluorescence; MOF, microstructured optical fibres; SPR, surface plasmon resonance; DDI, direct DNA immobilisation; PEG, polyethylene glycol; SAF, supercritical angle fluorescence; DPI, dual polarisation interferometry; SAM, self-assembling monolayer.

close contact with the epitope on the antigen. Use of a spacer (e.g. dextran-based hydrogels or other 3D surfaces) facilitates flexibility and rotation of the fragments increasing the chances of the antigen epitope and the antibody coming into contact (Fig. 3.3).

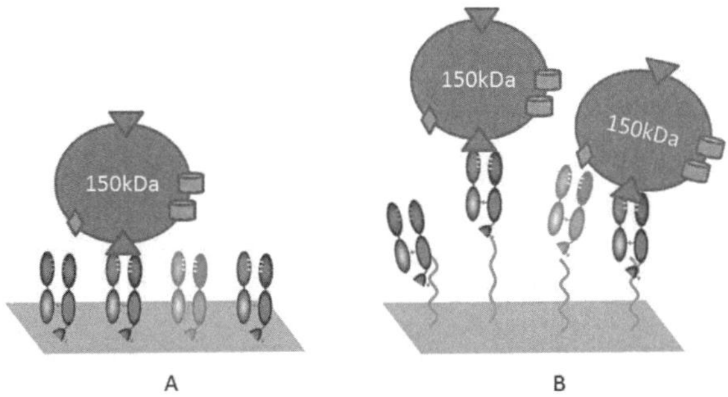

Figure 3.3 Steric hindrance of a planar surface. (A) Polyclonal antibodies with specificities for different epitopes (represented here as different shapes) on the antigen are immobilised on a planar surface. However, not all antibodies have access to their relative cognate epitope for binding. (B) Conversely, in the hydrogel approach, ordered immobilisation is achievable but it imparts potentially extended conformations and permits rotation/movement, thus increasing the odds of multiple antigen-binding events and the propensity for avidity effects.

3.4 Antibody Conjugation to Quantum Dots

Conjugation of antibodies to labels is also of considerable importance. For example, the interest in using quantum dots (QDs) or an ever expanding range of labelled nanoparticles is substantial. The structure and application of QDs was described in Chapter 1 of this book. However, poor solubility of QDs in physiologically relevant buffers, stability and retention of antibody function following linkage are significant challenges for their widespread use. The use of chemical linkers for QD functionalisation using antibodies demonstrated that the type of coupling chemistry and linker may have significant effects on the antibody function. Lee and co-workers successfully applied anti-EGFR antibodies and the use of long chain heterobifunctional linkers (LC-SPDP and sulpho-SMCC) to pegylated QDs for imaging. Although primarily directed towards in vitro/in vivo imaging the approach highlights the key aspect of retaining antibody binding, and the long chain linkers were selected in order to reduce the stress on the antibody and to preserve antigen-binding activity [61]. Conjugating antibodies to nanostructures such as QDs introduces other issues, including separation of the unbound antibody from the preparation and ordered orientation of the antibody. Goldman and co-workers developed a multiplexed QD. Using a leucine zipper fusion of the IgG binding domain of protein G, the QD were functionalised with antibodies. The maltose-binding protein (MPB) was prepared with the same leucine zipper and facilitated removal of the functionalised QDs using amylose affinity resins. In this approach crosslinking and aggregation of the QD was minimalised the functionality of the antibody was retained [62]. For the cardiovascular marker brain natriuretic peptide (BNP) Maeng and co-workers developed an orientated scFv amperometric assay. The scFv expressed in yeast were orientated via the HIS-tag on gold surfaces via disulphide-NTA. In the developed system, the linear range appears to be in the 1–10,000 fg mL^{-1} range and would represent a significant advance in sensitivity, for a portable system with commercial potential [63].

3.5 Aspects and Case Studies of Antibody Immobilisation

Recombinant antibody technology is increasingly coming to the fore as the preferred approach for the generation of highly specific, tailored, biorecognition elements. Increasingly more examples of recombinant antibodies developed with applicability for environmental analysis, diagnostics and therapeutics (to name but a few) have emerged and so the much anticipated expansion of recombinant antibody pools is being realised. Many challenges remain for their ordered orientation as typically reducing the area of the antibody reduces the number of available reactive sites for conjugation. However, numerous strategies developed through research have identified approaches for ordered immobilisation of recombinant antibody fragments but this is typically achieved via random functionalisation that can affect antibody-antigen activity. Townsend and co-workers demonstrated that the structural format of the recombinant antibody fragment and chip functionalisation have effects on an assay for a small illicit drug conjugate. This illustrates that the format and the antibody impact the assay sensitivity in SPR-based analysis [64]. The utility of fusion proteins as mediators for immobilisation was demonstrated for a number of applications for truly ordered orientation. For the purposes of rapid chromatography, Blank and co-workers favoured the use of chitin-binding domains (CBDs). The fusion of antibody and CBDs allowed immobilisation on chitin-coated beads directly from crude bacterial lysates. Higher stability of the immobilised antibody was achieved using a number of CBDs per antibody molecule after first mutating a naturally occurring cysteine in the CBD to achieve maximal bacterial expression [65]. Such an approach could be used for antibody immobilisation on immunoassay surfaces and combines rapid purification with rapid functionalisation. Kwon and co-workers demonstrated the potential of cutinase-mediated SAMs for antibody arrays which maintained antibody reactivity. In that study, the serine esterase forms a site-specific covalent adduct with the surface bound phosphonate ligand [66].

In SPR-based analyses a number of proteins were immobilised and were also shown to be effective in a fluorescence-based microarray. The authors demonstrated an operational strategy for preparing the associated chips with controllable antibody density. Scholler and co-workers utilised yeast mating to generate in vitro biotinylated antibody fragments. These 'biobodies' were generated by first screening a library for anti-HE4 scFv (ovarian cancer marker) followed by mating with haploid yeast carrying a biotin ligase sequence. The generated constructs were readily used on biotinylated alkaloid-based surfaces which took advantage of the multiple biotin-binding sites available on streptavidin to capture the biobodies for characterisation [67]. In a similar approach, Even-Desrumeaux and co-workers developed a bead-based sandwich assay using novel single-domain antibody fragments (sdAbs), which are the V_{HH} domain antibodies from camelids. In this study, in vivo biotinylation was achieved in *E. coli* facilitating direct spotting of bacterial lysates for sandwich assay development for the purposes of developing high-throughput antibody-based diagnostic arrays. This bead-based approach has potential for multiplexing and is an attractive approach for low-density clinical-diagnostic arrays [68].

'Tunable' immunosorbents for the detection of atrazine contamination were described and take advantage of reversible phase transitions from soluble to aggregate with change in temperature. Kim and co-workers fused the elastin-like polypeptide (EPL) to a single chain antibody (scAb) which facilitated phase separation of the fused antibody bound to the atrazine antigen in a competitive assay format without the need to immobilise any elements of the assay. The assay carried out using the fusion was 10-fold more sensitive than the same assay carried out using the scAb alone [69]. This approach circumvents the need to chemically conjugate polymers to the antibody. However, in this case the ELP was fused the N-terminus of the scAb. To orientate the linker away from the binding site perhaps a C-terminal fusion to the human Ck chain would be of interest especially if developed for assays involving larger antigens such as proteins.

The SNAP-tag takes advantage of rapid, specific coupling by O(6)-alkyllguanine DNA alkyltransferase recombinantly expressed with the antibody, such that substrates containing O(6)-benzylguanine are covalently bonded via a thioether bond. The approach demonstrated by Kampmeier and co-workers aimed to broaden the utility of small antibody fragments by virtue of conjugation without compromising binding. This approach has been successfully demonstrated in a number of settings from introduction of flurophores for imaging to fluorescence activated cell sorting (FACS), in addition to labelling of non-antibody ligands (e.g. CD40L) [70].

Exploitation of the reactivity of free cysteines is a useful approach for ordered immobilisation. Brockmann and co-workers engineered a free cysteine into both scFv and Fab constructs to develop an ordered fragment assay for the thyroid stimulating hormone (TSH). The free cysteine was reacted with maleimide PEO_2-biotin and assembled on the surface through interaction with streptavidin. The surface-bound scFv and Fab molecules enabled sensitive detection of TSH in comparison to an intact monoclonal. The reason may be that more scFv and Fab can be captured per unit area of the functionalised surface, in comparison to the full-length antibody, thus allowing for the capture of a higher amount of antigen. In this case an 'all-in-one assay' was carried out with good detection limits [71]. Liu and co-workers utilised the free cysteine for a scFv-based Au nanoparticle aggregation. In this case the cysteine was engineered within the linker region of the scFv [72]. The aggregation of the scFv-stabilised nanoparticles allowed colourimetric detection and could potentially be applied in a lateral-flow type immunoassay using other antigen-specific scFv.

Another interesting site-specific approach exploits the so-called 21st amino acid, selenocysteine (Sec) which is a cysteine analogue that replaces the sulphur-containing thiol with a selenium-containing selenol group [73–75]. In this case issues regarding the low levels of expression of soluble proteins with free cysteine residues in *E. coli* are overcome. In recombinant proteins the targeted incorporation of Sec is achieved using the UGA codon downstream of a cis-like structure which in mammalian systems is known as the selenocysteine insertion sequence (SECIS), whereas in prokaryotic systems the Sel operon is also required. This allows conservation of other important cysteine residues and permits inclusion of a targeted/orientated reactive handle. Hofer and others have expressed Fc-Sec variants to demonstrate the utility of such antibody derivatives in mammalian systems [74–76]. In this fashion maleimide chemistry was shown to selectively target Sec for biotin derivatisation in the presence of DTT and not to conjugate with free cysteine under the same conditions [77]. Hofer and co-workers demonstrated the approach with intact IgG-sec and Fab-sec constructs expressed recombinantly for conjugation to a number of molecules with therapeutic, proteomic and diagnostic applications [76]. In this approach biotin-iodoacetamide and biotin-maleimide were conjugated to the antibody-sec recombinants. Rader and co-workers used dual cysteine and selenocysteine to allow decoration of scFv-Fc constructs with particular applicability to antibody-drug conjugates (ADCs) [74, 75]. The antibody-antigen-binding was also not disrupted in these cases. The inclusion of a Sec is advantageous as it facilitates site-specific conjugation without reduction or modification, has a high nucleophilic reactivity (>90% efficiency of conjugation), conserves natural disulphide bonds and has controllable stoichiometry. Given that the chemistry required for conjugation exists for numerous fluorphores and surfaces the incorporation of such proteins into immunoassay platforms appears to have potential.

The deployment of recombinant antibodies on immunoassay surfaces is gathering momentum as the selected antibodies are becoming truly ultra-sensitive and tailored towards such assay formats [78]. The recombinant antibodies are not necessarily taken from parental monoclonal antibodies, but from immune repertoires from practically any species and naïve sources. These recombinant antibodies, engineered to be of high-affinity and targeting crucial epitopes of many important disease targets, are rapidly engineered to overcome the issues associated with random immobilisation. Thus, the surfaces are becoming more homogenous and contain high capacities of functionally intact bio-recognition molecules to support the development of higher sensitivity immunoassays.

3.6 Conclusions and Future Perspectives

Proteins are fragile molecules and antibodies, in their role as biorecognition elements, must be treated under conditions that favour retention of their activity and promote immobilisation with adequate densities in correct orientations in order to support the development of novel immunoassays. Phage, ribosome and yeast display are generating novel antibodies for diagnostics. These recombinant formats are advantageous. Once established, they can be produced and engineered relatively cheaply. Novel substrate surface chemistries and conjugation approaches are advancing our ability to deploy these reagents, however, there is no one leading approach which marries all the analytical requirements that are essential for developing immunoassays. Advancing our knowledge of surface chemistries and integrating surface science, and biology and chemistry with a focus on developing physiologically relevant bio-materials is crucial to produce the next generation of immunoassays.

Considerable advances have been made to improve immunodiagnostic approaches that have focussed on surface preparation, microfluidic design, antibody immobilisation strategies and signal enhancement approaches. As discussed, the antibody immobilisation strategy is a key component of the process that makes a significant contribution to the assay performance. These advances coupled with the availability of high quality, highly specific antibodies to a range of important indicators of human and animal health have the potential to lead to the next generation of immune-diagnostic devices.

References

1. Kusnezow, W., and Hoheisel, J.D. (2003). Solid supports for microarray immunoassays, *J Mol Recognit*, **16**, pp. 165–176.
2. Angenendt, P. (2005). Progress in protein and antibody microarray technology, *Drug Discov Today*, **10**, pp. 503–511.
3. Liu, Y.S., and Li, C.M. (2012). Advanced immobilization and amplification for high performance protein chips, *Anal Lett*, **45**, pp. 130–155.
4. Bonroy, K., Frederix, F., Reekmans, G., Dewolf, E., De Palma, R., Borghs, G., Declerck, P., and Goddeeris, B. (2006). Comparison of random and oriented immobilisation of antibody fragments on mixed self-assembled monolayers, *J Immunol Methods*, **312**, pp. 167–181.
5. Wong, L.S., Khan, F., and Micklefield, J. (2009). Selective covalent protein immobilization: strategies and applications, *Chem Rev*, **109**, pp. 4025–4053.
6. Jung, Y., Jeong, J.Y., and Chung, B.H. (2008). Recent advances in immobilization methods of antibodies on solid supports, *Analyst*, **133**, pp. 697–701.
7. Abuknesha, R.A., Jeganathan, F., Wu, J., and Baalawy, Z. (2009). Labeling of biotin antibodies with horseradish peroxidase using cyanuric chloride, *Nat Protoc*, **4**, pp. 452–460.
8. Engin, S., Trouillet, V., Franz, C.M., Welle, A., Bruns, M., and Wedlich, D. (2010). Benzylguanine thiol self-assembled monolayers for the immobilization of SNAP-tag proteins on microcontact-printed surface structures, *Langmuir*, **26**, pp. 6097–6101.
9. Gaberc-Porekar, V., and Menart, V. (2005). Potential for using histidine tags in purification of proteins at large scale, *Chem Eng Technol*, **28**, pp. 1306–1314.
10. Wang, J.Y., and Chao, Y.P. (2006). Immobilization of cells with surface-displayed chitin-binding domain, *Appl Environ Microbiol*, **72**, pp. 927–931.
11. Schmid, A.H., Stanca, S.E., Thakur, M.S., Thampi, K.R., and Suri, C.R. (2006). Site-directed antibody immobilization on gold substrate for

surface plasmon resonance sensors, *Sens Actuators B-Chem*, **113**, pp. 297–303.

12. Park, T.J., Park, J.P., Lee, S.J., Hong, H.J., and Lee, S.Y. (2006). Polyhydroxyalkanoate chip for the specific immobilization of recombinant proteins and its applications in immunodiagnostics, *Biotechnol Bioprocess Eng*, **11**, pp. 173–177.
13. Zhong, M., Fang, J., and Wei, Y.N. (2010). Site specific and reversible protein immobilization facilitated by a DNA binding fusion tag, *Bioconjug Chem*, **21**, pp. 1177–1182.
14. MacCraith, B.D., and Peleretcky, L. (2010). Luminescence-based sensor using protuberance to direct light, U.S. Patent, 7,655,475.
15. Gerdtsson, A.S., Dexlin-Mellby, L., Delfani, P., Berglund, E., Borrebaeck, C.A.K., and Wingren, C. (2016). Evaluation of solid supports for slide- and well-based recombinant antibody microarrays, *Microarrays* (Basel, Switzerland), **5**, p. 16.
16. Dixit, C.K., and Kaushik, A. (2012). Nano-structured arrays for multiplex analyses and Lab-on-a-Chip applications, *Biochem Biophys Res Commun*, **419**, pp. 316–320.
17. Spencer, N.D. (2011). Tailoring Surfaces: Modifying Surface Composition and Structure for Applications in Tribology, Biology and Catalysis. IISc Centenary Lecture Series, Vol. 5, World Scientific Publishing.
18. Peterson, S., Gattermayer, M., and Biesalski, M. (2011). Hold on at the Right Spot: Bioactive Surfaces for the Design of Live-Cell Micropatterns, 1st ed., Vol. 240, Springer-Verlag Berlin Heidelberg.
19. Ertl, G. (2009). Reactions at Solid Surfaces. Wiley and Sons, NJ.
20. Sung, D., Shin, D.H., and Jon, S. (2011). Toward immunoassay chips: Facile immobilization of antibodies on cyclic olefin copolymer substrates through pre-activated polymer adlayers, *Biosens Bioelectron*, **26**, pp. 3967–3972.
21. Bhaskara, R.M., and Srinivasan, N. (2011). Stability of domain structures in multi-domain proteins, *Sci Rep*, **1**, p. 40.
22. Siow, K.S., Britcher, L., Kumar, S., and Griesser, H.J. (2006). Plasma methods for the generation of chemically reactive surfaces for biomolecule immobilization and cell colonization - a review, *Plasma Process Polym*, **3**, pp. 392–418.
23. Bech, L., Meylheuc, T., Lepoittevin, B., and Roger, P. (2007). Chemical surface modification of poly(ethylene terephthalate) fibers by aminolysis and grafting of carbohydrates, *J Polym Sci Part A-Polym Chem*, **45**, pp. 2172–2183.

24. Gandhiraman, R.P., Le, N.C., Dixit, C.K., Volcke, C., Doyle, C., Gubala, V., Uppal, S., Monaghan, R., James, B., O'Kennedy, R., Daniels, S., and Williams, D.E. (2011). Multi-layered plasma-polymerized chips for SPR-based detection, *ACS Appl Mater Interfaces*, **3**, pp. 4640–4648.

25. Dixit, C.K., Vashist, S.K., MacCraith, B.D., and O'Kennedy, R. (2011). Multisubstrate-compatible ELISA procedures for rapid and high-sensitivity immunoassays, *Nat Protoc*, **6**, pp. 439–445.

26. Nagase, K., Kumazaki, M., Kanazawa, H., Kobayashi, J., Kikuci, A., Akiyama, Y., Annaka, M., and Okano, T. (2010). Thermoresponsive polymer brush surfaces with hydrophobic groups for all-aqueous chromatography, *ACS Appl Mater Interfaces*, **2**, pp. 1247–1253.

27. Zhou, J., Ellis, A.V., and Voelcker, N.H. (2010). Recent developments in PDMS surface modification for microfluidic devices, *Electrophoresis*, **31**, pp. 2–16.

28. Huang, T.S., Tzeng, Y., Liu, Y.K., Chen, Y.K., Walker, K.R., Guntupalli, R., and Liu, C. (2004). Immobilization of antibodies and bacterial binding on nanodiamond and carbon nanotubes for biosensor applications, *Diam Relat Mater*, **13**, pp. 1098–1102.

29. Vermeer, A.W., and Norde, W. (2000). The thermal stability of immunoglobulin: unfolding and aggregation of a multi-domain protein, *Biophys J*, **78**, pp. 394–404.

30. Vermeer, A.W., and Norde, W. (2000). CD spectroscopy of proteins adsorbed at flat hydrophilic quartz and hydrophobic teflon surfaces, *J Colloid Interface Sci*, **225**, pp. 394–397.

31. Vermeer, A.W., Norde, W., and van Amerongen, A. (2000). The unfolding/denaturation of immunogammaglobulin of isotype 2b and its F(ab) and F(c) fragments, *Biophys J*, **79**, pp. 2150–2154.

32. Vermeer, A.W.P., Bremer, M.G.E.G., and Norde, W. (1998). Structural changes of IgG induced by heat treatment and by adsorption onto a hydrophobic Teflon surface studied by circular dichroism spectroscopy, *Biochim Biophys Acta - Gen Subj*, **1425**, pp. 1–12.

33. Buijs, J., Norde, W., and Lichtenbelt, J.W.T. (1996). Changes in the secondary structure of adsorbed IgG and F(ab')(2) studied by FTIR spectroscopy, *Langmuir*, **12**, pp. 1605–1613.

34. Arlett, J.L., Myers, E.B., and Roukes, M.L. (2011). Comparative advantages of mechanical biosensors, *Nat Nanotechnol*, **6**, pp. 203–215.

35. Kato, F., Ogi, H., Yanagida, T., Nishikawa, S., Hirao, M., and Nishiyama, M. (2012). Resonance acoustic microbalance with naked-embedded

quartz (RAMNE-Q) biosensor fabricated by microelectromechanical-system process, *Biosens Bioelectron*, **33**, pp. 139–145.

36. Pakiari, A.H., and Jamshidi, Z. (2007). Interaction of amino acids with gold and silver clusters, *J Phys Chem A*, **111**, pp. 4391–4396.
37. Vashist, S.K., Dixit, C.K., MacCraith, B.D., and O'Kennedy, R. (2011). Effect of antibody immobilization strategies on the analytical performance of a surface plasmon resonance-based immunoassay, *Analyst*, **136**, pp. 4431–4436.
38. Kim, D., Karns, K., Tia, S.Q., He, M., and Herr, A.E. (2012). Electrostatic protein immobilization using charged polyacrylamide gels and cationic detergent microfluidic western blotting, *Anal Chem*, **84**, pp. 2533–2540.
39. de la Escosura-Muñiz, A., and Merkoçi, A. (2010). Electrochemical detection of proteins using nanoparticles: applications to diagnostics, *Expert Opin Med Diagn*, **4**, pp. 21–37.
40. Masereel, B., Dinguizli, M., Bouzin, C., Moniotte, N., Feron, O., Gallez, B., Borght, T.V., Michiels, C., and Lucas, S. (2011). Antibody immobilization on gold nanoparticles coated layer-by-layer with polyelectrolytes, *J Nanoparticle Res*, **13**, pp. 1573–1580.
41. Aissaoui, N., Bergaoui, L., Landoulsi, J., Lambert, J.F., and Boujday, S. (2012). Silane layers on silicon surfaces: mechanism of interaction, stability, and influence on protein adsorption, *Langmuir*, **28**, pp. 656–665.
42. O'Mahony, C.C., Gubala, V., Gandhiraman, R.P., Daniels, S., Yuk, J.S., MacCraith, B.D., and Williams, D.E. (2012). Improving the sensitivity of immunoassays with PEG-COOH-like film prepared by plasma-based technique, *J Biomed Mater Res Part A*, **100A**, pp. 230–235.
43. Alf, M.E., Asatekin, A., Barr, M.C., Baxamusa, S.H., Chelawat, H., Ozaydin-Ince, G., Petruczok, C.D., Sreenivasan, R., Tenhaeff, W.E., Trujillo, N.J., Vaddiraju, S., Xu, J., and Gleason, K.K. (2010). Chemical vapor deposition of conformal, functional, and responsive polymer films, *Adv Mater*, **22**, pp. 1993–2027.
44. Shen, M., Rusling, J.F., and Dixit, C.K. (2016). Site-selective orientated immobilization of antibodies and conjugates for immunodiagnostics development, *Methods,* doi: 10.1016/j.ymeth.2016.11.010.
45. Shriver-Lake, L.C., Donner, B., Edelstein, R., Breslin, K., Bhatia, S.K., and Ligler, F.S. (1997). Antibody immobilization using heterobifunctional crosslinkers, *Biosens Bioelectron*, **12**, pp. 1101–1106.
46. Shmanai, V.V., Nikolayeva, T.A., Vinokurova, L.G., and Litoshka, A.A. (2001). Oriented antibody immobilization to polystyrene macro-

carriers for immunoassay modified with hydrazide derivatives of poly(meth)acrylic acid, *BMC Biotechnol*, **1**, p. 4.

47. Vikholm-Lundin, I. (2005). Immunosensing based on site-directed immobilization of antibody fragments and polymers that reduce nonspecific binding, *Langmuir*, **21**, pp. 6473–6477.
48. Brogan, K.L., Wolfe, K.N., Jones, P.A., and Schoenfisch, M.H. (2003). Direct oriented immobilization of F(ab') antibody fragments on gold, *Anal Chim Acta*, **496**, pp. 73–80.
49. Makaraviciute, A., and Ramanaviciene, A. (2013). Site-directed antibody immobilization techniques for immunosensors, *Biosens Bioelectron*, **50**, pp. 460–471.
50. Tedeschi, L., Domenici, C., Ahluwalia, A., Baldini, F., and Mencaglia, A. (2003). Antibody immobilisation on fibre optic TIRF sensors, *Biosens Bioelectron*, **19**, pp. 85–93.
51. Ruan, Y., Foo, T.C., Warren-Smith, S., Hoffmann, P., Moore, R.C., Ebendorff-Heidepriem, H., and Monro, T.M. (2008). Antibody immobilization within glass microstructured fibers: a route to sensitive and selective biosensors, *Opt Express*, **16**, pp. 18514–18523.
52. Peluso, P., Wilson, D.S., Do, D., Tran, H., Venkatasubbaiah, M., Quincy, D., Heidecker, B., Poindexter, K., Tolani, N., Phelan, M., Witte, K., Jung, L.S., Wagner, P., and Nock, S. (2003). Optimizing antibody immobilization strategies for the construction of protein microarrays, *Anal Biochem*, **312**, pp. 113–124.
53. Lee, W., Oh, B.K., Lee, W.H., and Choi, J.W. (2005). Immobilization of antibody fragment for immunosensor application based on surface plasmon resonance, *Colloids Surf B-Biointerfaces*, **40**, pp. 143–148.
54. Jung, Y., Lee, J.M., Jung, H., and Chung, B.H. (2007). Self-directed and self-oriented immobilization of antibody by protein G-DNA conjugate, *Anal Chem*, **79**, pp. 6534–6541.
55. Jung, Y.W., Kang, H.J., Lee, J.M., Jung, S.O., Yun, W.S., Chung, S.J., and Chung, B.H. (2008). Controlled antibody immobilization onto immunoanalytical platforms by synthetic peptide, *Anal Biochem*, **374**, pp. 99–105.
56. Boltovets, P.M., Boyko, V.R., Kostikov, I.Y., Dyachenko, N.S., Snopok, B.A., and Shirshov, Y.M. (2002). Simple method for plant virus detection: effect of antibody immobilization technique, *J Virol Methods*, **105**, pp. 141–146.
57. Wacker, R., Schroder, H., and Niemeyer, C.M. (2004). Performance of antibody microarrays fabricated by either DNA-directed immobilization,

direct spotting, or streptavidin-biotin attachment: a comparative study, *Anal Biochem*, **330**, pp. 281–287.

58. Boozer, C., Ladd, J., Chen, S.F., and Jiang, S.T. (2006). DNA-directed protein immobilization for simultaneous detection of multiple analytes by surface plasmon resonance biosensor, *Anal Chem*, **78**, pp. 1515–1519.
59. Song, H.Y., Zhou, X., Hobley, J., and Su, X. (2012). Comparative study of random and oriented antibody immobilization as measured by dual polarization interferometry and surface plasmon resonance spectroscopy, *Langmuir*, **28**, pp. 997–1004.
60. Kausaite-Minkstimiene, A., Ramanaviciene, A., Kirlyte, J., and Ramanavicius, A. (2010). Comparative study of random and oriented antibody immobilization techniques on the binding capacity of immunosensor, *Anal Chem*, **82**, pp. 6401–6408.
61. Lee, J., Choi, Y., Kim, K., Hong, S., Park, H.-Y., Lee, T., Cheon, G.J., and Song, R. (2010). Characterization and cancer cell specific binding properties of anti-EGFR antibody conjugated quantum dots, *Bioconjug Chem*, **21**, pp. 940–946.
62. Goldman, E.R., Clapp, A.R., Anderson, G.P., Uyeda, H.T., Mauro, J.M., Medintz, I.L., and Mattoussi, H. (2004). Multiplexed toxin analysis using four colors of quantum dot fluororeagents, *Anal Chem*, **76**, pp. 684–688.
63. Maeng, B.H., Choi, J., Sa, Y.S., Shin, J.H., and Kim, Y.H. (2012). Functional expression of recombinant anti-BNP scFv in methylotrophic yeast *Pichia pastoris* and application as a recognition molecule in electrochemical sensors, *World J Microbiol Biotechnol*, **28**, pp. 1027–1034.
64. Townsend, S., Finlay, W.J., Hearty, S., and O'Kennedy, R. (2006). Optimizing recombinant antibody function in SPR immunosensing. The influence of antibody structural format and chip surface chemistry on assay sensitivity, *Biosens Bioelectron*, **22**, pp. 268–274.
65. Blank, K., Lindner, P., Diefenbach, B., and Pluckthun, A. (2002). Self-immobilizing recombinant antibody fragments for immunoaffinity chromatography: generic, parallel, and scalable protein purification, *Protein Expr Purif*, **24**, pp. 313–322.
66. Kwon, Y., Han, Z., Karatan, E., Mrksich, M., and Kay, B.K. (2004). Antibody arrays prepared by cutinase-mediated immobilization on self-assembled monolayers, *Anal Chem*, **76**, pp. 5713–5720.
67. Scholler, N., Garvik, B., Quarles, T., Jiang, S., and Urban, N. (2006). Method for generation of in vivo biotinylated recombinant antibodies by yeast mating, *J Immunol Methods*, **317**, pp. 132–143.

68. Even-Desrumeaux, K., Baty, D., and Chames, P. (2010). Strong and oriented immobilization of single domain antibodies from crude bacterial lysates for high-throughput compatible cost-effective antibody array generation, *Mol Biosyst*, **6**, pp. 2241–2248.

69. Kim, J.Y., Mulchandani, A., and Chen, W. (2003). An immunoassay for atrazine using tunable immunosorbent, *Anal Biochem*, **322**, pp. 251–256.

70. Kampmeier, F., Ribbert, M., Nachreiner, T., Dembski, S., Beaufils, F., Brecht, A., and Barth, S. (2009). Site-specific, covalent labeling of recombinant antibody fragments via fusion to an engineered version of 6-O-alkylguanine DNA alkyltransferase, *Bioconjug Chem*, **20**, pp. 1010–1015.

71. Brockmann, E.C., Vehniainen, M., and Pettersson, K. (2010). Use of high-capacity surface with oriented recombinant antibody fragments in a 5-min immunoassay for thyroid-stimulating hormone, *Anal Biochem*, **396**, pp. 242–249.

72. Liu, Y., Mernaugh, R.L., and Zeng, X. (2009). Single chain fragment variable recombinant antibody functionalized gold nanoparticles for a highly sensitive colorimetric immunoassay, *Biosens Bioelectron*, **24**, pp. 2853–2857.

73. Johansson, L., Gafvelin, G., and Arner, E.S. (2005). Selenocysteine in proteins-properties and biotechnological use, *Biochim Biophys Acta*, **1726**, pp. 1–13.

74. Li, X., Patterson, J.T., Sarkar, M., Pedzisa, L., Kodadek, T., Roush, W.R., and Rader, C. (2015). Site-specific dual antibody conjugation via engineered cysteine and selenocysteine residues., *Bioconjug Chem*, **26**, pp. 2243–2248.

75. Li, X., Yang, J., and Rader, C. (2014). Antibody conjugation via one and two C-terminal selenocysteines., *Methods*, **65**, pp. 133–138.

76. Hofer, T., Skeffington, L.R., Chapman, C.M., and Rader, C. (2009). Molecularly defined antibody conjugation through a selenocysteine interface, *Biochemistry*, **48**, pp. 12047–12057.

77. Hofer, T., Thomas, J.D., Burke Jr., T.R., and Rader, C. (2008). An engineered selenocysteine defines a unique class of antibody derivatives, *Proc Natl Acad Sci U S A*, **105**, pp. 12451–12456.

78. Conroy, P.J., Hearty, S., Leonard, P., and O'Kennedy, R.J. (2009). Antibody production, design and use for biosensor-based applications, *Semin Cell Dev Biol*, **20**, pp. 10–26.

Chapter 4

Immunoassay Validation

Paul Leonard
Vaccinogen Inc., 949 Fell street, 2nd Floor, Baltimore, MD 21231, USA
pleonard@vaccinogeninc.com

This chapter is designed to provide a short primer for the design, development and **validation** of immunoassays. It is intended to guide researchers, managers and analysts from both academic and industrial laboratories through the strategies and recommendations for the validation of new immunoassay methods. While it provides lists of parameters that should be tested and evaluated, it contains by no means an exhaustive list and, therefore, the reader should determine on a case-by-case basis if their assays require further experimental design and testing to that suggested here. The chapter is laid out in such a manner that one can systematically perform experiments in a logical fashion lending to validation of an assay with continuous documenting and recording of the required data for a validation report. Preliminary assay development considerations such as antibody production and selection are also discussed, though these are covered in depth earlier in Chapter 2 of this book. In addition to the author's own experience, the reasoning behind this overview has stemmed from a review of recent publications

Immunoassays: Development, Applications and Future Trends
Edited by Richard O'Kennedy and Caroline Murphy

ISBN 978-981-4669-97-9 (Hardcover), 978-1-315-20654-7 (eBook)
www.panstanford.com

and regulatory guidelines, all of which are listed at the end of this contribution.

4.1 Why Is Validation Necessary?

Imagine the emotional stress of sitting in a doctor's office after having being told you have tested positive for a serious, life-threatening illness, only to find out weeks later that the test result was false. Of even greater concern, now imagine you have tested negative for this life-threatening illness, only to discover months later that you actually have the disease and it has now progressed to an advanced life-threatening stage. Fortunately for us, regulations and quality standards that have an impact on analytical laboratories require methods to be validated [1, 2], ensuring that misdiagnosis cases, whether **false positive** or **false negative**, rarely occur. While the extent of guidelines for validation [1, 3–10] requirements provided by the different regulatory organisations (e.g., U.S. FDA, ICH, PIC/S, USP, ISO/IEC 170025) varies widely, the overall objective is always to achieve valid analytical test results [2]. The laboratory using a given method is responsible for ensuring that it is adequately validated, and, if necessary, equipped sufficiently for carrying out further work to supplement existing data. For example, where a method has been validated by a standards approving organisation, such as AOAC International, the user will normally need only to establish performance data for their own use of the method [3].

4.2 Assay Validation Overview

In its most generic form, an immunoassay is an analytical method dependent on the specific binding of an antibody with its target analyte. Detection is achieved by the addition of a signal-generating component (reporter label), which gives a response to the target analyte [11]. The objective of immunoassay validation is to be able to define an assay in terms of statistically quantifiable parameters with measured confidence. The designation of *validated assay* is only merited when it has been defined in terms of its capacity to classify samples with regard to the presence or absence of a particular analyte [12]. Bioanalytical method validation includes all the procedures that demonstrate that a particular method used for quantitative measurement of analytes in a given biological matrix, such as blood, plasma, serum, urine, sweat or milk, is reliable and reproducible for the intended use [8]. The fundamental parameters for this validation include but are not limited to (1) **accuracy**, (2) **precision**, (3) **selectivity**, (4) **reproducibility**, and (5) stability. The validation process (see Fig. 4.1) involves documenting, through the use of specific laboratory investigations, that the performance characteristics of the method are suitable and reliable for the intended analytical applications. The acceptability of analytical data corresponds directly to the criteria used to validate the method.

4.2.1 Planning 'It Takes Time to Save Time'

It is by no means a coincidence that the first 'P' in Mintzberg's 5Ps for better strategy is planning [13]. Planning is fundamental to any project as proper planning prevents poor performance. Immunoassays can involve many different components of varying degrees of complexity, all of which can introduce variance into the assay. Successful immunoassay validation therefore requires a well-defined master plan to ensure consistent and efficient execution of the validation project. The validation plan should be written before the initiation of a validation project and prior to commencement of validation experiments. This plan can be a stand-alone document or can be contained in an appropriate laboratory notebook. The documentation should include a description of the intended use of the immunoassay under consideration and a summary of the performance parameters to be validated. These should include, but may not be limited to, precision, accuracy, range of quantification, standard curve, **specificity** and selectivity, linearity, reproducibility and robustness [14]. One way to save time in assay development is to spend time planning. By answering the antibody selection questions listed below (Table 4.1) and by following step-by-step the subsequent sections in this chapter, one should reach their desired goal in reduced time and with the benefits of a well-proven assay.

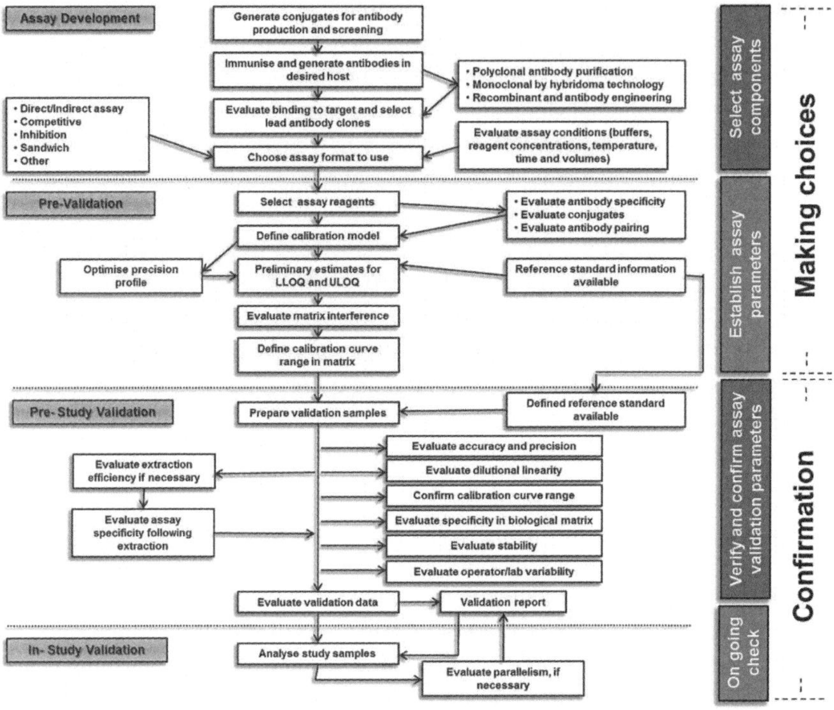

Figure 4.1 Schematic overview of the steps involved in the development, verification and validation of a typical immunoassay (adapted from [15]). Developing an assay usually starts with the assay development and pre-validation steps shown above. These sections involve what one may call the 'making choices' part of developing an assay and is where one defines the assay parameters. If the assay meets the analytical requirements determined a priori, a pre-study validation can be performed to verify that the assay is suitable for its intended purpose. This section involves 'confirming you made the right choice' as it is dependent on the decisions made previously such as the calibration model and sample range used. The in-study validation is performed as a continuous validation of an approved assay and is required to check that this assay still functions as intended.

4.3 Assay Development

Method feasibility studies address the likelihood that an assay will be able to achieve its intended purpose and whether the performance characteristics of the assay are appropriate for the

Table 4.1 Important considerations to be made prior to antibody selection and assay development

Questions that one should ask before starting	How your answers could define your plan
What is the assay for?	If the assay is desired for a disease, then antibodies against a specific marker for that disease will be needed. Selection of species appropriate antibodies (e.g. chicken antibodies) may need to be considered to eliminate or reduce heterophilic antibody interaction such as human anti-mouse antibody (HAMA) effects [16].
Where will the test be used? (e.g. point-of-care or in a lab)	If the test is going to be POC, then considerations should be taken as temperature fluctuations and short assay times can influence the process of selecting the optimal antibody [17].
What type of test will it be? (e.g. LFIA, ELISA, Biosensor?)	The antibody may have to be immobilised or conjugated to a particle or enzyme. This can affect the choice of antibody format and selection strategy used. Antibodies should be selected that retain their functionality when immobilised on the assay platform.
What will the matrix be?	This will affect how the antibody should be selected and characterised. The antibody should perform well in the sample matrix and should be tested in this matrix prior to assay development.
Is there an extraction process?	The extraction process will influence the selection of the antibody (so it works well in extraction buffer) and also the performance of the test. How accurate, precise and reproducible is the extraction method? This will impact on your overall assay procedure performance. How will the samples be taken and how will that affect the assay? For example, an assay for heart disease will probably use serum of patients undergoing treatment who will have contaminants like heparin or warfarin in their blood. Will these interfere with antibody performance?
What are the analyte properties? (size, stability, pH, etc.)	If the analyte is less than 10 kDa it may need to be conjugated prior to immunisation. If it is a drug that easily metabolises it might be better to design an assay for a stable metabolic form. If it is a protein antigen and forms breakdown products that could interfere with the assay, it would be advantageous to only select antibodies against a stable or disease-specific epitope.

(*Contd.*)

Table 4.1 (*Continued*)

Questions that one should ask before starting	How your answers could define your plan
What is the current MRL or clinically relevant 'cut-off' level?	Knowing these values will help determine if antibody affinity maturation or selection of a new antibody is needed. It will also determine if assay re-design to improve performance is needed (e.g. more sensitive signal label, more sensitive reader or detection method, larger sample volume or the use of an analyte concentration step).
Is there a test already available?	Can it be used for comparison and selectivity studies? What is the gold standard technology currently in use? Can your assay be compared side by side?
What assay format?	A sandwich assay will require a minimum of two antibodies directed against different epitopes. A direct assay will require labelling if not using a 'label-free' platform. Analyte size will often determine assay format.
What is the desired assay time?	The 'quicker the better' is the growing trend with the development of POC devices [16]. The desired time will influence having a direct or indirect assay format. It will also influence the antibody selection strategy. For a POC device, a selection should be based on antibody 'on-rate' and not 'off-rate'. However, if developing an assay with a longer time-course, the antibody 'on-rate' and 'off-rate' should be taken into careful consideration during the antibody selection strategy.

needs of the study [18]. Method development and optimisation activities should result in an assay that the analyst believes is 'ready for validation', meaning that there is a significant amount of development data indicating potential reliability of the assay and suitability for its intended purpose [18]. Information on the following should be generated during assay development: critical assay reagent selection and stability, assay format selection (antibodies, diluents, plates, detection system etc.), standard curve model selection, matrix selection, specificity of the reagents, sample preparation and preliminary performance evaluation [19]. The goal of the development phase for immunoassays is to establish a method that can consistently produce a reliable result culminating in a validation plan with established target acceptance criteria for accuracy and precision [14]. Therefore, assay development is probably the most critical section as errors made here such as the use of an inappropriate immunogen, poor quality antibody (low affinity, tendency to cross react, unstable), suboptimal assay format, incorrect concentrations used and suboptimal test components and conditions will significantly affect the overall assay performance. While many analysts embarking on an immunoassay validation project may be presented with many if not all source materials such as antibodies to develop the assay, sometimes one has to source suitable reagents or even produce these reagents 'in-house'. In the latter case, it is important to take into account the following considerations:

4.3.1 Immunogen for Antibody Production and Screening

Time spent choosing a good immunogen will save a lot of assay development time and produce a better quality immunoassay. The immunogen should ideally be pure and structurally identical to the target analyte. If looking to develop an assay for a protein analyte, the immunogen could be the whole protein or a peptide sequence shown to originate from a highly specific region of that protein. A study of the target analyte and its properties should be performed a priori to aid in designing an immunisation strategy that will produce a highly specific antibody. If developing a hapten–carrier conjugate for immunisation, a panel of conjugates should be produced to aid the screening process.

4.3.2 Antibody Production

If within scope of the project, it is best to develop a tailored antibody for a desired assay rather just developing an assay with an antibody that one has, which in many cases could have suboptimal performance on the assay platform or format. I always suggest 'starting at the finish line' by asking one-self what is the assay for? Where will it be tested? What will the matrix be? What specificity and **sensitivity** is needed? In answering these and other questions (see Table 4.1) before proceeding to an antibody production campaign, the immunogen and selection strategies can be refined to provide the best approach for yielding high quality antibodies suitable for incorporation into the desired immunoassay and platform. While polyclonal and monoclonal antibodies are currently the most commonly utilised antibodies for diagnostics, recombinant antibodies are growing in importance [20]. The advantage of recombinant antibody selection methods such as using phage display as a selection methodology provides a facile route to biasing enriched antibody pools for enhanced performance in the desired assay matrix (e.g. blood, serum, food extract or buffer with low percentage organic solvent such as PBS with 5% (v/v) methanol), temperature (phage can be selected at a range of temperatures to suit the assay needs), pH, sensitivity (introducing stringency biases higher affinity clones) and even time (e.g. select for faster association rates).

4.3.3 Assay Format

A lot of consideration should be put into choosing the format for the assay. Factors that will affect this may include size (haptens are generally not suited to sandwich assays), labelling (direct or indirect assays), stability (antibody stability and analyte stability) and platform. In many cases it may be a matter of empirically testing a couple of assay formats and evaluating the best one. Irrespective of the assay format chosen, optimisation of buffers and conditions should be performed. This section should contain

- information on the choice of format (possibly with comparative data of different formats)

- evaluation of buffers and coating concentrations
- empirical testing of optimum antibody concentrations, volumes and incubation times
- preliminary assay sample range estimation

4.4 Pre-validation

Once the best antibody (or antibody panel) has been selected and assay conditions defined, a pre-validation study can be performed. The section is where the assay will be defined in terms of calibration model, LOD, LLOQ, sample range, reproducibility and robustness. While it is always important to document laboratory experiments it is extremely important to track and record all assay steps fastidiously from this point on. Any data outliers or protocol deviations should be recorded and explained. It is good practice to type up a protocol (standard operating procedure (SOP) style) listing all materials used, how they were made up and a step-by-step breakdown of the protocol.

4.4.1 Select Assay Reagents

It is important at this stage to prepare enough reagents that will be sufficient for the whole validation study. All calibration samples (analyte samples) and antibody (preferably highly purified to reduce possible assay interference) should be well characterised a priori. Having to produce and purify more analyte or antibody mid validation will necessitate re-optimisation of concentrations and conditions that could affect the reproducibility of the assay. These reagents should be stored so that repeat use does not affect the integrity of the sample (i.e. stored in aliquots at -20°C or preferably at -80°C).

4.4.2 Evaluate Assay Conditions

Ligand binding assays are methods that depend on specific binding of an analyte to a biomolecule. Typically these are reversible binding events governed by the laws of mass action [21]. Suitable assay optimisation should be undertaken to ensure that the assay is performing to its maximum capabilities. For example, **minimum dilution**, coating concentration, conjugate concentration, washing conditions and incubation times should be evaluated empirically.

4.4.3 Define Calibration Model

The selection and preparation of the calibration curve are central in the design, validation and application of all quantitative assay methods. Calibration curves prepared from heterogeneous, impure, and/or poorly characterised analytes are more likely to yield greater uncertainty and higher variability [22]. The calibration model chosen should be the model that gives the best fit to your data. A suboptimal curve fitting will increase assay percentage error and more than likely increase the concentration at which the limit of quantification can be defined. Ligand binding assays (LBA) measure the signal of a series of interactions that follow the law of mass action, resulting in a nonlinear and often sigmoidal standard curve. The **response error relationship** is not constant (heteroscedastic); therefore, the highest precision does not necessarily coincide with the highest sensitivity [23]. Due to this heteroscedastic nature of the response variance, four- and five-**parameter logistic** calibration models are often used to fit the LBA standard curves [24].

- As standard concentrations should not be changed once assay **validation** has begun, a greater number of standard points and replicates should be included during method development and pre-validation to facilitate an early detailed investigation of the concentration–response relationship [19].
- It is recommended that at least 3 **runs** be used to establish the calibration model with at least 8 non-anchor standards run in duplicate. The acceptance of the model must be verified by evaluating the relative **bias** between the back-calculated and **nominal concentration** of the calibration. The use of the correlation coefficient is not recommended for confirmation of the **regression model** [23]. For a model to be acceptable, it is suggested that the mean %RE of calibrators within the anticipated **validated range** be

generally no more than 10% [15]. In some cases, if differences in bias and precision are practically unimportant, it may be preferable to choose a simpler model over a more accurate but complex model. In general, the simplest model that adequately describes the concentration response should be used [1].

- Curve fitting without appropriate weighting for unequal standard deviations can produce suboptimal results and incorrect assessment of the true assay performance (e.g. inferior sensitivity and limited assay range) [22]. As precision varies according to concentration, it is therefore better if a curve-fitting program weights the calibrator points so that the more precise ones influence the curve fitting most. In most weighted regression procedures, the weight applied to each point is the reciprocal of the variance of the response metameter used. This means that the smaller the variance is, the larger the weight is, thereby forcing the curve fitting routine to concentrate on those points on the **calibration curve** having greatest precision [24].

4.4.4 Evaluate Selectivity and Specificity

A challenge in interpreting results derived from immunoassays is the understanding of what exactly the assay is detecting. Fundamental to this is the knowledge of antibody specificity (cross reactivity analysis with related compounds) and selectivity (the assay's ability to solely measure the target analyte in the presence of other protein constituents in the sample). Experiments designed to determine the antibody's specificity can involve assessing their cross-reactivity with similar compounds. When feasible, it is suggested that the sample matrix is spiked with physiochemically similar compounds or variants of the target analyte. Selectivity is the easier of the two parameters to assess experimentally. After the assay format is relatively fixed, multiple lots of the sample matrix should be spiked near the **lower limit of quantification** and the **recovery** of the analyte calculated. This will aid in finally selecting a lower limit of quantification, before initiating assay validation. An additional experiment to understand selectivity involves spiking both the diluent and the matrix with standard curve **calibrators** to detect **matrix effects** at all concentrations across the range of calibration [14].

- Selectivity
  - The ability of the assay to selectively identify the target analyte in the preference of interfering substances (e.g. complex matrix like blood)
  - The selected or identified analyte should be verified by a validated reference method if available
- Specificity
  - Specific non-specificity (**interference** from substances physiochemically similar to the analyte). Cross-reactivity of endogenous compounds should be evaluated individually and in combination with the analyte of interest
  - Non-specific non-specificity (matrix effects unrelated to the analyte). The standard curve in biological matrix should be compared to standard curve in buffer to detect matrix effects

4.4.5 Preliminary Estimates for LLOQ and ULOQ

Assay dynamic range, also known as the 'reportable range' extends from the lower limits of quantification (LLOQ) to the upper limits of quantification (ULOQ). Within these limits, the analyte is measurable with acceptable levels of accuracy, precision and **total error** [22]. It is important to understand that the LLOQ and ULOQ are selected because they define the true, accepted limits of the standard curve. Standard curve points below or above the LLOQ and ULOQ, respectively, are considered extrapolated and cannot be used to report sample concentrations. LLOQ is the lowest concentration of the standard curve that can be measured with acceptable accuracy and precision [8]. Early in development, back-calculated standard values may be used to generate a preliminary estimate of the range of quantification. Later, spiked samples are used to refine the estimated range. At this stage, it is useful to include more points in

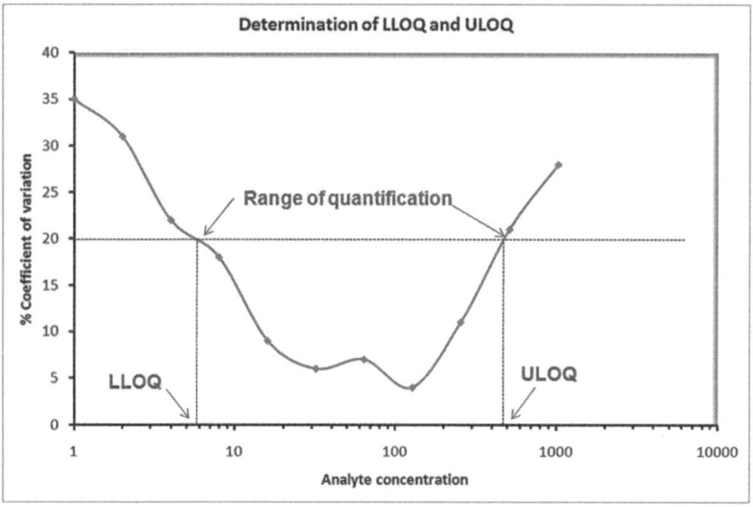

Figure 4.2 Example curve of a typical precision profile that can be used for the calculation of the lower and upper limits of quantification. It is necessary to obtain the data for the precision profile from multiple runs over time rather than using one set of data due to the high inter-assay variance over the intra-assay variance.

the areas of the anticipated LLOQ and ULOQ. A plot (Fig. 4.2) of the precision profile can be helpful in assessing the prospective limits of quantification [23].

Lower Limit of Quantification (LLOQ) is the lowest standard that the following conditions are met [10].

- The analyte response at the LLOQ should be at least 5 times the response compared to the blank response
- Analyte response should be identifiable and reproducible with a precision of 20% and accuracy of 80–120%

4.4.6 Preliminary Estimates of Precision and Accuracy

Method precision and **accuracy** (see Fig. 4.3) are performance characteristics that describe the magnitude of random errors (variation) and systematic error (mean bias) associated with repeated measurements of the same homogeneous (spiked) sample under specified conditions. Method precision and accuracy for

LBAs should be evaluated by analysing **validation samples** (QC samples) that are prepared in the same biological matrix as the anticipated study samples. During pre-validation and pre-study validation, measurements are made over multiple assay **batch** runs with replicate determinations in each run. In line with ICH guidelines [5, 10], precision is subdivided into short-term (within-run precision or intrabatch) and **intermediate precisions** (between run or interbatch), which measure precision with time, and may involve different analysts, equipment and reagents [2]. Method accuracy, intrabatch (within run) precision, and interbatch (between-run) precision should be established preliminarily during pre-validation and confirmed in pre-study validation. Design and analysis recommendations for precision and accuracy assessments of LBAs for **macromolecules** are summarised in Table 4.2 [19].

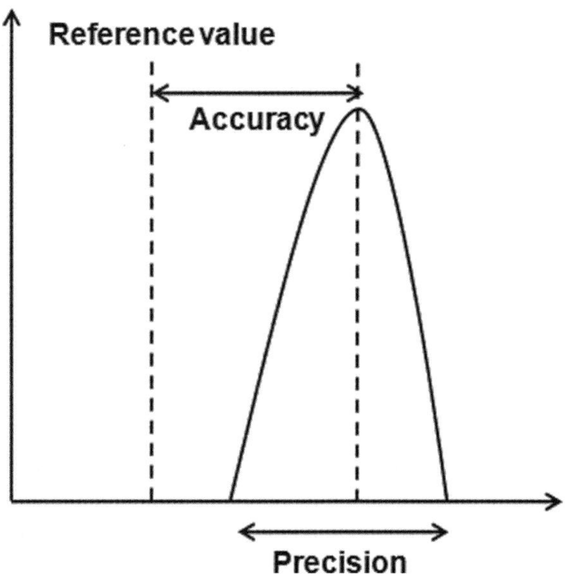

Figure 4.3 Diagramatic representation of the relationship between accuracy and precision. Accuracy is the relationship of test values to 'true' value of analyte concentration, while precision is a measure of the spread of repeated measurement results and depends on the distribution of random errors.

Table 4.2 Precision and accuracy assessment criteria. Recommended analysis and acceptance criteria apply to each sample concentration analysed. Adapted from Deserve et al., 2003 [19]

Assessment topic		Pre-validation	Pre-study validation	In-study validation
DESIGN				
1. Number of batch runs		≥3	≥6	1
2. Number of sample concentrations		≥8	≥ 5	≥3
3. Concentration levels		Span calibrator range	LLOQ, LQC, MQC, HQC, ULOQ	LQC, MQC, HQC
4. Number of replicate results/batch		≥2	≥2	≥2
ANALYSIS				
5. Compute statistics to target limits	(a) Bias	± 20 (25 at LLOQ)	±20 (25 at LLOQ)	–
	(b) Intrabatch precision (%CV)	≤20 (25 at LLOQ)	≤20 (25 at LLOQ)	–
	(c) Interbatch precision (%CV)	≤20 (25 at LLOQ)	≤20 (25 at LLOQ)	–
	(d) Total error (%RE)	–	–	±30
ACCEPTANCE CRITERIA				
Part 1: Apply limits separately		Calculated bias and precision satisfy 5a,5b and 5c above.		"4-6-30 rule"
Part 2: Combined limit		Bias %RE + Interbatch precision %CV ≤30		

Note: please refer to glossary for definition of terms.

Experimental tips:

- Perform 3 batch runs (3 separate assays) with at least 8 samples (more is better) in duplicate (or triplicate) for interbatch and 5–6 replicates for intrabatch studies.
- Analyse precision of replicate results ($\geq$5 replicates for intrabatch and $\geq$2 replicates for interbatch) by calculation of the **coefficient of variation.**
- Apply best calibration curve to mean data and determine the assay accuracy by back calculating the predicated concentration of the known standards (see Fig. 4.4).
- Use this data to estimate LLOQ and ULOQ described in the previous section.

4.4.7 Estimation of the Assay Limit of Detection (LOD)

The terms limit of blank (LOB), **limit of detection** (LOD) and lower limit of quantification (LLOQ) describe the smallest concentration of a molecule that can be reliably measured by an analytical procedure. To establish these parameters an assay analyst should test a large number of sample replicates to increase the robustness and the statistical confidence of the estimate. LOB and LOD are important for tests to discriminate between the presence or absence of an analyse, while LLOQ is necessary to reliably measure low levels of analytes (i.e. LOD = qualitative data and LLOQ = both qualitative and quantitative data) [26]. In essence, the limit of detection is the point at which a measured value is larger than the uncertainty associated with it. It is the lowest concentration of analyte in a sample that can be detected but not necessarily quantified [2]. LOD is often confused with the sensitivity of the assay method. The sensitivity of an analytical method is the capability of the method to discriminate small differences in concentration or mass of the test analyte. In practical terms, sensitivity is the slope of the calibration curve (see Fig. 4.5) that is obtained by plotting the response against the analyte concentration [2].

LOD is a well-established parameter used to characterise an analytical confirmatory method. It can be defined as the lowest analyte concentration likely to be reliably distinguished from the

A

	Intraday			Interday		
Concentration (cells/ml)	Back-calculated concentration (cells/ml)	CV's %	% Accuracies	Back-calculated concentration (cells/ml)	CV's %	% Accuracies
1.00×10^{10}	6.37×10^{10}	3.76	136.34	5.77×10^{9}	8.16	142.26
5.00×10^{9}	5.20×10^{9}	3.16	96.07	5.27×10^{9}	7.51	94.65
2.50×10^{9}	2.50×10^{9}	3.68	99.87	2.51×10^{9}	7.66	99.59
1.25×10^{9}	1.54×10^{9}	3.36	76.93	1.32×10^{9}	7.28	94.20
6.25×10^{8}	7.02×10^{8}	3.97	87.71	6.66×10^{8}	6.48	93.43
3.13×10^{8}	2.87×10^{8}	2.87	108.28	3.04×10^{8}	6.78	102.56
1.56×10^{8}	1.69×10^{8}	3.81	91.99	1.56×10^{8}	8.69	100.28
7.81×10^{7}	6.54×10^{7}	3.20	116.31	7.87×10^{7}	4.65	99.21
3.91×10^{7}	3.99×10^{7}	5.72	97.91	3.96×10^{7}	5.06	98.60
1.95×10^{7}	2.35×10^{7}	3.80	79.84	1.97×10^{7}	3.60	99.30
9.77×10^{6}	8.19×10^{6}	2.83	116.17	8.60×10^{6}	4.18	111.97
4.88×10^{6}	5.74×10^{6}	3.45	82.52	5.14×10^{6}	4.72	94.69
2.44×10^{6}	2.38×10^{6}	3.25	102.54	3.20×10^{6}	4.96	68.88
1.22×10^{6}	6.78×10^{5}	4.37	144.46	1.29×10^{6}	4.04	94.72
6.10×10^{5}	6.04×10^{5}	1.30	101.09	4.01×10^{5}	3.79	134.28
3.05×10^{5}	5.18×10^{5}	5.11	30.31	4.72×10^{5}	3.57	45.23
1.53×10^{5}	2.29×10^{5}	3.11	49.98	4.04×10^{4}	5.57	173.51
7.63×10^{4}	6.94×10^{4}	2.30	199.09	9.47×10^{4}	3.01	75.90
3.81×10^{4}	-	1.41	-	-	1.41	-

B

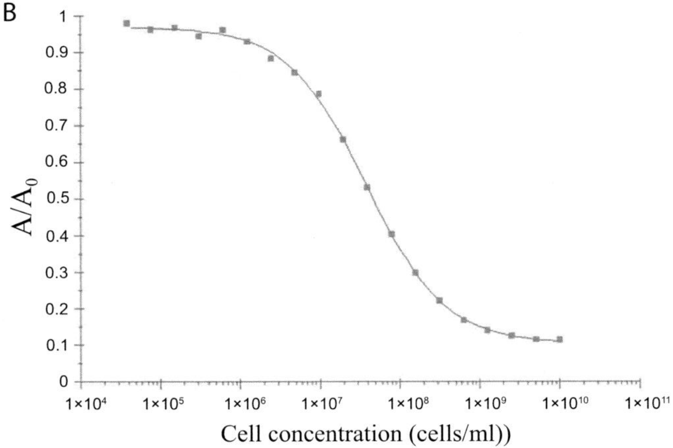

Figure 4.4 Example of assay accuracy and precision calculated from an immunoassay for *Listeria monocytogenenes* [25]. (A) Interday assay calibration curve for the anti-*Listeria monocytogenes* antibody. A 4-parameter equation was fitted to the data set using BIAevaluation 3.1 software. The inter-assay means coefficients of variance are tabulated in 5B. Each point on the curve is the mean of five replicate measurements over five days. (B) Coefficients of variance (a quantitative measure of precision) was calculated using the equation $\%CV = (SD/Mean) \times 100$ where for intraday studies, the standard deviation (SD) is computed from replicate (5 replicates) analyses within a single validation run and for intermediate precision (interday), the SD is computed from replicate (3 replicates) analyses over 5 validation runs on 5 separate days. Cells containing a dash indicate that no value could be obtained as the data point did not fit the calibration curve. A/A_0 is the normalised absorbance, where A_0 represents the value when no cells are present.

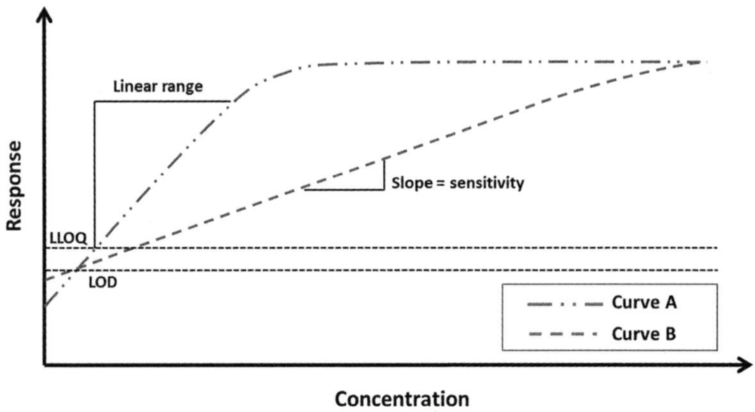

Figure 4.5 Example plot demonstrating assay sensitivity and limit of detection. Both curves A and B have the same LOD but have very different sensitivities to differences in analyte concentration. Curve A has a narrower linear range than curve B but is much more sensitive across this range. Adapted from Huber 2010 [2].

limit of the blank (LOB) and at which detection is feasible. It is therefore greater than LOB. A typical approach to estimate LOD consists of measuring replicates, usually $n = 20$, of a zero calibrator or blank sample, determining the mean value and SD, and calculating LOD as the mean +2 SD. Variations of this approach use the mean plus 3, 4, or even 10 SDs to provide a more conservative LOD [26]. This is a simple and quick method. The weakness is that there is no objective evidence to prove that a low concentration of analyte will indeed produce a signal distinguishable from a blank (zero concentration) sample.

An alternative approach recommend by Armbruster and Pry [26] and adopted by our group [27] utilises analysis of samples containing small but known concentrations of the substance of interest. The advantage of this empirical approach is that objective data is used to compare the analytical response of blank and low concentration samples to determine conclusively what concentration of analyte is necessary to distinguish its presence from its absence. A recommended practical number of LOB and LOD samples to be used by a manufacturer to establish these parameters is 60, while a laboratory verifying a manufacturer's LOD (and possibly the

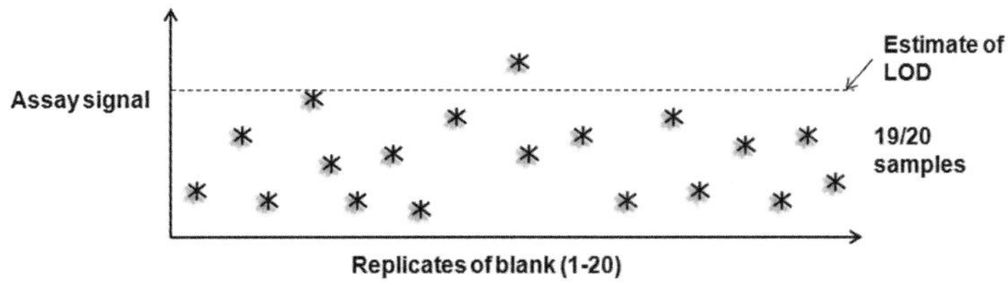

Figure 4.6 Example of experimental determination of the LOD for an assay.

LOB) is 20. Once a provisional LOD is established, it can be confirmed by examining the observed values for samples containing the LOD concentration. Some LOD sample values are expected to be less than the estimated LOD (Fig. 4.6), but with parametric approaches using mean plus using 1.645 SD, where 1.645 is the 95th percentile of the normal distribution no more than 5% of the values should be less than the LOB [28]. If the observed LOD sample values meet this criterion, the LOD is considered established or verified. If more than 5% (roughly 1 out of 20 observations) of the LOD sample values fall below LOB, the LOD is too low and must be re-estimated (i.e. by testing a sample of higher concentration that will generate a higher mean and SD and thus a higher LOD).

Experimental tip:

- Analyse (20–60) blank samples and determine the limit of the blank using ***LOB = mean blank + 1.645(SD blank).***
- Analyse (20–60 replicates) samples at and above the LOB to verify that they are distinguishable from the blank 19/20 times.
- Calculate the LOD with the lowest analyte concentration distinguishable from the blank 19/20 times using ***LOD = LOB + 1.645(SD low conc. sample).***

4.4.8 Reference Method

If available, a reference assay or analytical technique should be purchased or sourced so the assay that one is preparing can be compared to a previously validated method. This adds weight to the validation of the new assay and allows one to directly compare any assay improvements. It also helps prove antibody selectivity as the recovered (or detected) analyte can be verified using the standard method.

4.4.9 Validation Samples and Method Definition

Before pre-study validation experiments are performed, all reagents should be prepared and documented. A typed-up protocol (SOP style) should be prepared and any deviation from this documented with reasons. Ideally validation samples should be spiked real samples (example pooled negative patient blood [10–20 donors] with spiked analyte or extracted drug from tissue source with known drug concentration). A reference standard is very important here to verify analyte concentration. The juncture between pre-validation and **pre-study validation** is where one could potentially differentiate between standard curve and calibration curve (even though these terms are usually used synonymously). Up to now a standard curve will have been developed with a large range of standards, all of which help to define the curve fitting, LOD and LLOQ. For pre-study validation a smaller range of samples (well calibrated i.e. calibration samples) are required that span the range of the assay. Therefore, the calibration curve will be fitted to a small number of calibration samples using the curve fitting determined with the standard curve. The calibration samples should include low, medium and high concentration samples and samples at the LOD and LLOQ. A blank should also be included.

4.4.10 Evaluate Extraction Efficiency/Effects

How an analyte is extracted from tissue (e.g. drug extracted from meat) or how a blood sample is taken and stored can affect assay sensitivity and accuracy. Inefficient extraction will lower the overall functional sensitivity of the assay. For example, the developed assay may be able to quantify down to 1 ng/mL but if the extraction procedure is only 10% efficient the practical assay sensitivity is 10 ng/mL as 90% of the sample is lost. Blood samples are usually taken and stored in tubes with anti-coagulants, which may affect the assay. In addition, patients undergoing treatment for cardiovascular disease may be on heparin or warfarin treatment that may affect the ability of the assay to accurately detect the analyte. These factors should be investigated as they can influence assay robustness. Early, consistent application of predefined sample collection and handling techniques is especially important when such manipulation might affect sample and/or analyte integrity [22].

Experimental tip (extraction efficiency):

- Prepare analyte standards and spike tissue with samples. Also spike final extraction buffer with sample (this is the 100% sample without any loss).
- Extract the analyte (usually a drug) from the tissue according to the recommended protocol.
- Analyse extracted samples and spiked samples using the optimised assay conditions from the pre-validation along with calibration standards.
- Calculate the extraction efficiency as (conc. of extracted sample/conc. of spiked sample) $\times$ 100.

Experimental tip (effect of blood sample variation):

- Prepare blood samples with physiologically relevant concentrations of possible contaminants using a factoral approach (i.e. addition of EDTA, heparin and warfarin separately and in combinations plus a negative blood sample with no contaminants). Also spike the extraction buffer with sample (this is the 100% sample without any loss).
- Spike the analyte (usually a protein) into the blood samples prepared above.
- Analyse the blood samples and spiked samples using the optimised assay conditions from the **pre-validation** along with calibration standards.
- Calculate the effect on assay efficiency as (conc. of analyte blood sample/conc. of analyte in blood containing no contaminants) $\times$ 100.

4.5 Pre-study Validation

The aim of this section of the validation process is to confirm that the assay continues to perform as per predefined specifications in each study run (i.e. to ensure the assay remains 'in control') [22]. It involves determining the assay reproducibility, robustness, stability and **linearity** while also examining how other factors such as sample extraction and storage and small changes in protocol/reagents can affect the assay. One is in effect testing how far the assay can be pushed before it no longer meets the predefined requirements for its use such as precision and accuracy. In addition to testing for stability, extraction efficiency and robustness, pre-study validation involves the repeated measurements of calibration samples to determine if the assay can be reproduced within an acceptable predefined level of error. Method validation is an iterative and evolving process, therefore, the performance characteristics discussed in the exploratory pre-validation section should also be included in the pre-study validation. For the purpose of clarity, only additional parameters such as stability, linearity, robustness and the assay validation report will be discussed here. Similar to the pre-validation studies above, both the degree of confidence and number of validation parameters needed to be addressed will depend on one's own application, one's regulatory agency's requirements and regulatory guidelines for that field of use.

4.5.1 Stability

Assay stability is a function of the storage conditions, the chemical properties of the analyte (and assay functional chemistry), the **matrix** and the container system. Conditions used in stability experiments should reflect situations likely to be encountered during actual sample handling and analysis such as [8]:

- Freeze and thaw stability (analyte stability should be determined after three freeze and thaw cycles. At least three aliquots at each of the low and high concentrations should be stored at the intended storage)

- Short-term temperature stability (three aliquots of each of the low and high concentrations should be thawed at room temperature from 4–24 hours and analysed)
- Long-term temperature stability
- Stock solution stability (the stability of the stock solutions and internal standards should be evaluated at room temperature for at least 6 hours)
- Post-preparative stability (stable during processing time)

Experimental tip:

Freeze and thaw stability (at −20°C and/or −80°C)

- Prepare 18 aliquots (at sufficient volume to analyse in duplicate in the assay) of high concentration samples (near ULOQ) and 18 aliquots of low concentration samples (near LLOQ) and label 3 aliquots FT1, 3 aliquots FT2, 3 aliquots FT3, 3 aliquots FT4, 3 aliquots FT5 and 3 aliquots FT6 for each high and low sample (FT refers to freeze/thaw).
- Freeze all aliquots long enough to ensure they are completely frozen. Then thaw FT2-FT6 at room temperate until completely thawed.
- Repeat the process for FT3-FT6, then FT4-FT6, etc., until FT6 has been frozen six times.
- Analyse all the aliquots on the same assay plate and compare stability.

Short-term storage stability

- Repeat as above for FT stability except after freezing all the samples remove different batches at 0, 2, 4, 8, 12, and 24 hours before analysis (i.e. take out a sample before going home, first thing in the morning, 4 hours later, 4 hours later, 2 hours later and run the assay). The times here can be changed or shortened to suit the working day.

4.5.2 Evaluate Dilutional Linearity

This analysis should be performed to prove that high concentration samples (samples reading higher than the ULOQ) can be diluted and read on the assay where multiplying by the dilution factor yields the actual high sample concentration. This is similar to assay **parallelism** whereby instead of using spiked samples, high concentration 'real' samples (i.e. diseased patient or highly contaminated food) are used.

4.5.3 Evaluate Assay Robustness and Ruggedness

Measuring how sensitive one's assay is to changes in procedure and environment provides vital information on assay robustness and **ruggedness**. The assay robustness refers to factors that might influence the assay like changes in buffer, incubation times, matrix, pH, light exposure while ruggedness relates to how routine changes such as operator, instrument, batch size affect the assay [12]. The actual batch size for a routine sample analysis run is frequently overlooked but is often an impactful ruggedness measurement that should be addressed [14]. These parameters are very closely related and often both robustness and ruggedness experiments are treated as one. The level of robustness/ruggedness needed for each assay will depend on assay type and location, where for example, a POC test will have to be very robust, an automated assay will not have to demonstrate as much robustness. The factors to evaluate should represent possible deviations from protocol that might happen once the assay is 'out of your hands'. Parameters such as change in operator or lab, changes in incubation times, buffer pH and temperature should be analysed.

4.5.4 Assay Validation Report and Documentation

A complete account of the performance of the bioanalytical method should be provided in the final report for both method validation and study sample analysis [29]. During assay development, changes occur in the selection of critical reagents, the assay format, and the understanding of the drug product during the method development phase. These factors, which would be part of the final selection criteria, require some form of documentation, typically in a lab notebook or binder. As the assay matures during development and the expected format is defined, this too should be documented. With the final format in place, these parameters should be captured in a draft method standard operating procedure (SOP) or an analytical procedure [23].

The pre-study validation plan guides the validation process and relies on an analytical procedure or method SOP, which may be still in final draft or may be approved. All validation experiments should be documented in a laboratory notebook (or as per the individual company policies). As the validation comes to completion, the details of the experiments and the data that contribute to the validation must be compiled in a validation report. It is important to summarise all the runs to accurately illustrate the assay performance. The pre-study validation data should, to some extent, predict what to expect during sample analysis ('in-study' validation). Since stability data are frequently obtained over time, the validation report should be updated periodically as new data are generated.

4.6 Summary

Immunoassays are extremely useful analytical techniques for the rapid analysis of analytes in a broad range of matrices. This chapter has addressed some of the key elements involved in validating an immunoassay. However, depending on the desired field of use, regulatory influences and approval criteria, an immunoassay analyst may need to validate their assay using all or just some of the parameters discussed in this chapter. Irrespective of the validation parameters incorporated, the assay should be 'fit-for-purpose' and be able to perform as it is intended to do. It is hoped that this chapter, along with the excellent literature cited in the reference section, can help improve one's probability of success and ensure optimal assay performance.

References

1. Huber, L., ed. Validation and Qualification in Analytical Laboratories. 2nd ed. 2007, Informa Healthcare: New York.
2. Huber, L., ed. Validation of Analytical Methods, A Primer. Vol. 2. 2010, Agilent Technologies: Santa Clara, CA.

3. Eurachem, The Fitness for Purpose of Analytical Methods: A Laboratory Guide to Method Validation and Related Topics, 1998.
4. Thompson, M., S.L.R. Ellison, and R. Wood, Harmonized guidelines for single-laboratory validation of methods of analysis: (IUPAC technical report). *Pure Appl Chem*, 2002. **74**(5):835–855.
5. International Council for Harmonisation (IHC)-Q2A, Guideline for Industry: Text on Validation of Analytical Procedures. 1995.
6. LGC, In-House Method Validation: A Guide for Chemical Laboratories. 2003.
7. United States Food and Drug Administration, Guidance for Industry (draft): Analytical Procedures and Methods Validation: Chemistry, Manufacturing and Controls and Documentation. 2000.
8. United States Food and Drug Administration, Guidance for Industry, Bioanalytical Method Validation. 2001.
9. AOAC, How to Meet ISO 17025 Requirements for Methods Verification, 2007.
10. International Council for Harmonisation (IHC)-Q2B, Guidance for Industry: Validation of Analytical Procedures: Methodology, 1996.
11. Lipton, C.R., et al., Guidelines for the validation and use of immunoassays for determination of introduced proteins in biotechnology enhanced crops and derived food ingredients. *Food Agric Immunol*, 2000. **12**(2):153–164.
12. Crowther, J.R., ed. Validation of Diagnostic Tests in The ELISA Guidebook. Vol. 149. 2001, Humana Press Inc.: Totowa, NJ.
13. Mintzberg, H., ed. 5Ps for Strategy in the Strategy Process. 1992, Prentice-Hall International Editions: Upper Saddle River, NJ. pp. 12–19.
14. Kelley, M., and DeSilva, B., Analytical considerations for immunoassays for macromolecules, in *Handbook of Pharmaceutical Biotechnology*, ed. S.C. Gad. 2007, John Wiley and Sons: New York. pp. 573–584.
15. Findlay, J.W.A., et al., Validation of immunoassays for bioanalysis: a pharmaceutical industry perspective. *J Pharm Biomed Anal*, 2000. **21**(6):1249–1273.
16. McDonnell, B., et al., Cardiac biomarkers and the case for point-of-care testing. *Clin Biochem*, 2009. **42**(7–8):549–561.
17. Leonard, P., C.J. Hayes, and R. O'Kennedy, Rapid temperature-dependent antibody ranking using Biacore A100. *Anal Biochem*, 2011. **409**(2):290–292.

18. Shankar, G., et al., Recommendations for the validation of immunoassays used for detection of host antibodies against biotechnology products. *J Pharm Biomed Anal*, 2008. **48**(5):1267–1281.
19. DeSilva, B., et al., Recommendations for the bioanalytical method validation of ligand-binding assays to support pharmacokinetic assessments of macromolecules. *Pharm Res*, 2003. **20**(11):1885–1900.
20. Hearty, S. and R. O'Kennedy, Exploiting recombinant antibodies in point-of-care (POC) diagnostics: the combinatorial advantage. *Bioeng Bugs*, 2011. **2**(3):182–186.
21. Miller, K.J., et al., Workshop on bioanalytical methods validation for macromolecules: Summary report. *Pharm Res*, 2001. **18**(9):1373–1383.
22. Lee, J.W., et al., Fit-for-purpose method development and validation for successful biomarker measurement. *Pharm Res*, 2006. **23**(2):312–328.
23. Kelley, M. and B. DeSilva, Key elements of bioanalytical method validation for macromolecules. *AAPS J*, 2007. **9**(2):E156–E163.
24. Nix, B., and Wild, D., Calibration curve fitting, in *The Immunoassay Handbook*. 3rd ed., ed. D. Wild. 2005, Elsevier: Oxford, UK. pp. 235–244.
25. Leonard, P., Production of antibodies for use in a biosensor-based assay for *Listeria monocytogenes*. 2003, Dublin City University: Ireland.
26. Armbruster, D.A. and T. Pry, Limit of blank, limit of detection and limit of quantitation. *Clin Biochem Rev*, 2008. **29**(Suppl 1):S49–S52.
27. Fitzgerald, J., et al., Light-chain shuffling from an antigen-biased phage pool allows 185-fold improvement of an anti-halofuginone single-chain variable fragment. *Anal Biochem*, 2011. **410**(1):27–33.
28. Mire-Sluis, A.R., et al., Recommendations for the design and optimization of immunoassays used in the detection of host antibodies against biotechnology products. *J Immunol Methods*, 2004. **289**(1–2):1–16.
29. Viswanathan, C.T., et al., Workshop/conference report—Quantitative bioanalytical methods validation and implementation: Best practices for chromatographic and ligand binding assays. *AAPS J*, 2007. **9**(1):E30–E42.

Chapter 5

Lab-on-a-Chip Immunoassay Systems

Barry Byrne and Louise M. Barrett

Biomedical Diagnostics Institute and National Centre for Sensor Research, Dublin City University, Collins Avenue, Glasnevin, Dublin 9, Ireland

barry.byrne@dcu.ie

Immunoassays have become the gold-standard technique for detecting a panel of biologically and medically important antigens. Furthermore, recent trends have seen the integration of biomedical engineering and immunoassay development for the production of miniaturised, microfluidic platforms capable of detecting relevant analytes in a rapid, sensitive and reliable manner. Here, we examine the current state of the art of these 'lab-on-a-chip' immunoassay systems, with particular emphasis placed on four key areas, namely (i) available substrates, (ii) microfluidic platform design and fabrication, (iii) strategies for the delivery and mixing of analytical reagents and (iv) the integration of antibodies as biorecognition elements. While a comprehensive discussion of all currently available 'lab-on-a-chip' immunoassay platforms is beyond the remit of this chapter to demonstrate the immense potential for sensitive detection and the scope for multiplexed analysis, we highlight key examples which focus on the detection of bacterial and fungal pathogens, toxins and selected disease markers of cardiovascular disease (CVD).

Immunoassays: Development, Applications and Future Trends

Edited by Richard O'Kennedy and Caroline Murphy

ISBN 978-981-4669-97-9 (Hardcover), 978-1-315-20654-7 (eBook)

www.panstanford.com

5.1 Introduction

Through the use of methodologies described in Chapter 2 of this book [1] and elsewhere [2–5], monoclonal, polyclonal and recombinant antibodies can be produced with high-affinity and specificity for their desired target. The versatility of such approaches is illustrated by the fact that these biorecognition elements can be directed towards a panel of structurally diverse antigens, ranging from large, complex proteinaceous entities (e.g. disease biomarkers, surface-residing antigenic determinants) to smaller, hapten-like molecules such as toxins. Furthermore, through the implementation of rigorous screening strategies it is possible to positively identify candidate antibodies which selectively bind to the target with high-affinity, and permit differentiation from other antigens which share some structural homology. Hence, antibody-based assays, or immunoassays, represent an important enabling technology for reliably detecting analytes of interest which may be present in trace amounts in complex sample matrices.

With the evolution and enhancement of immunoanalysis platforms, particular emphasis has been placed on the development of miniaturised configurations where the assay is performed using networks of enclosed channels whose dimensions are in the micron scale. In such formats, analytical samples (e.g. blood, bacterial suspensions, buffer containing analytes of interest) exhibit laminar flow properties where fluidic streams flow in parallel to one another, with mixing typically occurring by diffusion [6]. Such microfluidic or 'lab-on-a-chip' platforms have many advantages over conventional immunoassays, such as those performed in a 96/384-well format. Firstly, the reduced dimensions of integrated channels result in a significant decrease in the amount of reagents that are needed to undertake immunoanalysis. This can be a key consideration where expensive consumable reagents (e.g. purified antigens, fluorescently labelled detection antibodies) are required for use. The second key advantage relates to the increased surface-to-volume ratios afforded by these miniaturised structures, which in turn mediates faster antibody/antigen interactions and consequently, more rapid analysis. Many microfluidic platforms have also been modified to integrate automation strategies, such as for liquid handling, which can contribute significantly towards improving assay throughput and reproducibility.

5.2 Substrates Used for Microfluidic Chip Design

A panel of different substrates are available for selection when designing and fabricating microfluidic platforms. These include silicon, glass and polymers [7–9]. When selecting a material for use in a 'lab-on-a-chip' immunoassay, an important consideration is to choose a substrate which allows the intended assay to be performed in a reliable and cost-effective manner, without having any detrimental effect on any of the assay components by not exhibiting any toxicity-related properties. Furthermore, the material selected must be compatible with the detection strategy to be applied. For example, in the case of an immunoassay where fluorescently labelled detection antibodies are to be integrated, it is imperative that the material does not have any inherent fluorescent properties which could interfere with analysis. Furthermore, the material should easily allow microfluidic channels to be integrated for the benefit of sample transfer and mixing (if applicable), and should also be ideally suited towards mass-transfer of analytical components [10, 11].

Silicon has excellent thermal conductivity properties and its potential use as a substrate for 'lab-on-a-chip' applications has been enhanced by the considerable advances that have been made in the semiconductor industry, with reference to microstructure and fabrication technologies for developing complex microfluidic structures [12, 13]. While in many instances this is advantageous, the use of silicon is often limited by the opacity of this material, which can complicate optical detection. In contrast, glass is a transparent material with well-defined surface chemistries and suitable electro-osmotic flow (EOF) characteristics. While the latter is a key consideration for devices intended for use in diagnostic applications, the use of glass in microfluidic applications has been limited primarily by the associated cost. Hence, recent trends have seen more cost-effective materials with comparable physical qualities being selected for use instead (Fig. 5.1). Here,

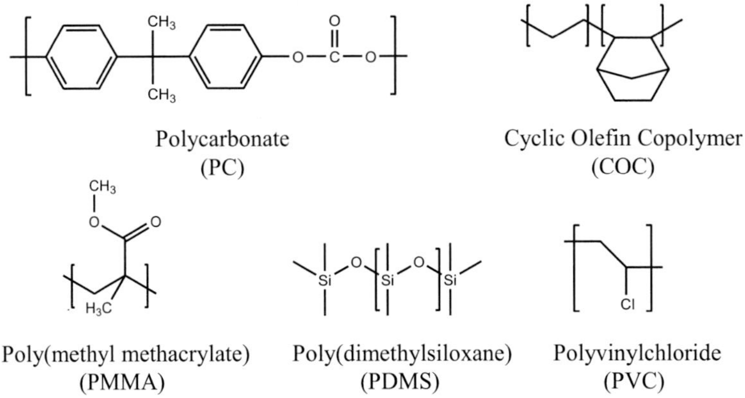

Figure 5.1 Chemical structures of polymers available for 'lab-on-a-chip' immunoassays.

we focus primarily on two polymers, namely poly(dimethylsiloxane) (PDMS) and poly(methyl methacrylate) (PMMA), and discuss their applications in 'lab-on-a-chip' immunodiagnostic assays.

PDMS is almost universally selected for use as a polymer when fabricating microfluidic platforms for use in 'lab-on-a-chip' immunoassays. This inert, stable elastomer is a cost-effective material which is transparent in the visible/UV region and does not fluoresce. Hence, PDMS has ideal optical properties for use in immunoanalysis, specifically for assays incorporating fluorescently labelled detection antibodies. This non-toxic polymer is also impermeable to water, which infers that it is ideally suited for use in assays using biological analytes, such as proteins and antibodies [6]. Finally, a key advantage of PDMS is that it can easily be moulded. This is permitted by the fact that this polymer naturally exists in a highly coiled structure that can stretch, which results in the polymer recoiling. Hence, this polymer can easily be moulded to a desired configuration using methodologies described in more detail below.

PDMS is comprised of repeating units of $–O\text{-}Si\text{-}(CH_3)_2–$ groups (Fig. 5.1), with methyl (–CH3) groups conferring hydrophobicity [10]. In many cases, this surface property may have a deleterious effect on assay performance, and may render microchannels susceptible to the trapping of air bubbles. For example, hydrophobic material which may be present in the analytical matrix may non-specifically bind to the substrate and leach into the PDMS. Furthermore, the presence of organic solvents can result in swelling. Hence, many 'lab-on-a-chip' assays that utilise PDMS modify the surface to improve its hydrophilicity, and also to stabilise its electro-osmotic flow (EOF) properties. To achieve this, one can use two different modification strategies, namely gas-phase processing (e.g. plasma oxidation) and wet-chemical modification (e.g. layer-by-layer deposition). In some instances, these can be combined, depending on the specific application [12]. During this process, surface hydrophilicity can be determined by water contact angle measurements, where a decrease in this value represents an increase in hydrophilicity. Plasma oxidation uses gases (e.g. oxygen, nitrogen and hydrogen) for functionalising the PDMS surface, with native methyl ($Si\text{-}CH_3$) groups replaced with more hydrophilic silanols (Si-OH) [14]. Once this process has been completed, plasma-treated channels can be kept hydrophilic by the addition of polar organic solvents/water. Interestingly, silanol groups can be functionalised to facilitate the capture of proteins, which are integral components of immunoassays (e.g. antibodies/antigens). Bernard et al. [15] demonstrated the feasibility of this approach by silanising oxidised PDMS with an amino-terminated silane, namely aminopropyltriethoxysilane, which in turn presented a reactive surface for cross-linking antibodies via covalent derivatisation. This affinity contact-printed surface permitted the immunocapture of the neuron-glia cell adhesion molecule (NgCAM) from cell culture lysates and tissue homogenates, thus demonstrating the efficacy of this approach. An alternative gas phase processing strategy is chemical vapour deposition (CVD), which is a three-stage (sublimation, pyrolysis and deposition) chemical process which produces a thin film on a substrate surface through the deposition of gaseous molecules which react on the surface [16].

While PDMS is a highly effective polymer with excellent characteristics for use in microfluidic applications, the high permeability for oxygen suggests that it may not be ideally suited to oxygen-sensitive applications [17]. Hence, in many cases PMMA (Fig. 5.1) is selected as an alternative polymer. Similarly to PDMS, this low-cost material has ideal optical and mechanical properties, and can be decomposed to methyl methacrylate (MMA) by heating at a high temperature, suggesting that this can be re-moulded to form new microfluidic structures [18–20]. In contrast to PDMS, this polymer is generally regarded to be the least hydrophobic plastic available for use and hence, does not require additional treatments to enhance its hydrophilicity [21].

5.3 Microfluidic Channel Design and Fabrication

For the rapid prototyping of PDMS-based microfluidic platforms (Fig. 5.2), a computer-aided design (CAD) program is routinely selected for use to design the microstructures of a 'lab-on-a-chip' device. A number of commercially available platforms can be selected (e.g. AutoCAD, DraftSight, SolidWorks and Creo) which provide a schematic representation of the final microfluidic channel. When designing such a structure, one should consider the following: (i) the size of the analytical platform, (ii) the number of channels required for use and (iii) the channel dimensions, with emphasis on length, width and height. In most cases, at least one well (for sample insertion) and channel should be supplied for each analytical reagent. Channels should ideally be as short as possible to minimise the transport distance, but should be of sufficient length to avoid cross-contamination between different reagents due to putative minor fluctuations in flow driving force [22]. Finally, when designing such prototypes, it is also appropriate to integrate a waste-collection channel for facilitating the easy removal of waste materials, for example unbound antibody and wash solutions. Next, the finalised CAD file is printed onto a transparent film with a high-resolution image setter, and the resultant transparency functions as a photomask in contact photolithography, where the image to be printed is obtained through the illumination of a photomask in direct contact with a photoresist-covered substrate. For example, Su-8 is an epoxy-based and photo-curable material which can be exposed to ultraviolet (UV) light to polymerise exposed regions. Un-polymerised photoresist can subsequently be removed, which results in the channel structure being retained on the wafer. This in turn can be selected as a master mould for

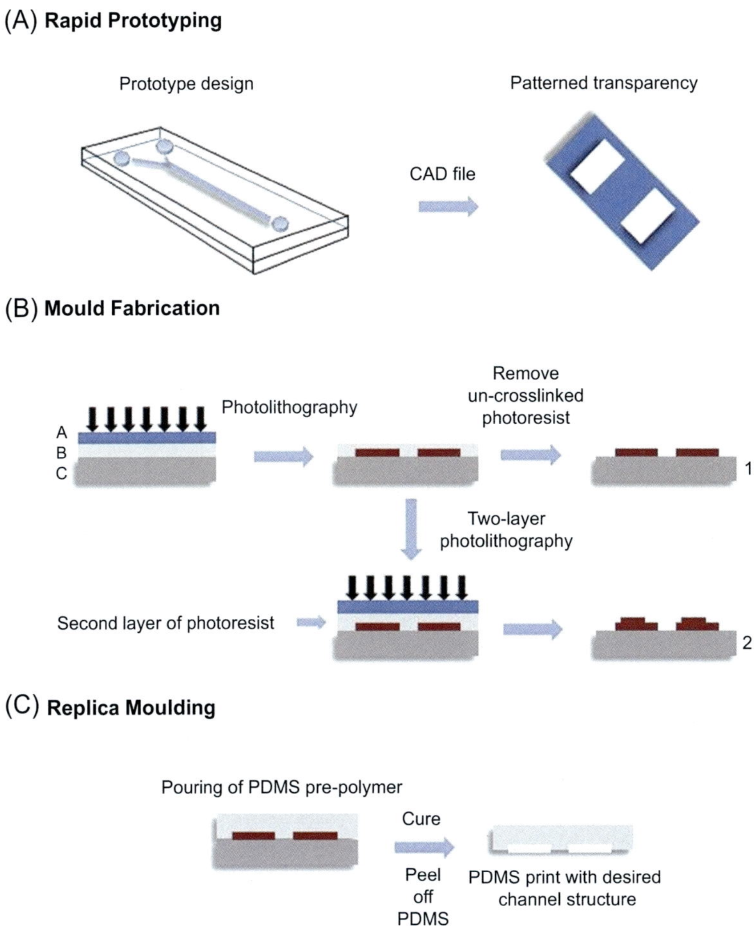

Figure 5.2 Schematic representation of the processes involved in PDMS rapid prototyping, mould fabrication and replica moulding (adapted from [10]). For mould fabrication, layers A, B and C are photomask, photoresist and silicon, respectively, with light represented by black arrows. 1 and 2 are re-usable masters.

the preparation of additional PDMS chips. Notably, it is feasible to repeat this process using two-level photolithography which allows multi-layered structures to be assembled (Fig. 5.2B). After the fabrication of a master 'mould,' a layer of fluorinated functional group-containing silane can be deposited to prevent irreversible bonding between the PDMS and the silicon wafer. The master mould also facilitates the replica moulding of additional chips [10].

For PDMS replica moulding (Fig. 5.2C), Sylgard 184 PDMS is commonly employed as a heat-curable pre-polymer. The PDMS microchannel device can then be cast by pouring the mixture (pre-polymer and a curing agent) over the mould, which can be housed within a structure such as a petri dish. Here, it is essential that all air bubbles are removed, and this can be facilitated by de-gassing in a vacuum desiccator. Curing can take place at temperatures of up to 75°C, and after this process the replica can easily be retained and cut into rectangular slabs containing individual platforms with a scalpel. When the chip is removed from the mould, it is often sealed with a suitable substrate either reversibly (e.g. PDMS to glass) or irreversibly (plasma oxidation or bonding of cured PDMS to fully cured PDMS). The former process can be performed at room temperature and is a relatively fast procedure. However, this cannot be performed under high pressure (>30 kPa) [23]. In contrast, irreversible sealing can be performed on a number of different substrates (e.g. glass, silicon), but not with polycarbonate (PC) or PMMA [24]. The low thermal conductivity of PDMS means that careful consideration should be given to the thickness of the layer. In cases where this is too thick, high temperatures may have a detrimental effect on flow properties, and hence impair the immunoreaction [22].

For PMMA microfluidic chips, channel plates may be fabricated by using methodologies including hot embossing, room temperature imprinting and injection moulding. Hot embossing, the most frequently selected method for PMMA chip fabrication [25, 26], involves placing a PMMA chip on a metal or silicon mould which contains raised microfluidic channel imprints. Both structures are subsequently mounted in an embossing system (e.g. Rowland) and treated under controlled temperature and pressure conditions. The embossing force is maintained until the temperature falls below 105°C, which is representative of PMMA's glass transition temperature. At this point, the channelled PMMA chip is removed from the mould [18].

Injection moulding is an alternative methodology for producing multiple PMMA-based microdevices [27]. This process involves the injection of molten PMMA (under high pressure) into a mould cavity containing a master mould, e.g. of silicon. The cavity is subsequently allowed to cool, which in turn facilitates the removal of the microfluidic device from the mould [18]. Other approaches for fabricating PMMA microfluidic chips include laser ablation [28], room temperature imprinting [29] and in situ polymerisation [30]. Once a PMMA microfluidic device has been assembled, a key consideration is to ensure that microchannels are closed without having a detrimental effect on the conformation of the device. This can be overcome by using thermal or solvent-based bonding [18].

In addition to using silicon or nickel-based moulds, more cost-effective alternatives exist for PMMA prototyping, and it is possible to custom-design master moulds for hot embossing applications. Fiorini and colleagues [17] describe the rapid prototyping of PDMS moulds for creating PMMA microfluidic devices. More recently, Yao and colleagues [31] developed a cost-effective and disposable mould based on agar hydrogel for synthesising PMMA chips. Here, molten agar hydrogel was used as an interface between a glass plate and PMMA bearing a negative relief of the microstructure. Upon cooling, the PMMA template can be removed, leaving a hydrogel template with the positive relief which can subsequently be applied for the production of additional prototypes.

5.4 Analyte Delivery, Mixing and Washing

Conventional heterogeneous immunoassays, as performed in microtitre plates with 96 or more sample wells, typically require at least six sequential steps, namely (i) sample preparation, (ii) introduction of assay components (e.g. antigens, antibodies) via pipetting, (iii) incubation, (iv) washing with buffers such as phosphate-buffered saline (PBS), used to remove unbound antibodies, (v) substrate delivery and (vi) detection (e.g. colourimetric/fluorescent). These processes are similar for 'lab-on-a-chip' applications, and the implementation of innovative strategies for analyte delivery and subsequent washing was shown to improve immunoassay sensitivity and performance [32, 33].

In many cases, the delivery of reagent solutions through the microfluidic channels can be accomplished by pressure-driven flow. Lin et al. [34] selected a 1.0 mL syringe with a 30-gauge needle and inserted this directly into the microchannel at the end furthest from the waste channel. Here, it was possible to sequentially introduce analytical solutions in a controlled manner. Furthermore, an additional syringe was then used to remove liquid from the waste reservoir. For ELISA-based analysis where, the antigen is to be directly immobilised on the surface, this can be performed by pipetting into the well and passively immobilising overnight (e.g. at room temperature or at 4°C). The same group [35] demonstrated the ability to capture lysate antigens by injecting into individual microchannels of a PDMS microdevice, with the antigen, in this case of the bacterial strains *Helicobacter pylori* and *Escherichia coli* O157:H7, captured by passive immobilisation. Similarly to conventional assays, unbound antigen was removed by washing in phosphate-buffered saline (PBS).

In spite of the reduced dimensions of microfluidic devices, analytes can be transport-limited in microchannels, especially if they are at low concentrations [36]. Furthermore, it is not always feasible to further reduce channel dimensions to accommodate this, as it may be conducive to an increase in fluidic resistance and impaired mass transport. Hence, alternative strategies can be developed to overcome this issue. Hofmann and colleagues [37] developed a microchip-based flow confinement system for permitting the rapid delivery of minute analytical volumes to a PDMS surface for effectively capturing antibodies. Under laminar flow conditions, the sample is maintained as a thin layer in close proximity with the surface, which results in an increase in velocity. To demonstrate the efficacy of this flow confinement method, a silicon nitride waveguide was selected as a substrate for capturing rabbit IgG in the presence of trifluoromethylaryldiazirine dextran, and a fluorescent detection antibody (cyanine 5, Cy5-labelled anti-rabbit IgG) was hydrodynamically pumped through the channel at different flow rates to regulate the degree of flow confinement. While the authors did conclude that this novel method did significantly reduce the amount of analytical reagents needed to perform an immunoassay by over 90%, they also noted that the loss of analyte into the confining layer via diffusion was a limiting factor. Notwithstanding this apparent limitation, the integration of this and other delivery systems, e.g. positive dielectrophoresis (DEP), discussed in more detail below, for concentrating and sorting bacterial cells [38], are important considerations for improving 'lab-on-a-chip' immunoassay performance.

An alternative strategy for improving analyte capture is based on the integration of mixing elements into the microfluidic device. Golden and co-workers [39] embossed patterned grooves in the top of PDMS microchannels by using soft lithography. The key advantage here is that the fluid traversing through the channel is redirected to improve delivery of the target analyte to the surface of the device from the bulk fluid. Furthermore, this was demonstrated to prevent the depletion of analytes at the boundary layer. As a demonstration of the ability of this enhanced mixing to improve immunoassay performance, a neutravidin-coated microscope slide was inserted into the microfluidic device and used as a substrate for the capture of a biotinylated primary antibody (rabbit anti-botulinum toxin IgG). The sandwich assay format involved the detection of botulinum toxin (250 $\mu g\ mL^{-1}$), with a CY5-labelled secondary antibody used for detection purposes. Comparative analysis between native and grooved channels demonstrated that the latter configuration resulted in a 26% increase in fluorescent signal intensity, which was attributed to continuous mixing within the channel. More recently, a miniaturised microfabricated flow cytometer for permitting the multiplexed detection of bacterial cells and toxins was developed by Kim et al. [40]. While discussed in more detail below with reference to pathogen detection, a key design feature which contributed to the efficacy of this platform, was the ability to integrate hydrodynamic focussing to facilitate the single-file movement of particles through the microfluidic channels by sheathing, in a manner analogous to microflow cytometry. This was demonstrated by monitoring the flow of rhodamine dye through the channel by confocal microscopy. The PDMS platform was fabricated to include chevron-shaped grooves, which facilitated the movement of fluid from the sides of the channel to the centre, which in this case was conducive to three-dimensional sheathing. The focussing of the sample into a narrow-diameter area allowed greater interrogation by optical fibre-based detection and enhanced assay sensitivity.

It is also well established that the optimisation of washing steps can have a positive effect on immunoassay performance, and this also applies to 'lab-on-a-chip' applications. Mulvaney et al. [41] described a fluid-force discrimination (FFD)-based washing methodology for reducing non-specific absorption of analytes and conversely, increasing assay sensitivity. The principle behind FFD involves labelling analytes captured on the microassay surface with microbeads, with unbound beads removed by a controlled laminar flow. Increased analyte concentration, therefore, results in a greater number of beads being retained, and this can be verified by optical detection. In this example, the authors utilised beads coated with either antibodies or oligo(dT)$_{25}$ probes for the detection of proteinaceous (*Ricinus communis agglutinin* II, ricin A, troponin I and IgG) and nucleic acid-based targets (single-stranded DNA), respectively, and demonstrated femtomolar sensitivities for both targets. Furthermore, the ability of the FFD-based assay to simultaneously detect both analytes in parallel was also demonstrated.

5.5 Antibody Integration

'Lab-on-a-chip' immunoassay configurations can be either heterogeneous or homogeneous. Homogeneous immunoassays involve interactions between antibodies and antigens in solution, and for microfluidics-based immunoassays bound and unbound antibodies are typically discriminated by their electrophoretic mobility properties in microchannels [32]. In contrast, heterogeneous assays routinely use antibodies which are directly immobilised on the surface of the microdevice or alternatively, are cross-linked to micrometre sizes beads which are integrated within the device (Fig. 5.3).

The efficacy of the antibody immobilisation strategy has a profound effect on assay performance, with particular emphasis on sensitivity. The functional orientation of full-length antibodies by proteins A and G has been described in detail elsewhere [42], and these bioligands can be used in 'lab-on-a-chip' assay formats for

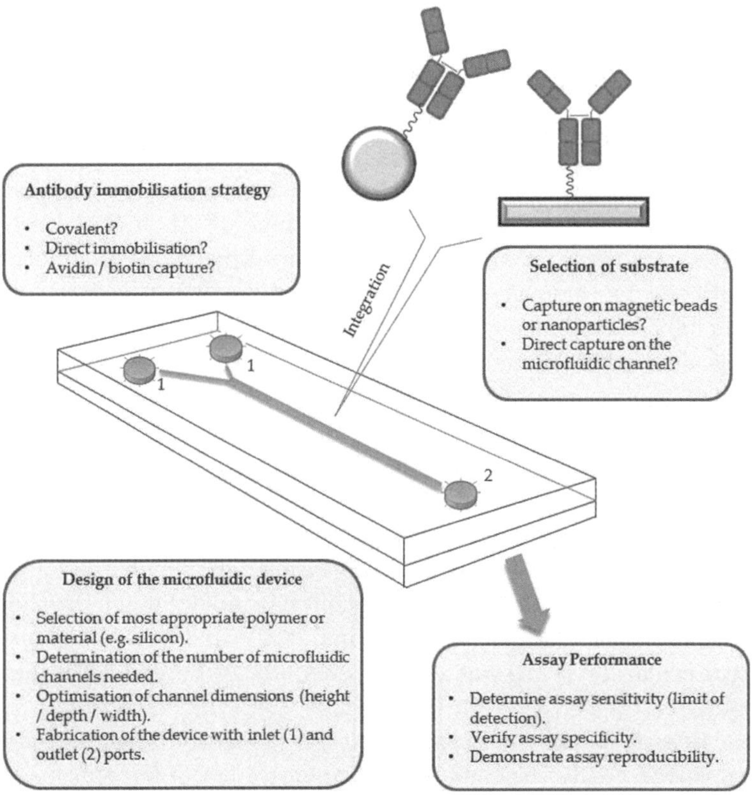

Figure 5.3 Schematic representation of homogeneous (bead-based) and heterogeneous immunoassay formats available for 'lab-on-a-chip' applications. The chip shown above is for representative purposes only; many other microfluidic designs incorporate multiple inlet ports and may permit multiplexed analysis. Examples are discussed in more detail in the text.

immobilising antibodies in a functional capacity. Vashist and colleagues [43] demonstrated that 1-ethyl-3-[3-dimethylaminopropyl] carbodiimide hydrochloride (EDC)/sulpho-N-hydroxysuccinimide (SNHS)-based covalent binding of a full-length anti- alpha-2-HS-glycoprotein (fetuin A) antibody resulted in greater antibody deposition on the surface when compared to random (passive immobilisation) and orientated (protein A) strategies, and resulted in greater assay sensitivity due to the complementarity-determining regions (CDRs) being functionally orientated.

The covalent attachment of antibodies for microfluidic applications can also be enhanced by using flexible linkers of varying sizes to circumvent problems associated with accessibility and steric hindrance. There are numerous linkers that can be selected for use, ranging from short (e.g. 3-aminopropyltriethoxysilane, APTES) branches to more flexible structures, such as those conferred by the use of polyethylenimine (PEI). In one early study, Yakovleva et al. [44] selected an anti-atrazine polyclonal antibody for biorecognition, and used three linker formats for immobilisation, namely APTES, PEI (linear and branched) and 3-glycidoxy propyltrimethoxysilane (GOPS). When assay sensitivities were comparatively analysed, it was found that the longer, PEI-based linkers had greater assay sensitivity than their shorter APTES-based counterparts (3.8 ng L^{-1} and 45 ng L^{-1} for linear PEI and APTES, respectively), suggesting that the enhanced flexibility was conducive to increased binding to the antigen, in this case atrazine.

The ability of PEI to effect an increase in IgG immobilisation on PMMA relative to other aminated chemicals, namely hexamethylenediamine (HMD), 1,3-diaminopropane (DAP) and poly(allylamine hydrochloride) (PAH) was also demonstrated by Bai and colleagues [45].

Here, the authors also concluded that the larger spacer distance conferred greater flexibility. In a demonstration of the efficacy of this immobilisation approach, the PMMA-based microfluidic assay was performed in parallel with an ELISA assay in a 96-well format. The smaller channel dimensions of the 'lab-on-a-chip' platform reduced the assay duration by tenfold, and the observed dynamic range of detection of analyte, in this case rat IgG, (5 ng mL^{-1}–1 μg mL^{-1}) was wider than for the conventional ELISA (2–100 ng mL^{-1}). An excellent example of patterned antibody deposition is described by Didar and colleagues [46], using a combination of microcontact printing and microfluidic patterning to deposit five antibodies on an APTES-functionalised glass surface by EDC/NHS coupling. The resulting microarray consisting of five functionally orientated antibodies, including anti-CD36, anti-CD31 and anti-CD34, clearly demonstrates the feasibility of using such approaches for generating surfaces capable of high-throughput immunoanalysis on a miniaturised platform.

Interestingly, several other unique immobilisation strategies have also been developed for microfluidic applications. Dong et al. [47] generated supported bilayer membranes by fusing vesicles which were comprised of 1,2-dioleoyl-sn-glycero-3-phosphoethanolamine and phosphatidylcholine, with oxidised PDMS microchannels to reduce non-specific binding. Biotinylated antibodies, in this case for Staphylococcus enterotoxin B (SEB), were captured by adding streptavidin to this lipid layer. It was noted that non-specific binding was reduced by over 100-fold when compared to untreated channels, and the assay had a sensitivity of 0.5 ng mL^{-1} which demonstrates the efficacy of this approach.

More recently, Liu and colleagues [48] used electrospinning to deposit polyvinylidene fluoride (PVDF) nanofibrous membranes onto a PDMS channel to enhance protein absorption. Here, these surfaces were used to capture full-length IgG antibodies from leporine, caprine and human hosts. While this appears to be a unique approach for immobilising biomolecules, the authors conclude that the use of such membranes could contribute to enhanced assay sensitivity.

Non-specific absorption to PDMS can also be used to effectively couple proteins, and one example demonstrates how this process can be enhanced through the use of hydrophobins, namely cysteine-rich proteins (7–15 kDa) which exhibit 'surfactant-like' qualities. These are derived from fungal sources including *Agaricus bisporus* and *Trichoderma reesei*, and are found on the outer surface of hyphal walls and conidia [49]. The ability of class II hydrophobins to self-assemble into amphiphilic membranes, such as at a PDMS-water interface, and improve hydrophilicity was demonstrated by Wang et al. [50]. The patterned hydrophobin PDMS surface was used to capture chicken IgG which was subsequently detected by a fluorescein isothiocyanate (FITC)-labelled secondary antibody derived from a leporine host. The enhanced 'wettability' of the surface was subsequently confirmed by X-ray photoelectron spectroscopy (XPS) and water contact angle measurements. Liu and colleagues [51] developed a PC-PDMS hybrid microchip which was used for the detection of influenza viral particles. Here, the authors captured primary (detection) antibodies on an epoxy-silica sol gel substrate. In addition to providing functionally orientated antibodies (covalently captured), the authors also noted that the integration of sol-gel in the fabrication process resulted in a strong bond between the PDMS substrate and polycarbonate support and critically, observed background fluorescence was low.

While the above strategies result in functionally orientated and immobilised antibodies, it should be emphasised that physical absorption can often have a deleterious effect on assay performance by essentially generating a heterogeneous surface where antibodies are orientated in a non-uniform manner. This can result in unfavourable orientation, denaturation and, in some cases, steric hindrance [2, 32]. Hence, when developing a 'lab-on-a-chip' immunoassay platform, this approach is not always ideal and strategies which present functionally orientated antibodies are more desirable.

5.6 Lab-on-a-Chip–Based Immunodetection: Applications

5.6.1 Bacterial Pathogens and Toxins

A key advantage of miniaturised microfluidic platforms is the ability to perform 'on-site' analysis in a reliable manner. For example, devices can be designed for use in environments where a suspected pathogen or toxin is believed to be present, and an antibody-based detection strategy is to be employed. Here, the analytical sample (e.g. water for toxin analysis or a food sample for pathogen detection) can be taken 'at-source' and directly tested with the portable platform. This is easily facilitated by the reduced size of such devices.

Pathogens are ubiquitous in nature and pose a considerable risk to the well-being of human and animal hosts, in addition to severely compromising the quality of agricultural produce intended for human consumption. Thus, it is imperative that bacterial and fungal pathogens and associated toxins are detected in a rapid, sensitive and specific manner [2]. The majority of these assays developed to date have focussed on the detection of the human pathogen *Escherichia coli* O157:H7. This enterohaemmorhagic Gram-negative rod is a causative agent of foodborne illness, and is potentially fatal. Transmission typically occurs via the faecal-oral route, and symptoms of infection include diarrhoea and nausea [52]. An early example of a 'lab-on-a-chip' immunoassay for detecting this strain is presented by Lin et al. [35], using PDMS as a microfluidic substrate. In contrast to assays where intact cells are selected as analytes, cells were harvested and lysed to release internal antigenic determinants, a strategy which is routinely performed in the presence of a protease-inhibitor to ensure epitope structural conformation is retained. A leporine host-derived polyclonal antibody conjugated with biotin was selected, with assay sensitivity enhanced through the use of a goat anti-biotin detection antibody conjugated with resonance-light scattering (RLS) gold nanoparticles (80 nm) which facilitated visualisation by electron microscopy. The advantage of using such particles is that they allow the scattering of incident white light to generate monochromatic white light, which can be visualised by dark-field microscopy. The authors were subsequently able to image the PDMS microchannels by a digital camera and dark-field zoom stereoscope, with custom-developed computational software used for monitoring colour changes resulting from binding events. The integration of the above components resulted in the development of a sensitive assay for *E. coli* O157:H7 antigens, which were detected at a concentration of between 6 and 600 ng μL^{-1} of sample. As a further demonstration of the efficacy of this assay platform, the authors were also able to detect *Helicobacter pylori*, a Gram negative, microaerophilic bacterium which is a causative agent of chronic gastritis in human hosts [53], at levels similar to that afforded by conventional ELISA.

More recently, a hand-held, portable platform for *E. coli* O157:H7 detection based on immunomagnetic detection was developed [54]. In contrast to the previous example which used PDMS [35], here the authors preferentially selected silicon nitride (Si_3N_4) over SU-8 and silicon dioxide (SiO_2) as a substrate for the direct immobilisation of antibodies, and intact bacterial cells were used for detection. The sandwich assay format incorporated a horseradish peroxidase (HRP)-labelled secondary antibody, derived from a leporine host, which was coated on superparamagnetic beads. These are commonly used in microfluidic immunoassays for conferring greater surface area to volume ratios, and also facilitate the delivery of antibodies to a desired location within a microfluidic device, e.g. by magnetic manipulation [32]. In this example, the biosensor detected and quantified small magnetic field variations resulting from the presence of the antigen-bound superparamagnetic beads under an external magnetic field, and this contributed towards an assay sensitivity of 1×10^5 colony-forming units (CFU) mL^{-1} for *E. coli* O157:H7, with minimal cross-reactivity seen for *Salmonella choleraesuis*, selected as a negative control strain [54].

While the packaging of antibodies into microfluidic channels works well for this particular assay, immobilising antibodies on beads may enhance assay performance by improving sensitivity. To demonstrate this, a one-step, microbead-based immunoseparation platform for the detection of the same pathogen was subsequently developed by Guan and colleagues [55]. Antibodies were covalently captured via EDC/NHS coupling on 50 μm glass beads, which were functionalised with a self-assembled layer of aminosilane. Using this strategy, it was possible to align the beads as a monolayer within a PDMS/glass channel (70 μm in height) by injection through an inlet valve under positive pressure with a syringe pump. An interesting aspect of this immunoassay is the detection mechanism, with pathogen concentrations determined by the presence of adenosine triphosphate (ATP), and luminous intensity resulting from the addition of bioluminescence detection reagents (luciferin-luciferase) was indicative of the presence of bacterial cells and detected by a photodetector. The efficacy of the assay was illustrated by the ability to rapidly (less than 20 min) and selectively detect between 1×10^1–1×10^5 cells of *E. coli* per μL. Furthermore, a key advantage of using such a detection mechanism is that only viable cells are detected. Hence, integrating such methods of detection with lab-on-a-chip immunoassays indicates the way forward for 'on-site' viable pathogen detection using reduced sample volumes.

When developing immunoassays for detecting bacterial pathogens, it is common for preliminary, proof-of-concept measurements to detect strains of interest propagated in the laboratory. However, the natural progression is to then demonstrate the ability to detect the pathogen in a complex matrix, such as a food sample, without the need for a pre-enrichment step in bacteriological media. In the above example, Guan et al. [55] detected *E. coli* O157:H7 in spiked fresh meat samples. More recently, a novel, portable, handheld platform for detecting this strain, in addition to *E. coli* K12 in iceberg lettuce (10 CFU mL^{-1}) in less than 6 min, was developed [56]. The assay was based on a particle immuno-agglutination format, where particles are coated with antibodies (or, in some other cases, antigens) and mixed with the analytical sample. Here, biorecognition events are conducive to particle aggregation. While ocular inspection can be used to visualise precipitates, light scattering can be used to detect positive signals in the absence of precipitation, which significantly increases assay sensitivity and reduces the amount of antigen required for use in an assay. Hence, microfluidics-based particle immuno-agglutination assays allow rapid and sensitive pathogen detection, often to a single-cell level [57]. Here, strain-specific rabbit polyclonal antibodies were immobilised on latex microparticles (920 nm), with uncoated particles used for reference purposes. Differential detection was permitted by using Mie light scattering, which maximised the light scatter intensity of agglutinated microparticles and reduced the scattering intensity of the analytical sample matrix. Hence, this portable device represents another excellent example of integrating microfluidic channels, antibodies and advanced detection strategies for facilitating rapid and sensitive bacterial detection.

A very recent example demonstrates how the integration of companion signal amplification strategies can be used to significantly improve on assay quality when detecting bacterial pathogens. Raja and colleagues [58] successfully integrated linear microreflectors in a transparent polymer layer, which functioned as an optical sensing surface, and incorporated magnetic particles to effect light blocking. Pre-concentrated sample was captured on an antibody-modified microfluidic substrate, and the efficacy of this elegant approach is demonstrated by the excellent assay sensitivity, specifically permitting the detection of 4,000 cells of *Rickettsia conorii*, the causative agent of Mediterranean Spotted Fever.

When detecting pathogens with miniaturised platforms, high-throughput analysis can be ideal in cases where multiple bacterial strains are to be detected simultaneously in an analytical sample, such as water. Dharmasiri and colleagues [59] developed a PMMA-based 'lab-on-a-chip' immunoassay platform which facilitated the analysis of eight individual samples through the fabrication of

9.5 mm long microchannels (15 μm in width and 80 μm in depth). A demonstration of the efficacy of this approach used a caprine host-derived polyclonal antibody covalently immobilised onto photoactivated PMMA using EDC/NHS coupling. Microscopy was used to visualise bound *E. coli* O157:H7 cells, which were subsequently removed from the microfluidic channel through the use of a commercially available, non-enzymatic dissociation buffer. Enumeration was facilitated by quantitative real-time polymerase chain reaction (qPCR), and the limit of the detection was between 6 and 10 CFU. Assay specificity was demonstrated using *Micrococcus luteus*, *Staphylococcus aureus* and *Bacillus subtilis* as control bacterial strains. While this assay demonstrates excellent sensitivity and specificity and represents a novel immunodiagnostic 'lab-on-a-chip' platform, the authors acknowledge the fact that the assay takes approximately 5 hours to complete, and requires external instrumentation. Hence, subsequent prototype developments would benefit from integrating PCR-based genotyping of this and other pathogens.

Bacterial pathogens may be present in trace amounts in analytical samples and therefore, assay sensitivity is of paramount importance. In 'lab-on-a-chip' immunodiagnostic platforms, this can be enhanced through the use of advanced detection methodologies, such as amperometric detection which routinely utilises an enzyme-based system that generates an electroactive product which can be oxidised or reduced at a working electrode, with changes resulting from biorecognition events monitored by changes in current [2]. An excellent example where this approach is used to detect *E. coli* K12 in milk (100 cells mL^{-1} analyte) is described by Laczka et al. [60]. Bacterial cells were initially detected using a polyclonal anti-*E. coli* antibody which was captured on streptavidin-coated magnetic particles. Next, electrochemical detection was permitted by monitoring the production of hydrogen peroxide (H_2O_2) by a horseradish peroxidase (HRP)-labelled detection antibody in the presence of hydroquinone. Upon injection into a microfluidic system at a rate of 50 μL/min, the enzyme product was pumped along the microchannel (PDMS) and detected amperometrically by a set of integrated microelectrodes. Careful design of the microfluidic components of the 'lab-on-a-chip' immunoassay platform can further enhance assay performance, minimising contact of the analytical sample with the electrode, which reduced the possibility of fouling.

'Lab-on-a-chip' immunoassays have also been developed for other bacterial pathogens. These include *Listeria monocytogenes*, a potentially life-threatening human pathogen and causative agent of listeriosis [61]. To detect this pathogen in de-ionised water, Yang et al. [38] developed an elegant microfluidic immunoassay where positive dielectrophoresis (DEP) was used to concentrate and sort bacterial cells. DEP operates on the principle of the electrokinetic motion of di-electrically polarised entities when placed in a non-uniform electrical field, and when applied for the purpose of cell separation this requires the dielectric properties of target cells to be different to that of non-target cells. As this is often not the case, DEP can be coupled with immunodetection, as shown here, to improve assay specificity. The microfluidic device developed consisted of an array of oxide-covered interdigitated titanium/platinum electrodes which were aligned on a silicon substrate enclosed within PDMS. A biotinylated monoclonal anti-Listeria antibody was immobilised on the silicon oxide (SiO_2) surface on top of the interdigitated electrode array by capture on a biotin-BSA/streptavidin DEP channel surface, and bacterial cells were introduced to the microfluidic structure using a syringe pump and a gas-tight luer-lock syringe. The efficacy of using DEP for *L. monocytogenes* sorting was demonstrated by the observation that approximately 90% of cells under continuous flow conditions were retained. Interestingly, when this pathogen was tested alongside other bacterial strains, including *Enterobacter aerogenes* and *Enterococcus faecalis*, it was noted that only antibody-captured bacterial cells were retained within the microfluidic channel when positive DEP was turned off. Furthermore, the immunodetection of Listeria cells was enhanced under DEP, with capture efficiencies of between 18 and 27% observed when bacterial cells (10^1–10^3 per 5 μL sample volume) were selected as analytes. Hence, the key advantage of integrating DEP with a 'lab-on-a-chip' immuno-diagnostic platform is the ability to separate and selectively capture cells with similar dielectric properties and dimensions, and this technology has considerable potential for microfluidic immunodiagnostics.

One of the key benefits of using microfluidics-based platforms is the ability to fabricate chips which permit parallel, multiplexed analysis, e.g. of bacterial cells and associated toxins. The latter include Staphylococcal enterotoxin B (SEB) [62] and cholera toxin [63], and due to the fact that they pose a considerable risk to human health, developing strategies for reliable and sensitive detection is also an important consideration. To demonstrate multiplexed analysis, the PDMS-based microfabricated immunoassay based on flow cytometry designed by Kim et al. [40], discussed earlier with reference to how the microfluidic design enhanced sample delivery, for the detection of bacterial cells (*E. coli*, Listeria spp. and Salmonella spp.) and toxins (SEB/cholera toxin and ricin). The sandwich assay format integrated fluorescently coded and carboxy-functionalised microspheres, to which individual pathogen or toxin-specific antibodies were covalently coupled. Signal amplification was facilitated by the use of biotinylated, phycoerythrin-labelled anti-streptavidin antibodies, with optical fibres being integrated into the chip to facilitate laser-based detection. Limits of detection for bacterial cells were between 1×10^3 and 1×10^5 CFU mL^{-1}. However, the ability to also integrate toxin-specific antibodies is a considerable advantage, which further demonstrates the potential of this and related platforms for multiplexed analysis of structurally diverse analytes. Toxin limits of detection for this study are summarised in Table 5.1, which also highlights other excellent examples of 'lab-on-a-chip' immunoassay-based bacterial toxin detection.

While the examples listed above deal with the detection of food-borne pathogens and toxins, there has also been an emphasis on the development of miniaturised platforms for detecting biological warfare agents, including bacterial spores. It is interesting to note that such analysis has also evolved from using large, multicomponent platforms, such as the early fluidics-based system described by McBride et al. [64] for the detection of *Bacillus anthracis* and *Yersinia pestis*, which was comprised of several independent, integrated modules (e.g. an aerosol collector and a multiplexed immunoassay flow cytometer detector) to multi-analyte, miniaturised microfluidic immunoassay formats. Many of these have been designed to alert civilian populations to a potential terrorist attack.

Table 5.1 'Lab-on-a-chip' immunoassay platforms for bacterial toxin detection

Assay format	Substrate	Analyte	Sensitivity	Ref.
Antibodies (1°, fluorescently-labelled 2°) bind to toxin captured on supported bilayer membrane-deposited ganglioside receptor molecules (GM1)	PDMS	Cholera toxin	8 fM	[65]
Direct binding of antibody and antigen off-chip. Addition to microfluidic platform.	Glass	Ricin Shiga Toxin 1 SEB	20 nM 500 pM 300 pM	[66]
Sandwich immunoassay format integrating antibody-coated microspheres with streptavidin-phycoerythrin labelling.	PDMS	Cholera toxin SEB Ricin	1.6 mg mL^{-1} 0.064 mg mL^{-1} 1.6 ng mL^{-1}	[40]
Integration of a microfluidic assay into a 96-well ELISA plate, with antibody-conjugated carbon nanotubes immobilised in individual wells.	PMMA	SEB	0.1 ng mL^{-1}	[67]
Electrochemical impedance spectroscopy (EIS)-based detection, with protein A-immobilised antibodies captured on a self-assembled monolayer.	PDMS	Cholera toxin	10 pM	[68]

A key example is the SpectroSens™ consumable cartridge developed by Cartwright and colleagues [69] which permits multiplexed detection of an array of eight of bio-hazardous agents, including the bacterial strains *B. anthracis, Bacillus atrophaeus, Franciscella tularensis* and *E. coli*. Similar to commercially available platforms such as Biacore™ (GE Healthcare) and Octet® (Fortébio) which are discussed in more detail elsewhere [70], this system measured changes in refractive index resulting from the interaction of antigens with pathogen and toxin-specific antibodies within spatially separated waveguide channels in 'real-time.' Through the use of carefully designed microfabrication, an eight-channel microfluidic device mounted in a PMMA cartridge was produced which allowed the detection of eight different analytes in a single assay. To prepare surfaces for use in this miniaturised assay, individual channels were initially cleaned with oxygen plasma, and the silanised surface was coupled with optical fibres for detection purposes. Detection antibodies were functionally orientated using protein A/G-captured primary antibodies. With reference to sample delivery, reagents were introduced to the microchannels via a syringe pump-based module, with the rate of sample introduction regulated computationally, and the subsequent addition of hazardous material, such as bacterial cells and toxins, facilitated by a peristaltic 'pump-based' 'stand-alone' module. The biomolecular interactions between analytes and immobilised antibodies were conducive to increases in refractive index. The ability to detect an array of bacterial and viral pathogens in parallel in less than 15 min clearly demonstrates the efficacy of this platform for the rapid detection of biological warfare agents, with ricin also detected at low concentration (250 ng mL^{-1}), and potentiates its use in defence monitoring [69].

5.6.2 Marine and Fungal Toxins

A critical analysis of the many antibody- and biosensor-based assays that are currently in existence for monitoring marine toxins (phycotoxins) and fungal toxins (mycotoxins) is provided elsewhere [2]. It should be emphasised that relatively few examples of microfluidic immunoassays have been developed to date for detecting such analytes, with key examples now discussed. Okadaic acid (OA) (Fig. 5.4) is a toxin produced as a secondary metabolite by *Dinophysis* and *Prorocentrum* dinoflagellates, and the consumption of OA-contaminated shellfish results in diarrheic shellfish poisoning (DSP) [71]. To detect this phycotoxin in mussel and scallop samples, a flow-based immunosensor was reported by Prieto-Simón and colleagues [72] based on the principle of kinetic exclusion. Here, a capillary flow cell was packed with OA-coated PMMA beads,

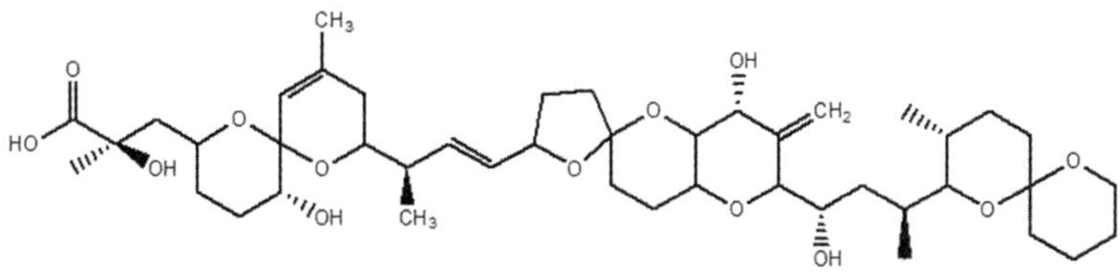

Okadaic Acid

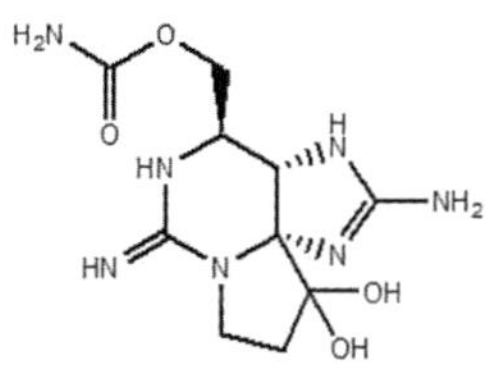

Saxitoxin

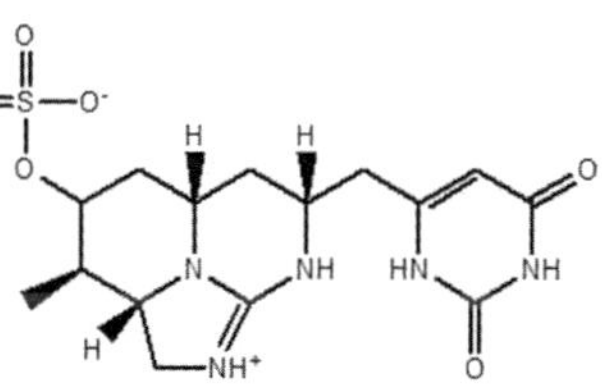

Cylindrospermopsin

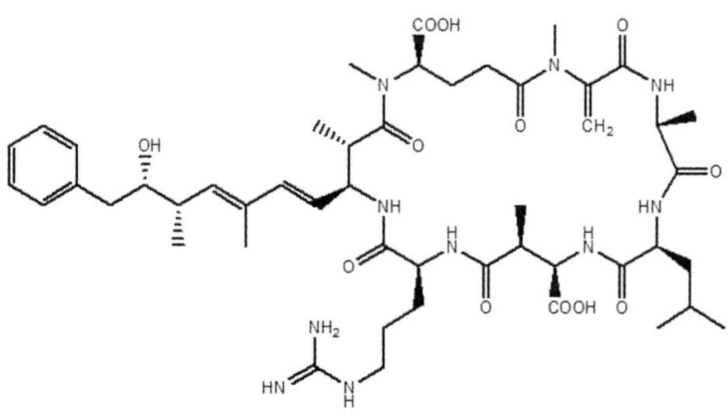

Microcystin LR

Figure 5.4 Chemical structures of marine toxins detected using 'lab-on-a-chip' immunoassay platform described in [61].

attached by either biotinylation or by conjugation with the large carrier protein ovalbumin (OVA), and a competitive immunoassay format using a monoclonal anti-OA antibody was employed. Such formats are routinely employed for the detection of small, hapten-like antigens [2]. A key output of this assay was the ability to detect toxin at limits of detection consistent with European legislative levels (0.3 μg L^{-1}).

Another key example which demonstrates the ability to detect algal toxins in a rapid, multiplexed and sensitive manner was described [73]. Three structurally diverse antigens (saxitoxin, cylindrospermopsin and microcystin LR; Fig. 5.4) were detected in parallel using a PDMS microfluidic device where protein A-coated microspheres (9 μM in diameter), used to capture toxin-specific antibodies, were packaged into specific microchannels. Using water as an analytical sample, assay sensitivity for each analyte was 0.02 ng mL^{-1}. While these two examples highlight the potential of using lab-on-a-chip immunodiagnostic platforms for marine and freshwater toxin analysis, the ability to use these for on-site detection of a panel of diverse targets will not be determined until additional prototypes are developed, implemented and qualified.

The detection of fungal toxins is also of great importance, due to their association with crop spoilage and their detrimental effect on human health. Similarly to the analysis of phycotoxins, this area is in its infancy, and key examples developed to date for the detection of mycotoxins such as ochratoxin A and citrinin are summarised in Table 5.2, with key relevant chemical structures shown in Fig. 5.5.

Another area in its infancy is the detection of fungal pathogens. To date, only one microfluidic immunoassay based on Plexiglas has been developed for detecting *Botrytis cinerea*, the causative agent of grey mould. However, the elegant microfluidic design, comprised of an immunosensor coupled with screen-printed carbon electrodes (SPCEs) for amperometric detection, and ability to sensitively detect this fungal pathogen in apple, grape and pear in the presence and absence of decay warrants mention. Antigen was captured on 3-aminopropyl-treated micromagnetic beads by glutaraldehyde coupling, with beads subsequently introduced into the microfluidic channels by a syringe pump. The assay format was similar to that used above for toxin detection, in that a monoclonal antibody

Table 5.2 'Lab-on-a-chip' immunoassay platforms for fungal toxin detection. Here, zearalenone, citrinin and ochratoxin A were detected in baby food, rice and apples, respectively. Note the platform used in [76] is a commercially available electrochemical flow cell package (ND, not disclosed)

Assay format	Substrate	Analyte	Sensitivity	Ref.
Anti-mycotoxin antibodies functionally orientated on protein-G-coated magnetic beads and used in a competitive immunoassay format.	Glass	Zearalenone	20 ppb	[75]
Competitive, amperometric immunoassay with ovalbumin-conjugated analyte immobilised on a glassy carbon electrode via an electro-deposited gold surface.	ND	Citrinin	0.1 ng mL^{-1}	[76]
Magnetic nanoparticle-based assay with anti-mycotoxin antibodies immobilised by glutaraldehyde coupling used to detect horseradish-peroxidase (HRP)-labelled antigen in solution.	PMMA	Ochratoxin A	0.05 μg Kg^{-1} apple	[77]

competed for free (fruit tissue) and immobilised antigen. The quantification of bound antibodies by a HRP-labelled detection antibody, and the subsequent oxidation of the enzymatic mediator 4-tert-butylcatechol (4-TBC) to 4-tert-butyl o-benzoquinone (4-TBBQ) in the presence of hydrogen peroxide (H_2O_2) was the basis of the detection mechanism. The electrochemical reduction back to 4-TBC was detected by the SPCEs, and the observed response current was inversely proportional to antigen concentration in the fruit sample. While somewhat lengthy (40 min), the assay had excellent sensitivity, correlating to 0.008 μg mL^{-1} [74].

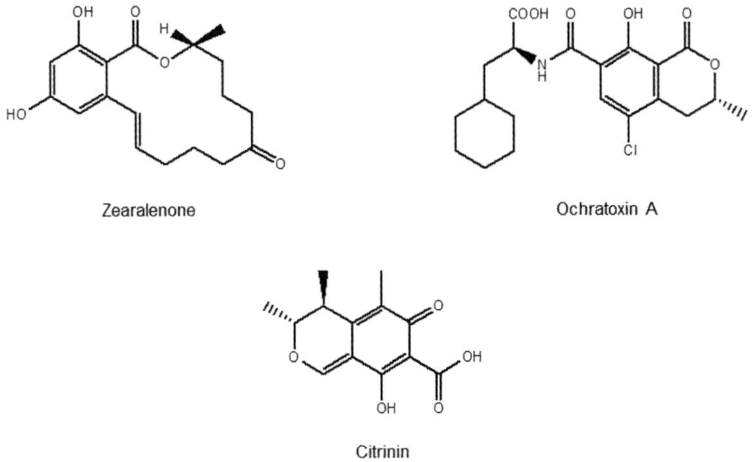

Figure 5.5 Chemical structures of fungal toxins detected using the 'lab-on-a-chip' immunoassay platform [75–77].

In summary, while relatively few examples of 'lab-on-a-chip' immunoassays for the detection of toxins and fungal pathogens currently exist, those discussed above demonstrate the immense potential of such platforms. The development of additional assays should permit the ability to screen agricultural produce pre- and post-harvest, which will be of considerable economic importance.

While the application of 'lab-on-a-chip' technology for the detection of mycotoxins is still developing, several key examples demonstrate the significant potential of applying this assay format for their detection [78–80]. Soares and and colleagues [80] describe an innovative 'point-of-use' platform compatible with multiplexing, which permits the detection of aflatoxin B1 (3 ng mL^{-1}), ochratoxin A (100 ng mL^{-1}) and deoxynivalenol (100 ng mL^{-1}) in less than 20 minutes based on chemiluminescent detection. Of notable importance is the successful integration of amorphous silicon photosensors below the microfluidic chip, which enhances signal detection and improves assay quality. Finally, a paper microfluidic competitive immunoassay was recently developed for the detection of aflatoxin B1, with a reported sensitivity of 1.31 ng mL^{-1} [79]. While this chapter has not focussed in detail on microfluidic paper-based analytical devices (PADs), it should be noted that this is an area of growing interest due to their ability to be used in fluorescent, chemiluminescent and colourimetric assay formats, while fabrication strategies such as photolithography are directly applicable for fabricating these low-cost devices.

5.7 Disease Markers and Their Detection Using Microfluidics-Based Devices

Disease biomarkers are analytes (typically proteinaceous), which are detected at elevated levels in a biological sample, such as blood, urine or saliva, during the onset and progression of disease. Their presence is indicative of the disease trait (e.g. risk factor), the disease state (e.g. pre-clinical or clinical) and the disease rate (progression) [81]. Cardiovascular disease (CVD) is a major killer which places a considerable financial burden on healthcare systems and accounts for approximately half of all deaths in the western world. Biomarkers of inflammation, ventricular overload, myocardial necrosis and myocardial ischemia can readily be detected in blood [82], and a selection of the 'lab-on-a-chip' immunodiagnostic platforms that have been developed to facilitate their detection is highlighted in Table 5.3. While this table is not exhaustive, in that it does not highlight every single microfluidic immunoassay developed to date for detecting CVD-related disease markers, it does focus on the detection of five targets of great clinical relevance. C-reactive protein (CRP) is a 125 kDa acute-phase reactant produced in the liver, and a well-established marker of inflammation. This highly stable protein is a member of the pentraxin family, and is comprised of five symmetric units (approximately 206 amino acids) which are covalently bound to one another [83]. Interestingly, Khreiss et al. [84] investigated the mechanism by which CRP activates endothelial cells and demonstrated that the loss of pentameric symmetry was conducive to the induction of interleukin-8 (IL-8) and monocyte chemoattractant protein-1 (MCP-1), which both play key roles in leucocyte recruitment. Furthermore, the observation that serum CRP concentrations increase by a factor of 10,000

Table 5.3 'Lab-on-a-chip' immunoassay platforms for the detection of biomarkers of cardiovascular disease.

Assay format	Substrate	Analyte	Sensitivity	Ref.
Rapid ($<$30 minutes) 'Immunostack'-based assay with microchannels initially filled with serum to bind CRP, which in turn is detected with primary and HRP-labelled secondary antibodies	Zeonex	CRP	0.1 mg L^{-1}	[86]
Three-step immunoassay using antibody-modified microrings, with tertiary antibodies conjugated to streptavidin-coated beads (100nm) for signal enhancement.	Silicon	CRP	3×10^{-5} μg mL^{-1}	[87]
Immobilisation of antibodies on a PDMS-gold nanoparticle composite film. Sandwich immunoassay integrating cadmium telluride and zinc selenide quantum dots. The electrochemical signal detected was proportional to the analyte concentration.	PDMS	TnI CRP	5 aM 307 aM	[88]
Fluorescence-based immunoassay on a two-channel, disposable chip. Capture of antigen/2°antibody complex by an immobilised primary antibody.	PS	Creatine Kinase Myoglobin	1.5 ng mL^{-1} 1.5 ng mL^{-1}	[91]
Electrochemical assay with an integrated interdigitated array gold electrode. Antibodies captured on protein-G deposited wells; antigen quantification determined by oxidation peak measurements based on production of para-aminophenol by detection antibody binding	PDMS	Troponin I	148 pg mL^{-1}	[92]
Magnetic bead-based sandwich immunoassay on an integrated, digital microfluidic cartridge. Antibodies coated on beads and pre-mixed with analyte. Analysis in less than 8 minutes.	Glass	Troponin I	5 ng mL^{-1}	[93]
Capture of antibodies on an amphiphilic polymer-coated layer by contact printing with a PDMS stamp. TnI detection by a sandwich immunoassay format incorporating fluorescent (Alexa 647) detection.	COC	Troponin I	10 ng mL^{-1}	[94]
Magnetic nanoparticle-based electrochemical immunosensor, with antibody-coated particles immobilised on an electrode. Amperometric responses measured after antibody-antigen interactions.	Gold	Pro-BNP	0.003 ng mL^{-1-}	[95]

during the acute-phase response [85] suggests that this biomarker is of great clinical significance. The lab-on-a-chip immunoassays summarised in Table 5.3 for CRP detection [86, 87] demonstrate how the integration of elegant microfluidic design and a sensitive antibody can be used to detect this biomarker, with blood selected as an analytical sample in the latter example.

While multiplexed analysis was described previously for pathogen [69] and toxin detection [40], the microfluidic platform developed by Zhou and colleagues for the detection of CRP and troponin I (TnI) is of great interest [88]. Cardiac troponin I (23.5 kDa) is widely accepted as being a gold standard for the specific diagnosis of myocardial infarction [89], and participates as part of a regulatory complex in striated cardiac muscle alongside troponins I (TnI) and C (TnC) which regulates skeletal and cardiac muscle contraction [90]. Elevated troponin levels have putative links with a number of secondary conditions, including congestive heart failure, chronic renal failure, pulmonary embolism and sepsis [82]. Hence, detecting this CVD biomarker of is clinical importance. The examples listed in Table 5.3 for TnI vary in their respective sensitivities (148 pg mL^{-1} to 10 ng mL^{-1}), although the example described by Zhou and colleagues [88] shows excellent (attomole) sensitivity, aided by quantum dot-based signal enhancement. Before the use of troponin, total creatine kinase (CK) was selected for the diagnosis of myocardial infarction. This enzyme is detected in heart and skeletal muscle and while it is a useful marker of re-infarction diagnosis [82], the clinical efficacy of CK somewhat is hindered by the fact that the levels of this enzyme in blood typically elevate late in the course of acute myocardial infarction. Furthermore, the presence of CK in skeletal muscle may present a false-positive result due to non-cardiac related injury which in turn can result in incorrect diagnosis [90]. Notwithstanding this apparent clinical limitation, it must be emphasised that a selection of commercially available platforms have been developed for the detection of the muscle brain fraction (CK-MB). These include PATHFAST (Mitsubishi Chemical Europe GmbH), Triage® Cardiac Panel (Biosite) and the Stratus CS STAT (Dade Behring Inc.) [82]. Furthermore, the rapid, disposable 'lab-on-a-chip' immunoassay developed by Ryu and colleagues [91] for CK-MB detection shows excellent sensitivity for this enzyme

(1.5 ng mL^{-1}). The dual-channel configuration of this platform also permits the detection of myoglobin, an iron and oxygen-binding protein (18 kDa) found in muscle which, alongside CK, TnI and TnT, is a clinically useful biomarker of myocardial necrosis [96]. A final example which perfectly demonstrates the use of 'lab-on-a-chip' immunoassay technology for cardiac marker detection is the spinit® platform, developed by Biosurfit (http://biosurfit.com/). This elegant microfluidic technology, encompassed within a centrifugal disc, facilitates sensitive detection of CRP using label-free detection (based on the principle of surface plasmon resonance, SPR). Here, immunorecognition is permitted through the integration of highly sensitive recombinant antibodies (anti-CRP), which detect this analyte in fingerprick blood samples in a highly sensitive manner. Notably, this technology is another exemplar of a technology integrating recombinant antibodies as biorecognition elements with microfluidic chip design for diagnostic applications. The company has recently expanded its product portfolio to determine whole blood cell counts using centrifugal microfluidic-based platforms.

5.8 Conclusions

In this chapter we have discussed the current status of 'lab-on-a-chip' immunoassay platforms, focussing on substrate selection, microfluidic design and antibody immobilisation. Furthermore, we have provided key examples which demonstrate the immense potential of such platforms for the detection of analytes of biological and medicinal importance. With reference to biomarkers, a comprehensive review of all available biomarkers and microfluidic systems is outside the scope of this chapter. However, several excellent reviews currently exist which discuss this topic [97–101], with emphasis on markers of CVD and cancer (e.g. circulating tumour cells, CTCs). When the terms *lab-on-a-chip immunosensor* and *biomarker* are entered into PubMed (http://www.ncbi.nlm.nih.gov/pubmed), over 400 examples can be found (based on a search conducted on the 29th of November, 2016), the earliest of these reported in 1997 [103]. Several recent examples have also expanded on how this technology can be applied for immunoassay applications, and have detailed enhancements made to increase sensitivity and specificity for targets of biological and diagnostic importance. For example, recent work described by Nwankire and colleagues [88] outlines a novel impedimetric assay, performed on a centrifugal microfluidic disc, which incorporates anti-epithelial cell adhesion molecule (EpCAM) antibodies for biorecognition of CTCs. This innovative 'electrochemical lab-on-a-disc' (eLoaD) technology incorporates rotationally activated valving strategies for controlling reagent release, including siphoning, capillary and centrifugo-pneumatic dissolvable films. Such features significantly enhance the ability of the immunoassay to detect the analyte of interest in a reliable and sensitive manner by proving the end-user with the ability to control reagent release. A second recent example also demonstrates how the integration of novel optical detection strategies, such as supercritical angle fluorescence (SAF), can be used to significantly improve assay sensitivity, in this case detecting human IgG in a bioprocess sample. This is a second key example of how valving technologies can be implemented to facilitate whole immunoassays to be performed on a single microfluidic device, thus satisfying the criteria for 'lab-on-a-disc.'

As a final example of a future trend in developing 'lab-on-a-chip' immunoassays, Singh and colleagues [104] describe the use of 3D printing to engineer a unique well-structure (referred to as the '3D well') which provides the end-user with an analytical substrate with greater surface area when compared with traditional 96-well ELISA plates. Upon fabrication, the authors demonstrated excellent assay performance in detecting autoantibodies to Rubella virus in serum samples, with >2 fold sensitivity when compared with conventional ELISA. Three dimensional printing is compatible with rapid prototyping, and has immense potential in the field of 'lab-on-a-chip' immunodiagnostics. While the authors comment on the potential application of such structures in microfluidic devices, we believe that there will be a notable increase in the number of microfluidic assays incorporating antibody-based biorecognition which contain elements fabricated using 3D printing by, for example, improving the sensing layers [105].

The observation that a significant number of the aforementioned manuscripts have been published since 2010 further suggests that this is an emerging research area which is destined to expand exponentially in the future, and will undoubtedly benefit from newly developed expertise in microfabrication, immunoassay development and detection. While examples to date for bacterial pathogen have focussed primarily on *E. coli* O157:H7, the potential to expand this current repertoire to include other pathogens of equal biological importance is entirely feasible, while the scope to develop additional platforms for multi-analyte and multiplexed, rapid analysis emphasises that lab-on-a-chip platforms signal the future of immunodiagnostic assays.

References

1. Hearty, S., and O'Kennedy, R. (2017). Recombinant antibodies for diagnostic applications: design considerations and structural correlates, chapter 2 in *Immunoassays: Development, Applications and Future Trends*, ed. R. O'Kennedy and C. Murphy. Singapore: Pan Stanford Publishing, pp. 37–58.
2. Byrne, B., Stack, E., Gilmartin, N., and O'Kennedy, R. (2009). Antibody-based sensors: principles, problems and potential for detection of pathogens and associated toxins. *Sensors*, **9**, 4407–4445.
3. O'Kennedy, R., Townsend, S., Donohoe, G.G., Leonard, P., Hearty, S., and Byrne, B. (2010). Speedy, small, sensitive and specific: reality of myth for future analytical methods. *Anal Lett*, **43**, 1630–1648.
4. Sharma, S., Byrne, H., and O'Kennedy, R.J. (2016). Antibodies and antibody-derived analytical biosensors. *Essays Biochem*, **60**(1), 9–18.
5. Kunert, R., and Reinhart, D. (2016). Advances in recombinant antibody manufacturing. *Appl Microbiol Biotechnol*, **100**(8), 3451–3461.
6. Sia, S.K., and Whitesides, G.M. (2003). Microfluidic devices fabricated in poly(dimethylsiloxane) for biological studies. *Electrophoresis*, **24**, 3563–3576.
7. Guber, A.E., Heckele, M., Herrmann, D., Maslija, A., Saile, V., Eichhorn, L., Gietzeld, T., Hoffmann, W., Hauser, P.C., Tanyanyiwa, J., Gerlach, A., Gottschlich, N., and Kneben, G. (2004). Microfluidic lab-on-a-chip

systems based on polymers:fabrication and application. *Chem Eng J*, **101**, 447–453.

8. Alrifaiy, A., Lindalh, O.A., and Ramser, K. (2012). Polymer-based microfluidic devices for pharmacy, biology and tissue engineering. *Polymers*, **4**, 1349–1398.
9. Nge, P.N., Rogers, C.L., and Woolley, A.T. (2013). Advances in microfluidic materials, functions, integration, and applications. *Chem Rev*, **113**(4), 2550–2583.
10. Ng, J.M.K., Gitlin, I., Stroock, A.D., and Whitesides, G.M. (2002). Components for integrated poly(dimethylsiloxane) microfluidic systems. *Electrophoresis*, **23**, 3461–3473.
11. Eribol, P., Uguz, A.K., and Ulgen, K.O. (2016). Screening applications in drug discovery based on microfluidic technology. *Biomicrofluidics*, **10**(1), 011502.
12. Zhou, J., Ellis, A.V., and Voelcker, N.H. (2010). Recent developments in PDMS surface modification for microfluidic devices. *Electrophoresis*, **31**, 2–16.
13. Fernández Gavela, A., Grajales García, D., Ramirez, J.C., and Lechuga, L.M. (2016). Last advances in silicon-based optical biosensors. *Sensors*, **16**(3), 285.
14. Chaudhury, M.K., and Whitesides, G.M. (1991) Direct measurement of interfacial interactions between semispherical lenses and flat sheets of Poly(dimethylsiloxane) and their chemical derivatives. *Langmuir*, **7**, 1013–1025.
15. Bernard, A., Fitzli, D., Sonderegger, P., Delamarche, E., Michel, B., Bossard, H.R., and Biebuyck, H. (2001). Affinity capture of proteins from solutions and their dissociation by contact printing. *Nat Biotechnol*, **19**, 866–869.
16. Makamba, H., Kim, J.H., Lim, K., Park, N., Hahn, J.H. (2003). Surface modification of poly(dimethylsiloxane) microchannels. *Electrophoresis*, **24**, 3607–3619.
17. Fiorini, G.S., Jeffries, G.D., Lim, D.S., Kuyper, C.L and Chiu, D.T. (2003). Fabrication of thermoset polyester microfluidic devices and embossing masters using rapid prototypes polydimethylsiloxane molds. *Lab Chip*, **3**(3), 158–163.
18. Chen, Y., Zhang, L., and Chen, G. (2008). Fabrication, modification, and application of poly(methyl methacrylate) microfluidic chips. *Electrophoresis*, **29**, 1801–1814.

19. Wongkaew, N., He, P., Kurth, V., Surareungchai, W., and Baeumner, A.J. (2013). Multi-channel PMMA microfluidic biosensor with integrated IDUAs for electrochemical detection. *Anal Bioanal Chem*, **405**(18), 5965–5974.
20. Han X., Liu, X., Tian, L., Zhang, H., and Gang Mao, Z. (2015). A non-photolithography fabrication for a microfluidic chip based on PMMA polymer. *Machines*, **3**, 107–122.
21. Yuan, C.H., and Shiea, J. (2001). Sequential electrospray analysis using sharp-tip channels fabricated on a plastic chip. *Anal Chem*, **73**(6), 1080–1083.
22. Gao, Y., Hu, G., Lin, F.Y.H., Sherman, P.M., and Li, D. (2005). An electrokinetically-controlled immunoassay for simultaneous detection of multiple microbial antigens. *Biomed Microdevices*, **7**(4), 301–312.
23. McDonald, J.C., Duffy, D.C., Anderson, J.R., Chiu, D.T., Wu, H., Schueller, O.J., and Whitesides, G.M. (2000). Fabrication of microfluidic systems in poly(dimethylsiloxane). *Electrophoresis*, **21**, 21–40.
24. Duffy, D.C., McDonald, J.C., Schueller, O.J.A., and Whitesides, G.M. (1998). Rapid prototyping of microfluidic systems in poly(dimethylsiloxane). *Anal Chem*, **70**, 4974–4984.
25. Martynova, L., Locascio, L.E., Gaitan, M., Kramer, G.W., Christensen, R.G., and MacCrehan, W.A. (1997). Fabrication of plastic microfluid channels by imprinting methods. *Anal Chem*, **69**(23), 4783–4789.
26. Peng, L., Deng, Y., Yi, P., and Lai, X. (2013). Micro hot embossing of thermoplastic polymers: a review. *J Micromech Microeng*, **24**(1), 013001.
27. McCormick, R.M., Nelson, R.J., Alonso-Amigo, M.G., Benvegnu, D.J., and Hooper, H.H. (1997). Microchannel electrophoretic separations of DNA in injection-molded plastic substrates. *Anal Chem*, **69**(14), 2626–2630.
28. Galloway, M., Stryjewski, W., Henry, A., Ford, S.M., Llopis, S., McCarley, R.L., and Soper, S.A. (2002). Contact conductivity detection in poly(methyl methacrylate)-based microfluidic devices for analysis of mono- and polyanionic molecules. *Anal Chem*, **74**(10), 2407–2415.
29. Xu, J.D., Locascio, L., Gaitan, M., and Lee, C.S. (2000). Room-temperature imprinting method for plastic microchannel fabrication. *Anal Chem*, **72**, 1930–1933.
30. Xu, G.X., Wang, J., Chen, Y., Zhang, L., Wang, D., and Chen, G. (2006). Fabrication of poly(methyl methacrylate) capillary electrophoresis microchips by *in situ* surface polymerization. *Lab Chip*, **6**(1), 145–148.

31. Yao, X., Chen, Z., and Chen, G. (2009). Fabrication of PMMA microfluidic chips using disposable agar hydrogel templates. *Electrophoresis*, **30**(24), 4225–4229.
32. Ng, A.H., Uddayasankar, U., and Wheeler, A.R. (2010). Immunoassays in microfluidic systems. *Anal Bioanal Chem*, **397**(3), 991–1007.
33. Chuang, C.H., Wu, T.F., Chen, C.H., Chang, K.C., Ju, J.W., Huang, Y.W., and Van Nhan, V. (2015). Lab on a chip for multiplexed immunoassays to detect bladder cancer using multifunctional dielectrophoretic manipulations. *Lab Chip*, **15**(14), 3056–3064.
34. Lin, F.Y., Sabri, M., Erickson, D., Alirezaie, J., Li, D., and Sherman, P.M. (2004). Development of a novel microfluidic immunoassay for the detection of *Helicobacter pylori*. *Analyst*, **129**(9), 823–828.
35. Lin, F.Y.H., Sabri, M., Alirezaie, J., Li, D., and Sherman, P.M. (2005). Development of a nanoparticle-labeled microfluidic immunoassay for detection of pathogenic microorganisms. *Clin Diag Lab Immunol*, **12**(3), 418–425.
36. Parsa, H., Chin, C.D., Mongkolwisetwara, P., Lee, B.W., Wang, J.J., and Sia, S.K. (2008). Effect of volume- and time-based constraints on capture of analytes in microfluidic heterogeneous immunoassays. *Lab Chip*, **8**(12), 2062–2070.
37. Hofmann, O., Voirin, G., Niedermann, P., and Manz, A. (2002). Three-dimensional microfluidic confinement for efficient sample delivery to biosensor surfaces. Application to immunoassays on planar optical waveguides. *Anal Chem*, **74**(20), 5243–5250.
38. Yang, L., Banada, P.P., Chatni, M.R., Seop Lim, K., Bhunia, A.K., Ladisch, M., and Bashir, R. (2006). A multifunctional micro-fluidic system for dielectrophoretic concentration coupled with immune-capture of low numbers of *Listeria monocytogenes*. *Lab Chip*, **6**, 896–905.
39. Golden, J.P., Floyd-Smith, T.M., Mott, D.R., and Ligler, F.S. (2007). Target delivery in a microfluidic immunosensor. *Biosens Bioelectron*, **22**(11), 2763–2767.
40. Kim, J.S., Anderson, G.P., Erickson, J.S., Golden, J.P., Nasir, M., and Ligler, F.S. (2009). Multiplexed detection of bacteria and toxins using a microflow cytometer. *Anal Chem*, **81**, 5426–5432.
41. Mulvaney, S.P., Cole, C.L., Kniller, M.D., Malito, M., Tamanaha, C.R., Rife, J.C., Stanton, M.W., and Whitman, L.J. (2007). Rapid, femtomolar bioassays in complex matrices combining microfluidics and magneto-electronics. *Biosens Bioelectron*, **23**(2), 191–200.

42. Peluso, P., Wilson, D.S., Do, D., Tran, H., Venkatasubbaiah, M., Quincy, D., Heidecker, B., Poindexter, K., Tolani, N., Phelan, M., Witte, K., Jung, L.S., Wagner, P., and Nock, S. (2003). Optimising antibody immobilisation strategies for the construction of protein microarrays. *Anal Biochem*, **312**(2), 113–124.
43. Vashist, S.K., Dixit, C.K., MacCraith, B.D., and O'Kennedy, R. (2011). Effect of antibody immobilisation strategies on the analytical performance of a surface plasmon resonance-based immunoassay. *Analyst*, **136**(21), 4431–4436.
44. Yakovleva, J., Davidsson, R., Bengtsson, M., Laurell, T., and Emnéus, J. (2003). Microfluidic enzyme immunosensors with immobilised protein A and G using chemiluminescence detection. *Biosens Bioelectron*, **19**(1), 21–34.
45. Bai, Y., Koh, C.G., Boreman, M., Juang, Y.J., Tang, I.C., Lee, L.J., and Yang, S.T. (2006). Surface modification for enhancing antibody binding on polymer-based microfluidic device for enzyme-linked immunosorbent assay. *Langmuir*, **22**(22), 9458–9467.
46. Didar, T.F., Foudeh, A.M., and Tabrizian, M. (2011). Patterning multiplex protein microarrays in a single microfluidic channel. *Anal Chem*, **84**, 1012–1018.
47. Dong, Y., Phillips, K.S., and Cheng, Q. (2006) Immunosensing of Staphylococcus enterotoxin B (SEB) in milk with PDMS microfluidic systems using reinforced supported bilayer membranes (R-SBMS). *Lab Chip*, **6**(5), 675–681.
48. Liu, Y., Yang, D., Yu, T., and Jiang, X. (2009). Incorporation of electrospun nanofibrous PVDF membranes into a microfluidic chip assembled by PDMS and scotch tape for immunoassays. *Electrophoresis*, **30**(18), 3269–3275.
49. Wösten, H.A.B. (2001). Hydrophobins: multipurpose proteins. *Annu Rev Microbiol*, **55**, 625–646.
50. Wang, R., Yang, Y.L., Qin, M., Wang, L.K., Yu, L., Shao, B., Qiao, M.Q., Wang, C., and Feng, X.Z. (2007). Biocompatible hydrophilic modifications of poly(dimethylsiloxane) using self-assembled hydrophobins. *Chem Mater*, **19**, 3227–3231.
51. Liu, J., Zhao, J., Petrochenko, P., Zheng, J., and Hewlett, I. (2016). Sensitive detection of influenza viruses with Europium nanoparticles on an epoxy silica sol-gel functionalised polycarbonate-polydimethysiloxane hybrid microchip. *Biosens Bioelectron*, **86**, 150–155.

52. Armstrong, G.L., Hollingsworth, J., and Morris Jr., J.G. 1996. Emerging foodborne pathogens: *Escherichia coli* O157:H7 as a model of entry of a new pathogen into the food supply of the developed world. *Epidem Rev*, **18**(1), 29–51.
53. Tomb, J.F., White, O., Kerlavage, A.R., Clayton, R.A., Sutton, G.G., Fleischmann, R.D., Ketchum, K.A., Klenk, H.P., Gill, S., Dougherty, B.A., Nelson, K., Quackenbush, J., Zhou, L., Kirkness, E.F., Peterson, S., Loftus, B., Richardson, D., Dodson, R., Khalak, H.G., Glodek, A., McKenney, K., Fitzgerald, L.M., Lee, N., Adams, M.D., Hickey, E.K., Berg, D.E., Gocayne, J.D., Utterback, T.R., Peterson, J.D., Kelley, J.M., Cotton, M.D., Weidman, J.M., Fujii, C., Bowman, C., Watthey, L., Wallin, E., Hayes, W.S., Borodovsky, M., Karp, P.D., Smith, H.O., Fraser, C.M., and Venter, J.C. (1997). The complete genome sequence of the gastric pathogen *Helicobacter pylori*. *Nature*, **388**(6642), 539–547.
54. Mujika, M., Arana, S., Castaño, E., Tijero, M., Vilares, R., Ruano-López, J.M., Cruz, A., Sainz, L., and Berganza, J. (2009). Magnetoresistive immunosensor for the detection of *Escherichia coli* O157:H7 including a microfluidic network. *Biosens Bioelectron*, **24**, 1253–1258.
55. Guan, X., Zhang, H.J., Bi, Y., Zhang, L., and Hao, D. (2010). Rapid detection of pathogens using antibody-coated microbeads with bioluminescence in microfluidic chips. *Biomed Microdevices*, **12**, 683–691.
56. You, D.J., Geshell, K.J., and Yoon, J.Y. (2011). Direct and sensitive detection of foodborne pathogens within fresh produce samples using a field-deployable handheld device. *Biosens Bioelectron*, **28**, 399–406.
57. Heinze, B.C., Song, J.Y., Lee, C.H., Najama, A., and Yoon, J.Y. (2009). Microfluidic immunosensor for rapid and sensitive detection of bovine viral diarrhoea virus. *Sensor Actuat B-Chem*, **138**, 491–496.
58. Raja, B., Pascente, C., Knoop, J., Shakarisak, D., Sherlock, T., Kemper, S., Kourentzi, K., Ranzi, R.F., Hatch, A.V., Olano, J., Peng, B.H., Ruchhoeft, P., and Willson, R. (2016). An embedded microretroreflector-based microfluidic immunoassay platform. *Lab Chip*, **16**(9), 1625–1635.
59. Dharmasiri, U., Witek, M.A., Adams, A.A., Osiri, J.K., Hupert, M.L., Bianchi, T.S., Roelke, D.L., and Soper, S.A. (2010). Enrichment and detection of *Escherichia coli* O157:H7 from water using an antibody-modified microfluidic chip. *Anal Chem*, **82**, 2844–2849.
60. Laczka, O., Maesa, J.M., Godino, N., del Campo, J., Fough-Hansen, M., Kutter, J.P., Snakeborg, D., Muñoz-Pascual, F., and Baldrich, E. (2011).

Improved bacteria detection by coupling magneto-immunocapture and amperometry at flow-channel microband electrodes. *Biosens Bioelectron*, **26**, 3633–3640.

61. Farber, J.M., and Peterkin, P.I. (1991). *Listeria monocytogenes*, a food-borne pathogen. *Microbiol Rev*, **55**(3), 476–511.
62. Ahanotu, E., Alvelo-Ceron, D., Ravita, T., and Gaunt, E. (2006). Staphylococcal enterotoxin B as a biological weapon: recognition, management and surveillance of Staphylococcal enterotoxin. *Appl Biosafety*, **11**(3), 120–126.
63. De Haan, L., and Hirst, T.R. (2004). Cholera toxin: a paradigm for multi-functional engagement of cellular mechanisms. *Mol Membr Biol*, **21**(2), 77–92.
64. McBride, M.T., Masquelier, D., Hindson, B.J., Marakewicz, A.J., Brown, S., Burris, K., Metz, T., Langlois, R.G., Tsang, K.W., Bryan, R., Anderson, D.A., Venkateswaran, K.S., Milanovich, F.P., and Colsten Jr., B.W. (2003). Autonomous detection of aerosolised *Bacillus anthracis* and *Yersinia pestis*. *Anal Chem*, **75**, 5293–5299.
65. Scott Phillips, K., and Cheng, Q. (2005). Microfluidic immunoassay for bacterial toxins with supported phospholipid bilayer membranes on poly(dimethylsiloxane). *Anal Chem*, **77**, 327–334.
66. Meagher, R.J., Hatch, A.V., Renzi, R.F., and Singh, A.K. (2008). An integrated microfluidic platform for sensitive and rapid detection of biological toxins. *Lab Chip*, **8**, 2046–2053.
67. Yang, M., Sun, S., Kostov, Y., and Rasooly, A. (2011). An automated point-of-care system for immunodetection of staphylococcal enterotoxin B. *Anal Biochem*, **416**, 74–81.
68. Chiraicò, M.S., Primiceri, E., D'Amone, E., Ionescu, R.E., Rinaldi, R., and Maruccio, G. (2011). EIS microfluidic chips for flow immunoassay and ultrasensitive cholera toxin detection. *Lab Chip*, **11**, 658–663.
69. Bhatta, D., Michel, A.A., Marti-Villalba, M., Emmerson, G.D., Sparrow, I.J.G., Perkins, E.A., McDonnell, M.B., Ely, R.W., and Cartwright, G.A. (2011). Optical microchip assay biosensor for multiplexed detection of bio-hazardous agents. *Biosens Bioelectron*, **30**, 78–86.
70. GE Healthcare. Biacore sensor surface handbook (web) (2005).
71. Tripuraneni, J., Koutsouris, A., Pestic, L., De Lanerolle, P., and Hecht, G. (1997). The toxin of diarrheic shellfish poisoning, Okadaic Acid, increases intestinal epithelial paracellular permeability. *Gastroenterology*, **112**(1), 100–108.

72. Prieto-Simón, B., Miyachi, H., Karube, I., and Saiki, H. (2010). High-sensitive flow-based kinetic exclusion assay for okadaic acid assessment in shellfish samples. *Biosens Bioelectron*, **25**, 1395–1401.

73. Zhang, J., Liu, S., Yang, P., and Sui, G. (2011). Rapid detection of algal toxins by microfluidic immunoassay. *Lab Chip*, **11**, 3516–3522.

74. Fernández-Baldo, M.A., Messina, G.A., Sanz, M.I., and Raba, J. (2010). Microfluidic immunosensor with micromagnetic beads coupled for carbon-based screen-printed electrodes (SPCEs) for determination of *Botrytis cineria* in tissue of fruits. *J Agric Food Chem*, **58**, 11201–11206.

75. Hervás, M., Ángel-López, M., and Escarpa, A. (2009). Electrochemical microfluidic chips coupled to magnetic bead-based ELISA to control allowable levels of zearalenone in baby foods using simplified calibration. *Lab Chip*, **134**, 2405–2411.

76. Arévalo, F.J., Granero, A.M., Fernández, H., Raba, J., and Zón, M.A. (2011). Citrinin (CIT) determination in rice samples using a micro fluidic electrochemical immunosensor. *Talanta*, **83**(3), 966–973.

77. Fernández-Baldo, M.A., Bertolino, F.A., Fernández, G., Messina, G.A., Sanz, M.I., and Raba, J. (2011). Determination of Ochratoxin A in apples contaminated with *Aspergillus ochraceus* by using a microfluidic competitive immunosensor with magnetic nanoparticles. *Analyst*, **136**, 2756–2762.

78. Uludag, Y., Esen, E., Kokturk, G., Ozer, H., Muhammad, T., Olcer, Z., Basegmez, HI, Simsek, S., Barut, S., Gok, M.Y., Akgun, M., and Altintas, Z. (2016). Lab-on-a-chip based biosensor for the real-time detection of aflatoxin. *Talanta*, **160**, 381–388.

79. Busa, L.S., Mohammadi, S., Maeki, M., Ishida, A., Tani, H., and Tokeshi, M. (2016). A competitive immunoassay system for microfluidic paper-based analytical detection of small size molecules. *Analyst*, **141**(24), 6598–6603.

80. Soares, R.R., Santos, D.R., Chu, V., Azevedo, A.M., Aires-Barros, M.R., and Conde, J.P. (2017). A point-of-use microfluidic device with integrated photodetector array for immunoassay multiplexing: detection of a panel of mycotoxins in multiple samples. *Biosens Bioelectron*, **87**, 823–831.

81. Vasan, R.S. (2006). Biomarkers of cardiovascular disease: molecular basis and practical considerations. *Circulation*, **113**(19), 2335–2362.

82. McDonnell, B., Hearty, S., Leonard, P., and O'Kennedy, R. (2009). Cardiac biomarkers and the case for point-of-care testing. *Clin Biochem*, **42**(7–8), 549–561.

83. Ablij, H., and Meinders, A. (2002). C-reactive protein: history and revival. *Eur J Intern Med*, **13**, 412–422.

84. Khreiss, T., Jozsef, L., Potempa, L.A., and Filep, J.G. (2004). Conformational rearrangement in C-reactive protein is required for proinflammatory actions on human endothelial cells. *Circulation*, **109**, 2016–2022.

85. Pepys, M.B., and Berger, A. (2001). The renaissance of C reactive protein. *BMJ*, **322**, 4–5.

86. Bhattacharyya, A., and Klapperich, C.M. (2007). Design and testing of a disposable microfluidic chemiluminescent immunoassay for disease biomarkers in human serum samples. *Biomed Microdevices*, **9**, 245–251.

87. Luchansky, M.S., Washburn, A.L., McClellan, M.S., and Bailey, R.C. (2011). Sensitive on-chip detection of a protein biomarker in human serum and plasma over an extended dynamic range using silicon photonic microring resonators and sub-micron beads. *Lab Chip*, **11**(12), 2042–2044.

88. Zhou, F., Lu, M., Wang, W., Bian, Z.P., Zhang, J.R., and Zhu, J.J. (2010). Electrochemical immunosensor for simultaneous detection of dual cardiac markers based on a poly(dimethylsiloxane)-gold nanoparticles composite microfluidic chip: A proof of principle. *Clin Chem*, **56**(11), 1701–1707.

89. Adams, J.E., Bodor, G.S., Davila-Roman, V.G., Delmez, J.A., Apple, F.S., Ladenson, J.H., and Jaffe, A.S. (1993). Cardiac troponin I. A marker with high specificity for cardiac injury. *Circulation*, **88**, 101–106.

90. Conroy, P.J., O'Kennedy, R., and Hearty, S. (2012). Cardiac troponin I: A case study in rational antibody design for human diagnostics. *Protein Eng Des Sel*, **25**(6), 295–305.

91. Ryu, G., Huang, J., Hofmann, O., Walshe, C.A., Sze, J.Y.Y., McClean, G.D., Mosley, A., Rattle, S.J., deMello, J.C., deMello, A.J., and Bradley, D.D.C. (2011). Highly-sensitive fluorescence detection system for microfluidic lab-on-a-chip. *Lab Chip*, **11**(9), 1664–1670.

92. Ko, S., Kim, B., Jo, S.S., Oh, S.Y., and Park, J.K. (2007). Electrochemical detection of cardiac troponin I using a microchip with the surface-functionalised poly(dimethylsiloxane) channel. *Biosens Bioelectron*, **23**, 51–59.

93. Sista, R., Hua, Z., Thwar, P., Sudarsan, A., Srinivasan, V., Eckhardt, A., Pollack, M., and Pamula, V. (2008). Development of a digital microfluidic platform for point-of-care testing. *Lab Chip*, **8**, 2091–2104.
94. Sung, D., Shin, D.H., and Jon, S. (2011). Toward immunoassay chips: facile immobilisation of antibodies on cyclic olefin copolymer substrates through pre-activated polymer adlayers. *Biosens Bioelectron*, **26**(9), 3967–3972.
95. Liang, W., Li, Y., Zhang, B., Zhang, Z., Chen, A., Qi, D., Yi, W., and Hu, C. (2012). A novel microfluidic immunoassay system based on electrochemical immunosensors: an application for the detection of NT-ProBNP in whole blood. *Biosens Bioelectron*, **31**(1), 480–485.
96. Antman, E., Bassand, J.P., Klein, W., Ohman, M., Lopez Sendon, J.L., Rydén, L., Simoons, M., and Tendera, M. (2000). Myocardial infarction redefined – a consensus document of the Joint European Society of Cardiology/American College of Cardiology Committee for the redefinition of myocardial infarction. *J Am Coll Cardiol*, **36**, 959–969.
97. Osiri, J.K., and Shadpour, H. (2010). Toward point-of-care microchip profiling of proteins. *Bioanalysis*, **2**(10), 1745–1754.
98. Karns, K., and Herr, A.E. (2011). Microfluidic homo- and heterogeneous immunoassays: a tool to accelerate protein biomarker development. *Bioanalysis*, **3**(19), 2161–2165.
99. Mohammed, M.I., and Desmulliez, M.P.Y. (2011). Lab-on-a-chip based immunosensor principles and technologies for the detection of cardiac biomarkers: a review. *Lab Chip*, **11**, 569–595.
100. Tarasow, T.M., Penny, L., Patwardhan, A., Hamren, S., McKenna, M.P., and Urdea, M.S. (2011). Microfluidic strategies applied to biomarker discovery and validation for multivariate diagnostics. *Bioanalysis*, **3**(19), 2233–2251.
101. Lianidou, E.S., and Markou, A. (2011). Circulating tumor cells in breast cancer: detection systems, molecular characterization and future challenges. *Clin Chem*, **57**(9), 1242–1255.
102. Key, G., Schreiber, A., Feldbrügge, R., Glatz, J.F., and Spener, F. (1997). An immunosensor for rapid estimation of the early heart infarction-marker FABP. *Acta Anaesthesiol Scand Suppl*, **111**, 289–292.
103. Nwankire, C.E., Venkatanarayanan, A., Glennon, T., Keyes, T.E., Forster, R.J., and Ducrée, J. (2015). Label-free impedance detection of cancer cells from whole blood on an integrated centrifugal microfluidic platform. *Biosens Bioelectron*, **68**, 382–389.

104. Singh, H., Shimojima, M., Shiratori, T., An, L.V., Sugamata, M., and Yang, M. (2015). Application of 3D printing technology in increasing the diagnostic performance of enzyme-linked immunosorbent assay (ELISA) for infectious diseases. *Sensors*, **15**(7), 16503–16515.
105. Mandon, C.A., Blum, L.J., and Marquette, C.A. (2016). Adding biomolecular recognition capability to 3D printed objects. *Anal Chem*, **88**(21), 10767–10772.

Chapter 6

Clinical Applications of Immunoassays

Karen Lawler[a] **and Gregor Kijanka**[b]

[a]*Royal College of Surgeons in Ireland, Dublin 15, Ireland*
[b]*Biomedical Diagnostics Institute, Dublin City University, Dublin 9, Ireland*
karenmlawler@physicians.ie, gregor.kijanka@dcu.ie

Immunoassays represent an invaluable tool for detection, confirmation and monitoring of disease in the clinical setting. Their major benefits are rapid assay times, simple handling and conclusive results, which can influence clinical decision-making and therefore have a direct impact on patient treatment. Human diseases are often accompanied by the presence of molecular factors such as **biomarkers**, which can be found in bodily fluids and tissues. Such factors may arise independently of clinical symptoms and can be therefore used as analyte biomarkers indicating the presence or absence of a disease. With the advances of bioanalytical methods in recent years, numerous disease-associated biomarker molecules have been identified and are now widely used with the aid of innovative immunoassays to detect the presence of disease. In this chapter we will discuss the clinical application of immunoassays in the detection of disease and their relevance in monitoring of some of the most common disease processes.

Immunoassays: Development, Applications and Future Trends
Edited by Richard O'Kennedy and Caroline Murphy

ISBN 978-981-4669-97-9 (Hardcover), 978-1-315-20654-7 (eBook)
www.panstanford.com

6.1 Clinical Specimen Analysis

The most commonly used clinical immunoassays are based on the analysis of small volumes of patient blood. As blood circulates, it accumulates molecular biomarkers secreted by diseased tissue, providing an excellent means of detecting disease. The major practical advantage of using blood for clinical analysis is its availability through minimally invasive blood collection techniques. Blood can be further processed into plasma or serum, which is often the preferred choice for analytical assays. In addition, simple finger pinprick blood withdrawal methods allow the use of minute volumes of blood required for emerging lab-on-chip-based immunoassays and **point-of-care** devices.

Other bodily fluids like urine, cerebrospinal fluid, amniotic fluid and saliva are also important sample sources for clinical analysis where blood cannot be used (Fig. 6.1). They are less frequently used in immunoassays due to the lack of clinically relevant biomarkers. However, occasionally they are superior to blood. Immunoassays utilising urine can be used for diagnosis of urinary tract diseases by measuring creatinine levels [1], multiple myeloma through Bence Jones proteins [2] or detection of drugs such as amphetamines, opiates and other performance-enhancing drugs [3]. However, the most widely used urine immunoassay is the pregnancy test, which

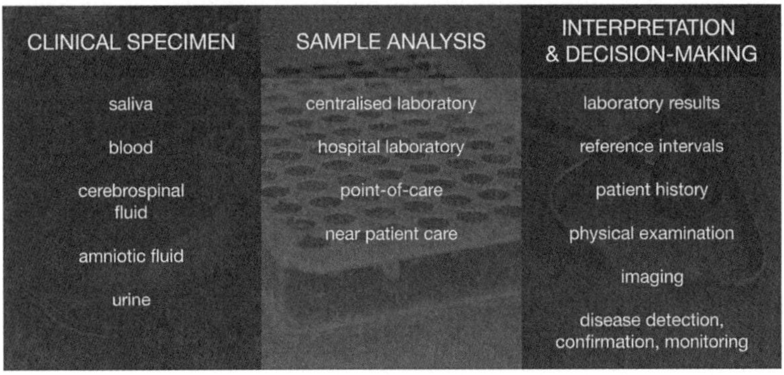

Figure 6.1 Clinical pathway from sample to clinical decision-making supported by immunoassays.

can detect pregnancy within two days of fertilisation based on the detection of human choriogonadotropin (hCG) [4]. Cerebrospinal fluid (CSF), which is more difficult to access and requires a lumbar puncture procedure, can be used to detect the presence of lactate or proteins such as alpha cryptococcal antigen, to test for meningitis, or more recently for cryptococcosis [5]. Amniotic fluid, which surrounds the foetus in the womb throughout the pregnancy, can be used for the analysis of congenital abnormalities. A sample of the amniotic fluid can be taken from the amniotic sac with a needle in a procedure called amniocentesis. Clinical immunoassays utilising amniotic fluid are applied for instance for analysis of alpha-fetoprotein (AFP) which indicates neural tube or abdominal wall defects and chromosomal conditions of the foetus [6]. Saliva is the most easily accessible bodily fluid and it can be used to measure cortisol concentrations for the diagnosis of hypercortisolism and adrenal insufficiency [7]. Since cortisol can directly diffuse into saliva, salivary cortisol immunoassays are more accurate than measuring free cortisol in serum.

Effective salivary assays are also used for the diagnosis of HIV infections, by measuring IgG antibodies specific to HIV1 antigen [8]. Interestingly, HIV1 antibody titers are high in saliva and its non-invasive sampling manner results in good acceptance and high uptake among tested individuals [9], demonstrating the relevance of all body fluids for clinical applications of immunoassays.

Clinical immunoassays are usually performed in small-, medium-, and high volume laboratories within hospitals or in independent centralised laboratories. Often, highly specialised core laboratories are established within large national hospitals and clinical samples are sent off from smaller peripheral hospitals or from general practitioner clinics for analysis in the core laboratory. Clinical laboratories, operated by highly trained staff, provide a wide range of services, rapid turnaround and accurate analysis of clinical samples to the highest standard. The laboratories are fitted with ever more advanced immunoassay equipment capable of multi-analyte, multi-sample analysis with throughput of up to several hundred samples per hour, capable of continuous random access operation. For further reading on clinical immunoassay automation, please refer to *The Immunoassay Handbook* by Wild [10]. With recent advances in micro-sale **lab-on-a-chip** technologies there is currently a strong trend towards the use of novel point-of-care (POC) immunoassay devices, which allow clinical sample analysis without a need for a laboratory facility. Sample analysis can be performed directly in the general practitioner's clinic, smaller hospitals and also in 'resource-poor' environments. POC immunoassay testing is suitable for 'near-patient' care and provides a faster turnaround [11, 12]. A patient tested by their general practitioner can be diagnosed immediately at the time of the first visit potentially reducing delays in treatment.

Clinical laboratories usually deliver results which need to be interpreted by the attending doctor. The diagnosis of a specific disease is largely based on a thorough patient history and physical examination. However, laboratory tests also play a major role in the diagnosis of disease (Fig. 6.2). Laboratory **reference intervals** are generally provided by immunoassay manufacturers. However, due to sample collection and treatment, patient cohort specifics,

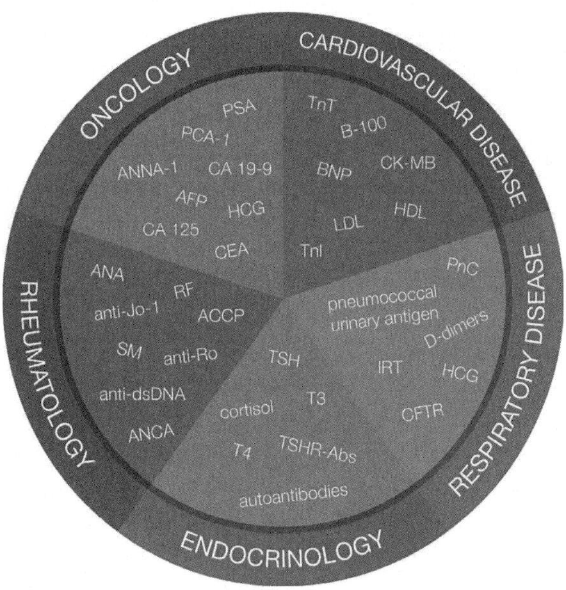

Figure 6.2 Markers of disease commonly used in detection, confirmation and monitoring of disease.

such as sex, age and race, can vary in many hospitals [13]. Clinical laboratories, therefore, should implement specific reference intervals, in addition to the manufacturer's recommendations, to improve the sensitivity and specificity of disease biomarkers [14].

6.2 Cardiovascular Disease

6.2.1 Ischemic Heart Disease and Cardiac Enzymes

A compromise of blood flow to the heart muscle results in the release of numerous cytosolic and structural proteins from cardiac myocytes. The initial rise and peak serum levels of these proteins is useful in diagnosing the extent of myocardial damage and if reversible or irreversible damage has occurred [15]. The most commonly assayed cardiac proteins include troponins, creatine kinase, myoglobin and lactate dehydrogenase. The timing, initial rise and peak levels of these cardiac proteins are shown in Table 6.1.

Cardiac troponin serum levels (TnT and TnI) are the most sensitive and specific markers of myocardial damage as they are found in higher abundance in heart muscle than other cardiac enzymes and, therefore, have a higher detectable concentration in serum following cardiac injury [16]. Serum levels rise within 3–12 hours from the onset of chest pain and peak at 24 hours before normalising by days 3–10. Peak values correlate with the extent of cardiac injury. It is important to note that a rise and/or fall in the troponin level over a fixed period of time is one of the criteria for the diagnosis of an acute myocardial infarction. A level greater than the 99th percentile value for the immunoassay is regarded as a positive result [17]. Although the troponins are specific for cardiac damage, there are variations in the sensitivity

Table 6.1 Presence of cardiac markers in blood

Marker	Initial rise	Peak	Return to normal
Troponin	3–12 h	3–10 days	3–10 days
Creatine kinase	4–8 h	18 h	2–3 days
Myoglobin	1–4 h	6–7 h	24 h
Lactate dehydrogenase	10 h	14 days	14 days

and specificity of the immunoassay used in the detection of troponin levels, and therefore local guidelines should be consulted prior to interpretation [18, 19]. The main reasons for this variation are a lack of standardisation, differences in antibody cross-reactivity to skeletal muscle and degradation products of TnI, and the presence of modified TnI and TnT which interferes with true assay values [20, 21]. Creatine kinase comprises three isoenzymes: CK-MM (found mainly in skeletal muscle), CK-BB (found mainly in brain) and CK-MB (found mainly in the heart). Most assays measure CK-MB mass, as it avoids the detection of macrokinases (CK linked to IgG and dimers of mitochondrial CK), which can interfere with enzyme activity assays [22]. A rise in CK-MB is relatively specific for cardiac muscle injury; however, because CK-MB can be released from skeletal muscle, it can lead to falsely elevated levels in chronic skeletal muscle diseases such as that seen in dermatomyositis and polymyositis, and therefore troponins are the preferred cardiac biomarker in acute coronary syndrome [23, 24].

Myoglobin is a small heme protein, which is released from damaged tissue. It lacks specificity for heart muscle and is falsely elevated after injury to other tissues and therefore is not used in the diagnosis of acute coronary syndrome [25]. Similarly as lactate dehydrogenase lacks specificity when compared to cardiac troponins, it is not routinely used in diagnosing cardiac disease [26].

6.2.2 Heart Failure and Brain Natriuretic Peptide

Brain natriuretic peptide (BNP), a cleavage product of the prohormone pro-BNP, is a hormone released predominantly from the heart and is closely related to left ventricular heart pressures. It is particularly useful in diagnosing heart failure where there is considerable myocardial stretch, and increased plasma BNP concentrations can be detected in both symptomatic and asymptomatic left ventricular heart failure patients [27]. In normal healthy individuals, the plasma concentration of BNP is approximately 10 pg L^{-1}. Immunoassays used in the measurement of BNP have a standard 'cut-off' value of >100 ng L^{-1} for a diagnosis of heart failure; however, values vary according to gender, body mass index (BMI) and age. A BNP of <50 ng L^{-1} can be used to rule out heart failure with a negative predictive value of 96% [28].

N-terminal pro-BNP (NT-proBNP), another cleavage product from the prohormone pro-BNP, can also be used in diagnosing heart failure. Of note, NT-proBNP is secreted in left ventricular heart failure in higher concentrations when compared to plasma BNP [29]. In immunoassays, a NT-proBNP level >900 pg L^{-1} has similar accuracy to the plasma BNP level of >100 ng L^{-1}; however, higher levels are detected in women, older individuals and those with renal failure.

Although both plasma BNP and NT-proBNP levels can be used in the diagnosis of heart failure, clinically, commercial immunoassays detect each hormone level in addition to the degradation product of proBNP and the respective hormone. Given the assay variation and impact of other clinical conditions, the use of serial BNPs is more informative in the management of patients with heart failure.

6.2.3 Serum Lipids and Lipoproteins

Serum lipids are carried to tissue in the form of lipoproteins for energy utilisation. There are five major classes of lipoproteins circulating in blood: chylomicrons, very-low-density lipoprotein (VLDL, carries mainly triglyceride), intermediate density lipoprotein (IDL), low-density lipoprotein (LDL, carries mainly cholesterol) and high-density lipoprotein (HDL, carries mainly phospholipid). Measurement of individual lipid profiles is of paramount importance in the management of a number of clinical conditions, including cardiovascular and cerebrovascular disease, diabetes mellitus and those with lipid abnormalities. Standard serum lipid profiling uses apolipoprotein immunoassays to measure the concentration of total, VLDL and HDL cholesterol. Apolipoproteins, which make up the protein fraction of the lipoproteins, consist of different variants specifically associated with the five lipoprotein classes. Elevated plasma levels of apolipoprotein B-100, predominantly found in low-density and very-low-density lipoprotein, are clinically relevant and are measured with immunoassay-based tests [30]. Clinical immunoassays are also used for the measurement of a modified form of LDL called lipoprotein (a) in serum to assess the risk of developing cardiovascular disease. However, size polymorphism of the lipoproteins leads to a large variation in immunoassay conformity and the use of reference reagents is therefore internationally recommended [31].

6.3 Respiratory Disease

6.3.1 Bacterial Respiratory Infections

Pneumonia is an inflammatory condition of the lung, which causes serious morbidity and mortality worldwide. The laboratory investigation of pneumonia includes microscopy, culture, bacterial identification, antibiotic susceptibility, serology and molecular techniques [32]. Sputum sampling is a quick and efficient way to culture specific strains of bacteria and is a non-invasive and relatively low-cost technique. However, it has a low sensitivity (35–60%), with high variability between readers. In addition, about 30–40% of community-acquired pneumonia patients do not produce sputum and hence identifying the infective bacterial strain is more problematic.

Certain bacterial antigens such as the pneumococcal and legionella can be detected through urine analysis and offer another non-invasive and simple test to identify specific infections [33]. Testing for bacterial urinary antigens is more sensitive and specific than use of the Gram stain and culture of sputum as commonly performed by most labs. The results are immediately available and remain valid even after the initiation of antibiotic therapy. Immunoassays used in the identification of some of the main bacterial pneumonia infections are discussed below.

6.3.1.1 *Streptococcus pneumonia*

Streptococcus pneumonia, commonly known as *pneumococcus*, is the most common cause of community-acquired pneumonia and is responsible for most respiratory infections requiring hospitalisation. Pneumococcal cell wall components can be detected in various bodily fluids, including blood, sputum and urine. The pneumococcal urinary antigen can be detected using immunochromatographic urinary assays with sensitivities of 70–90% and specificities of 80–100% [34]. The American Thoracic Society recommends the use of the pneumococcal antigen in patients who have failed outpatient antibiotic treatment, who require intensive care, have a history of alcohol abuse, a low white cell count, asplenia and in those who have a pleural effusion. Several serotypes, including 3, 6A, 6B, 9N and 19F, are associated with a poorer patient outcome. As pneumococcal resistance is increasing in incidence worldwide, identifying resistant strains using rapid detection methods will become a priority in the treatment of this disease.

6.3.1.2 Legionella species

Legionella is a common cause of both community- and hospital-acquired pneumonia. It is better known as Legionnaires' disease, which manifests as 'flu-like' symptoms preceding a dry cough and is of particular importance in immunocompromised patients, where the infection is most severe. Legionnaires' disease is often diagnosed by determining the *Legionella pneumophila* urinary antigen rather than by direct fluorescent antibody (DFA) staining or culture [35]. The urinary antigen test is an **enzyme immunoassay** with high specificity of >99% and sensitivity of 70–80% for Legionnaires' disease. One of the main disadvantages of this test is that it is only useful for the diagnosis of the *Legionella pneumophila* group 1 serogroup. Nonetheless, this serogroup accounts for 80% of Legionnaires' disease acquired in the community.

6.3.1.3 *Mycoplasma pneumonia*

Mycoplasmas are the smallest free-living organisms. *Mycoplasma pneumonia* commonly causes upper respiratory tract infections; however, it is also a common cause of pneumonia. *M. pneumonia* is commonly detected through IgM and IgG-based serological assays [33]. Antibody titers begin to rise approximately seven to nine days after infection and peak at three to four weeks. Enzyme immunoassay (EIA) techniques have been used with a sensitivity of 97.8% and specificity of 99.7%. A positive EIA result is best determined by comparing acute and convalescent phase sera two to three weeks apart. In general, a four-fold or greater increase in the titer of paired sera is indicative of infection. Novel antigen immunoassays have been developed and are best used for detection of *M. pneumoniae* in respiratory secretions; however, they have been largely replaced by polymerase chain reaction-based testing [36].

6.3.1.4 *Haemophilus influenzae*

Haemophilus influenzae is a gram negative bacteria which has both encapsulated and non-encapsulated forms. The most important serotype is *H. influenzae* serotype b (Hib), which was a frequent cause of bacterial meningitis prior to the introduction of the Hib conjugate vaccines in children. Clinical diagnosis of *H. influenza* is typically performed by bacterial culture, polymerase chain reaction (PCR) or **antibody-based latex particle agglutination test (LAT)** [37]. The LAT is a more sensitive method to detect *H. influenzae* than culture as this method relies on antigen rather than viable bacteria and, therefore, the results are not affected by prior antibiotic use.

6.3.1.5 *Chlamydia pneumonia*

Chlamydia pneumonia is an obligate intracellular bacterium, which has a complex growth-cycle involving elementary bodies (EB) and reticulate bodies (RB). Bacterial multiplication occurs in the intracellular RB phase and reverts to the infectious EB, which survives in the environment. Serological tests for *C. pneumonia* lack both the sensitivity and specificity for the organism as a positive serologic result can indicate either current or past infection. **Direct antigen testing (DAT)** and the polymerase chain reaction (PCR) appear to be the most promising advances for the diagnosis of *C. pneumonia* pneumonia [38].

6.3.2 Fungal Respiratory Infections

6.3.2.1 Aspergillus

Allergic bronchopulmonary aspergillosis (ABPA) results from a hypersensitivity reaction in the lung to the fungus *Aspergillus fumigatus*. In the early stages, the allergic response causes bronchoconstriction, which over time can lead to debilitating lung conditions such as bronchiectasis and fibrosis. The diagnosis of ABPA is based on a number of major diagnostic features including a history of asthma, lung infiltrates on chest x-ray, skin test reactivity to the aspergillus antigen, a raised eosinophil count and a host of different immunoassay-based tests. These immunoassays include measuring the precipitating antibodies to *A. fumigatus*, a raised serum IgE concentration and elevated specific serum IgE and IgG antibodies [39]. Initial evaluation involves a skin prick test for ABPA. If this test is deemed positive, serum IgE and precipitins to aspergillus are assayed. A serum IgE concentration of >1000 ng mL^{-1} together with a positive precipitins test and antibodies to *Aspergillus fumigatus* (IgE and IgG) would indicate a likely diagnosis of ABPA.

6.3.3 Viral Respiratory Infections

6.3.3.1 Influenza A and B

Influenza is a major cause of respiratory illness worldwide and is the most common viral cause of community-acquired pneumonia. Influenza viruses circulating in animals pose a major threat to human health, as seen in recent years with the H1N1 influenza A (swine flu) infection which was a declared a public health emergency of international concern by the World Health Organisation (WHO) in 2009. Diagnostic assays for the detection of influenza are discussed in Chapter 7 of this book.

6.3.4 Cystic Fibrosis

Cystic fibrosis (CF) is one of the commonest life-threatening autosomal recessive conditions primarily affecting Caucasian populations. It is caused by a mutation in the cystic fibrosis transmembrane conductance regulator (CFTR) gene on chromosome 7, which results in the expression of a dysfunctional chloride channel in exocrine tissue. This defect leads to abnormal transport of chloride and sodium across the epithelium leading to the formation of thick viscous secretions affecting the lung, pancreas, liver, intestine and the reproductive tract. Ultimately it is progressive lung disease, which is the major cause of morbidity and mortality in CF patients, as increased viscous secretions in the lung promote bacterial colonisation [40]. Diagnosis of CF is based on both biochemical and genetic testing. The sweat chloride test is the mainstay of laboratory confirmation. This test is performed using pilocarpine iontophoresis followed by chemical analysis of the secretions. A chloride concentration >60 mmol L^{-1} is required for a diagnosis of CF. A small quantity of a dried blood sample is now routinely used in screening newborns for CF and can identify approximately 95% of CF cases. This test is based on the detection of elevated immunoreactive trypsin (IRT) levels and can be quantified by either **radioimmunoassay** or by an **enzyme-linked immunoassay** [41].

6.3.5 Pulmonary Embolism and D-Dimers

Pulmonary embolism (PE) is a blood clot in one or more arteries in the lungs and usually arises from a venous thrombosis in the pelvis or legs. D-dimers, the degradation products of thrombi, can be used as an aid in the diagnosis of a PE. Although D-dimers have good sensitivity and negative predictive value, they have a poor specificity and positive predictive value. An elevated D-dimer level is not diagnostic of a PE as D-dimers are also increased in patients with renal failure, malignancy, and in those who have undergone recent surgery and hospitalisation. Multiple immunoassays have been developed to measure D-dimers including rapid ELISA methods [42].

A D-dimer level >500 ng mL^{-1} is taken to be significant; however, it is important that the patient's risks factors for thrombus formation, i.e. the pretest probability, are determined prior to interpretation of D-dimer values. While multiple assays are used in the measurement of D-Dimer levels, the evidence indicates that a D-dimer level <500 ng mL^{-1} by quantitative ELISA or semi-quantitative latex agglutination can exclude a PE in patients with a low to moderate risk of PE [42].

6.4 Endocrinology

6.4.1 Type 1 Diabetes Mellitus

Type 1 diabetes mellitus (DM) is an autoimmune disease where autoimmune destruction of insulin-secreting beta cells occurs in the pancreas. As a result, insulin production is negated preventing normal glucose homeostasis. Patients with type 1 DM require exogenous insulin for glucose maintenance and are at risk of diabetic ketoacidosis, a serious medical emergency requiring prompt treatment. No single test is available for diagnosing type 1 DM, although the presence of serum islet-specific autoantibodies, glutamic acid decarboxylase (GAD), insulinoma-associated protein 2 (IA2), the zinc transporter ZnT8 and insulin autoantibodies can be found in 85% of patients with type 1 DM [43]. Interestingly, these autoantibodies can be detected during the preclinical stage, thereby enabling surveillance of 'at-risk' patients [44]. Novel highly sensitive immunoassays have been developed which can detect insulin-specific DM-associated antibodies; nevertheless, their absence does not rule out a diagnosis of type 1 DM [45]. Research is currently under way to identify a panel of **autoantigens**, which may play an important role in the initiation, and progression of this autoimmune disease.

6.4.2 Thyroid Disease

Thyroid hormone abnormalities are usually due to thyroid gland dysfunction. Thyroid-stimulating hormone (TSH) stimulates the release of thyroxine (T4) and triiodothyronine (T3) from the thyroid gland, which exerts a negative feedback on TSH production. In hyperthyroidism, serum concentrations of TSH are low, while T4 and T3 are elevated. Conversely in hypothyroidism, serum concentrations of TSH are high, while T4 and T3 are low. Thyroid function is assessed by measuring the serum concentrations of TSH, total T4, total T3 and free T4 or T3. The normal range for TSH is 0.4 to 5 mU L^{-1}. Current methods used to measure TSH include chemiluminometric assays, which have very low detection limits (0.01 U L^{-1}) and can diagnose the mildest forms of hyperthyroidism [46]. Serum total T4 and T3 are usually measured by radioimmunoassay (RIA) or chemiluminometric assay, measuring both the bound and unbound T4 to the carrier protein thyroxine binding globulin (TBG). The unbound or free T4 or T3 is more useful in the interpretation of thyroid disease as TBG levels are altered in various conditions including pregnancy, drug use, hepatitis and malnutrition [47]. Autoimmunity also plays a major role in hypo- and hyperthyroidism and can be detected using immunoassays [48]. Anti-thyroglobulin autoantibodies are present in 60% of cases in a hypothyroid condition known as Hashimoto's thyroiditis, while anti-microsomal antibodies are present in 90%. In Graves' disease, thyroid stimulating hormone receptor antibodies (TSHR-Abs) stimulate the release of T4 and T3 leading to a hyperthyroid condition known as Graves' thyrotoxicosis. Almost all patients with Graves' disease have detectable TSHR-Abs, which can be measured using immunoassays; however, lower concentrations of both anti-thyroglobulin and anti-microsomal antibodies can also found in Graves' disease.

6.4.3 Adrenal Hormone and Cushing's Syndrome

The adrenal cortex produces a number of important steroids involved in cell metabolism. The secretion of cortisol is dependent on the release of adrenocorticotropic hormone (ACTH) from the pituitary gland, which stimulates cortisol and androgen production in the adrenal cortex and negatively regulates ACTH production. In a hormone disorder known as Cushing's syndrome, there is sustained over-production of cortisol with loss of the normal cortisol circadian rhythm. Excess cortisol leads to a change in body habitus (weight gain, 'moon faces' and 'buffalo hump'), susceptibility to recurrent infections and a host of other bone, skin and gonadal problems. The most common cause of excess cortisol is the ingestion of prescribed steroids. Other causes of Cushing's syndrome include an adrenal tumour, hypersecretion of ACTH from a pituitary tumour (Cushing's disease) or ectopic production of ACTH from a cancer.

Cortisol production can be assessed by measurement of cortisol in serum, urine or saliva. A variety of different immunoassays are used to measure cortisol, including **fluorometric assays, radio-**

receptor assays, radioimmunoassays and **high-performance liquid chromatography** (HPLC) or **mass spectrometry**. Of all assays used in the measurement of cortisol, HPLC, mass spectrometry or a combination of the two remain superior due to their high specificity for the cortisol molecule. Urinary cortisol measured over a 24-hour period provides an integrated measure of the serum free cortisol concentration [7].

First line tests used in the diagnosis of Cushing's syndrome include measuring urinary and salivary cortisol and performing a low dose dexamethasone suppression test. As excess cortisol leads to the production of lower ACTH levels and, hence, lower cortisol secretion from the adrenals, the ingestion of dexamethasone, a potent glucocorticoid, in suppression tests should produce a similar result if the patient has Cushing's syndrome. In the dexamethasone suppression test, patients take 1.0 mg of dexamethasone overnight and their serum cortisol is measured at 8 a.m. the following day [49]. The 2008 Endocrine Society guidelines suggest that a serum cortisol of $>$1.8 mcg dL^{-1} (50 nmol L^{-1}) should be used to diagnose Cushing's syndrome in the low dose dexamethasone suppression test, but, if patients fail to take the required steroid dose or if there is abnormal metabolism of the drug, significant error can occur in interpretation of the results.

Once a diagnosis of Cushing's syndrome is made, the next step involves localising a cause for the excess cortisol production. A high dose dexamethasone 48-hour suppression test is used to distinguish Cushing's disease from patients with ectopic sources of ACTH from secreting tumours [50]. In the 48-hour test patients take 0.5 mg of dexamethasone every 6 hours for 8 doses and bloods samples are taken 2–6 hours after the last dose. Urinary cortisol excretion should be $<$10 mcg per 24 hours on the second day and serum cortisol should be $<$5 mcg dL^{-1}.

6.5 Rheumatology

6.5.1 Rheumatoid Arthritis

Rheumatoid arthritis (RA) is a chronic symmetric inflammatory polyarthritis, typically affecting small joints; however, soft tissues and extra-articular structures are also involved in the inflammatory response. The diagnosis of RA is primarily based on the history and examination but a number of laboratory tests can help diagnose the condition [51].

Rheumatoid factors (RF) and anti-cyclic citrullinated peptide (aCCP) antibodies are the main markers used in the detection of RA. Rheumatoid factors are antibodies specific to the Fc portion of the IgG and are found to be positive in 75–80% of patients with RA [52]. However, most increased levels of RF are due to active inflammation (e.g. malaria, rubella, hepatitis C) or other chronic inflammatory conditions (e.g. Sjögren's syndrome, systemic lupus erythematosus). The detection of a high titer of RF IgM in a patient with a chronic inflammatory polyarthritis is highly suggestive of RA. In addition, RF can be used to assess disease severity and response to therapy [53]. Seropositive RA patients are more likely to have more aggressive disease and extra-articular manifestations.

Antibodies to anti-cyclic citrullinated peptide (aCCP) have a high specificity for RA and are particularly useful in patients who are seronegative for RF [54]. Standardised enzyme-linked immunosorbent assays (ELISA) are used in the detection of antibodies to CCP. In this test, arginine residues are replaced by citrulline in a mixture of CCP, which increases the sensitivity of the assay [55]. ACCP measurement can also be used to assess response to therapy, with lower titers present in patients with resolving inflammatory phases of arthritis.

6.5.2 Systemic Lupus Erythematosus

Systemic lupus erythematosus (SLE) is a chronic inflammatory multisystem disease characterised by periods of relapses and remissions. The clinical diagnosis is based on specific symptoms and signs associated with SLE in addition to a number of laboratory investigations. Routine inflammatory markers, positive tests for the antinuclear antibodies (ANA), antibodies to double stranded DNA (dsDNA) and the Smith (Sm) antigen are highly suggestive of SLE [56]. In addition to the clinical history and examination, several different serological markers are used to assess disease severity. In the active stage of SLE there is an initial rise in IgG dsDNA titers and a fall in complement factors such as CH50, C3 and C4, while persistently low levels of C1q are associated with marked renal pathology. More recently, antibodies to C1q and nucleosomes are being investigated as potential serological markers of disease severity and organ involvement in SLE. Although, these markers can be useful in monitoring the disease, it is important to note that not all patients with these markers have active SLE [57].

6.5.3 Systemic Sclerosis

Systemic sclerosis is a multisystem connective tissue disorder and is characterised by thickening and fibrosis of the skin (scleroderma). There are two disease patterns comprising diffuse cutaneous systemic sclerosis (dcSS) and limited cutaneous systemic sclerosis (lcSS) based on the extent of skin involvement. In dcSS, sclerotic skin is seen on the trunk and proximal limbs as well as face and distal limbs and is associated with a worse prognosis. In lcSS, scleroderma is restricted to the face, neck and limbs distal to the elbow and knee and generally has a better prognosis when compared to dcSS. Many patients with lcSS have the CREST syndrome, which is an acronym for calcinosis, Raynaud's disease, esophageal dysmotility, sclerodactyly and telangiectasia.

More than 95% of patients with systemic sclerosis have at least one detectable **autoantibody** [58]. Serological tests useful in confirming a diagnosis of systemic sclerosis includes antinuclear antibody (ANA) and specific tests for anti-topoisomerase I (anti-Scl-70), anti-centromere, anti-RNA polymerase III, and anti-beta2-glycoprotein I antibodies.

6.5.4 Sjögren's Syndrome

Sjögren's syndrome (SS) is a chronic inflammatory condition characterised by lymphocytic infiltration of exocrine glands. Decreased exocrine gland function can lead to dry eyes (keratoconjuctivitis) and dry mouth (xerostomia), i.e. the sicca complex. It is classified as either primary SS, which is not associated with other diseases, or secondary SS, commonly associated with rheumatological disease [59]. Antibodies to Ro or La antigens can be detected in primary

SS and the presence of anti-Ro is used as one of the criteria in diagnosing the disease. Most laboratories utilise solid phase assays including ELISA or antigen-coated fluorescent microspheres and flow cytometry-based assays to detect anti-Ro or anti-La [60]. The anti-Ro comprises of antibodies directed against Ro60 and Ro52, which are relatively specific for Sjögren's syndrome, are also found to a lesser degree in SLE and RA.

6.5.5 Vasculitis

Vasculitis is defined as an inflammatory disorder of blood vessels. It is classified according to the size of the vessel involved and the pattern of organ involvement. The presentation of vasculitis depends on the organs affected; however, many serological tests can be used as an aid in the diagnosis of vasculitis [61]. The detection of anti-nuclear antibody (ANA) indicates an underlying inflammatory process while anti-neutrophil cytoplasmic antibodies (ANCA), directed against proteinase 3 and myeloperoxidase is suggestive of small vessel vasculitis. ELISAs and indirect immunofluorescence assays are the current methods of detection of ANCA. The ELISA has a higher specificity but the preferred method is the indirect immunofluorescence assay, which has a higher sensitivity. Of note, it is important to emphasise that ANCA assays are not standardised and hence their sensitivity and specificity varies in different clinical settings.

6.5.6 Dermatomyositis and Polymyositis

Dermatomyositis (DM) and polymyositis (PM) are idiopathic inflammatory disorders of skeletal muscle. Although both inflammatory conditions share the same clinical feature of muscle weakness, dermatomyositis is also associated with cutaneous lesions. A muscle biopsy is the definitive test for establishing a diagnosis of inflammatory myositis. A variety of autoantibodies detected by immunoassay in patient sera are associated with the disease. Anti-nuclear antibodies (ANA) are present in over 80% of patients with DM and PM [62]. The detection of anti-Ro, anti-La, anti-Sm, anti-ribonucleoprotein (RNP) and anti-TIF1 antibodies are highly suggestive of an inflammatory muscle condition; however, these antibodies also overlap with other connective tissue diseases and an associated diagnosis of cancer [63, 64]. Cytoplasmic RNA synthetases and other cytoplasmic proteins, including ribonucleoproteins are known as myositis-specific autoantibodies and are found in 30% of patients with DM and PM. Anti-Jo-1 antibodies are the most common type of myositis-specific autoantibody and are associated with interstitial lung disease, Raynaud's phenomenon and arthritis [65]. Anti-SRP antibodies, primarily found in PM, are associated with a more severe myopathy with aggressive disease. In addition to autoantibodies, muscle enzyme analysis is important in diagnosing myopathy. Creatine kinase, lactate dehydrogenase, aldolase and the liver enzymes, aspartate aminotransferase and alanine aminotransferase are routinely measured with immunoassay. Muscle weakness with normal enzyme levels is more commonly seen in DM when compared to PM.

6.6 Oncology

Immunoassays for the detection of markers associated with cancer are common practice in oncology [66]. Tumour markers are frequently used for monitoring of disease and planning of treatment and to a lesser degree for diagnostic purposes. In this section, we will review clinically established tumour markers and the corresponding immunoassay tests.

6.6.1 Alpha-Fetoprotein

Alpha-fetoprotein (AFP) is a glycoprotein normally produced by the foetal liver; however, it is often elevated in the sera of patients with hepatocellular carcinoma (HCC), germ cell tumours and seminomas. Patients with serum levels greater than 500 ng mL^{-1} are considered high-risk for HCC, but, AFP levels may be normal in patients with small tumours ($\leq$3 cm). Normal AFP levels are set between 10 and

20 ng mL^{-1}, whereas intermediate serum concentrations indicate benign liver disease [67].

HCC arises in approximately 20% of patients with liver disease. Serum AFP levels greater than 20 ng mL^{-1} in immunoassays have a specificity and sensitivity of 80–94% and 41–65%, respectively, for the diagnosis of HCC. The negative predictive value of the test is at 98%; however, the positive predictive value is low at only 25% [68]. AFP immunoassays are also used as a prognostic biomarker for patients undergoing liver transplantation, in predicting recurrence of disease when AFP levels are $>$1000 ng mL^{-1} and for staging of testicular cancer germ cell tumours [69].

6.6.2 Prostate-Specific Antigen

Prostate-specific antigen (PSA) is a glycoprotein expressed in normal and neoplastic prostate tissue. PSA can 'leak' into blood due to the disruptions of the normal prostate gland architecture typically found in prostate cancer. Elevated levels of PSA in serum are indicative of prostate cancer; however, they can be also found in healthy men reflecting prostate size and age and ethnic background [70, 71]. PSA values of 4.0 ng mL^{-1} detect 21% of all prostate cancers and 51% of high-grade prostate cancers with an estimated specificity of 91% [72].

Although serum PSA is a validated marker in prostate cancer, tests are currently being developed to increase the sensitivity and specificity of PSA in immunoassays. Novel strategies to improve the accuracy of traditional tests were recently devised including serial PSA analysis, assessment of the accelerated rise of PSA levels in aging men with the cancer versus healthy aging men, and measurement of PSA levels in relation to the size of prostate gland size [73]. However, there is also a keen interest in developing novel immunoassays based on a better understanding of the molecular insights of PSA. Methods measuring free and bound PSA circulating in blood; complex PSA, which is bound to alpha-1-antichymotripsin; circulating fragments of the PSA precursor, specifically the (-2) proPSA isoform; and glycosylated isoforms of the antigen. For an extensive review PSA detection methods and novel developments please refer to Gilgunn et al. [74].

6.6.3 Carbohydrate Antigens

6.6.3.1 CA 125

CA 125 is a glycoprotein antigen elevated in serum of women with ovarian cancer [75]. Serum concentrations of $\geq$30 U mL^{-1} are predictive of increased ovarian cancer risk in asymptomatic postmenopausal women. Elevated CA 125 levels can be found in approximately half of women with early stage ovarian cancer and more often in advanced disease [76]. The specificity of the marker, however, is quite low and elevated serum levels can be found in 1% of healthy women but are also found in malignancies of the ovary, uterus, breast and in benign conditions, including endometriosis. Nonetheless, CA 125 immunoassays are commonly used for ovarian cancer screening and the validity of the marker is increased in serialised serum measurements [77].

6.6.3.2 CA 15-3 and CA 27-29

CA 15-3 and CA 27-29 are products of the MUC-1 gene and are both raised in breast cancer. The corresponding immunoassays are well characterised; however, the recent ASCO guidelines recommend both markers solely for monitoring selected patients with metastatic breast cancer [78].

6.6.3.3 CA 19-9

CA 19-9 is a carbohydrate antigen raised in pancreatic carcinoma, cholangiocarcinoma, hepatocellular cancer and to a lesser extent in colorectal, gastric and other cancers. CA 19-9 serum levels >37 U mL^{-1} have an overall sensitivity and specificity of approximately 80% and 90% in patents with pancreatic cancer [79]. In addition, combination immunoassays with the CA 125 marker are frequently used to differentiate between the clinically similar pancreatic carcinomas and pancreatic inflammation [80].

6.6.4 Carcinoembryonic Antigen

Carcinoembryonic antigen (CEA) is a glycoprotein normally expressed during foetal development. Although suppressed in adulthood, it can be re-expressed in certain cancers and secreted into circulation. Elevated serum CEA levels can be found in colorectal cancer, medullary thyroid cancer, cholangiocarcinomas and breast cancer [81]. However, CEA can also be elevated due to cigarette smoking and in other benign disorders such as gastritis, liver disease and diabetes. Due to its lack of specificity, CEA in not recommended as a diagnostic marker [82]; however, it is the only marker test routinely used for colorectal cancer surveillance and for predicting poorer prognosis at preoperative levels of above 5 ng mL^{-1} [83].

6.6.5 Beta-Human Chorionic Gonadotrophin

Human chorionic gonadotrophin (HCG) is produced by trophoblasts and secreted into the blood of patients with testicular cancer germ cell tumours. HCG is a dimer of a unique 145 amino acid beta-subunit and 92 amino acid alpha unit, which is also found in other pituitary hormones [73]. Clinical immunoassays target the unique beta unit and its isoforms, usually using two antibodies, one capture antibody and lanthanide or radioactively labelled antibody for immunometric analysis [84]. Elevated beta-HCG serum levels are found in 80–85% patients with non-seminomatous germ cell tumours and in 25% of patients with seminomas. Beta-HCG levels in these patients are approximately 20% above the normal levels of 5 to 10 IU L^{-1}. The assays are exceptionally sensitive (100%) and very specific with very rare false positive results [85]. Beta-HCG may be used in support of a testicular cancer diagnosis; however, its main benefit lies in staging of the disease [69].

6.6.6 Antibody-Associated Paraneoplastic Disease

Paraneoplastic disorders are rare, non-metastatic manifestations of tumours associated with serum antibodies specific to aberrantly expressed tumour antigens, which are normally expressed only by the nervous system [86]. Importantly, paraneoplastic disease can manifest prior to the onset of malignancy, thereby enabling the detection of occult tumours based on neurological symptoms and paraneoplastic antibodies [87]. Patients positive for ANNA-1 and CRMP-5 predominantly develop small cell lung cancer (SCLC) and thymomas; PCA-1 antibodies may predate breast, ovary and uterus cancers; PCA-2 and ANNA-3 antibodies may predate SCLC and non-small cell lung cancer (NSCLC); amphiphysin antibodies may predate SCLC and breast cancer and ANNA-2 antibodies may predate SCLC, NSCLC and breast cancer [88]. Research is currently underway to detect novel panels of autoantigens, which may play an important role as diagnostic markers in cancer [89, 90].

6.7 Conclusion

Immunoassays are indispensable in the clinical setting facilitating detection, monitoring and confirmation of many different disease processes. Limits of detection, sensitivity and specificity of disease markers must be validated in quality controlled laboratory centres to ensure reliable interpretation of results. Although such antibody-based laboratory tests are routinely used across all disease areas as described in this chapter, they often need to be interpreted in conjunction with patient history and clinical examination.

The global drive to identify novel markers, poses many challenges for immunoassay development, with the greatest potential in identifying disease through minimally invasive techniques. With more and more pressures being placed on secondary and tertiary referral centres, the primary care setting is becoming an attractive alternative for the implementation of point-of-care and miniaturised devices. A vast array of nano- and micro- technologies are currently being developed which utilise minimal amounts of patient sample and have the potential to be used at primary care level. With the advancement of bioanalytical methods and biomarker discovery, novel disease-associated molecular biomarkers will fuel the development of highly innovative sensitive immunoassays, identifying at risk patients in a more efficient and cost-effective manner.

References

1. Mattix, H.J., et al., Use of the albumin/creatinine ratio to detect microalbuminuria: implications of sex and race. *J Am Soc Nephrol*, 2002. **13**(4):1034–1039.
2. Bradwell, A.R., et al., Serum test for assessment of patients with Bence Jones myeloma. *Lancet*, 2003. **361**(9356):489–491.

3. Moeller, K.E., K.C. Lee, and J.C. Kissack, Urine drug screening: practical guide for clinicians. *Mayo Clin Proc*, 2008. **83**(1):66–76.
4. Montagnana, M., et al., Human chorionic gonadotropin in pregnancy diagnostics. *Clin Chim Acta*, 2011. **412**(17–18):1515–1520.
5. Binnicker, M.J., et al., Comparison of four assays for the detection of cryptococcal antigen. *Clin Vaccine Immunol*, 2012. **19**(12):1988–1990.
6. Jorgensen, F.S., et al., Alpha-fetoprotein and acetylcholinesterase activity in first- and early second-trimester amniotic fluid. *Prenat Diagn*, 1995. **15**(7):621–625.
7. Raff, H., P.J. Homar, and E.A. Burns, Comparison of two methods for measuring salivary cortisol. *Clin Chem*, 2002. **48**(1):207–208.
8. Malamud, D., Oral diagnostic testing for detecting human immunodeficiency virus-1 antibodies: a technology whose time has come. *Am J Med*, 1997. **102**(4A):9–14.
9. White, D.A., A.N. Scribner, and J.V. Huang, A comparison of patient acceptance of fingerstick whole blood and oral fluid rapid HIV screening in an emergency department. *J Acquir Immune Defic Syndr*, 2009. **52**(1):75–78.
10. The Immunoassay Handbook. Theory and applications of ligand binding, ELISA and related techniques, ed. D. Wild. 2013: Elsevier.
11. Glynn, M., et al., Centrifugo-magnetophoretic purification of CD4+ cells from whole blood towards future HIV/AIDS point-of-care applications. *J Lab Autom*, 2014. **19**(3):285–296.
12. Song, Y., et al., Point-of-care technologies for molecular diagnostics using a drop of blood. *Trends Biotechnol*, 2014. **32**(3):132–139.
13. Horowitz, G.L., Estimating reference intervals. *Am J Clin Pathol*, 2010. **133**(2):175–177.
14. Katayev, A., C. Balciza, and D.W. Seccombe, Establishing reference intervals for clinical laboratory test results: is there a better way? *Am J Clin Pathol*, 2010. **133**(2):180–186.
15. Jaffe, A.S., et al., It's time for a change to a troponin standard. *Circulation*, 2000. **102**(11):1216–1220.
16. White, H.D., Higher sensitivity troponin levels in the community: what do they mean and how will the diagnosis of myocardial infarction be made? *Am Heart J*, 2010. **159**(6):933–936.
17. Apple, F.S., et al., Plasma 99th percentile reference limits for cardiac troponin and creatine kinase MB mass for use with European Society of Cardiology/American College of Cardiology consensus recommendations. *Clin Chem*, 2003. **49**(8):1331–1336.

18. Ricchiuti, V., et al., Cardiac troponin T isoforms expressed in renal diseased skeletal muscle will not cause false-positive results by the second generation cardiac troponin T assay by Boehringer Mannheim. *Clin Chem*, 1998. **44**(9):1919–1924.
19. Heeschen, C., et al., Evaluation of a rapid whole blood ELISA for quantification of troponin I in patients with acute chest pain. *Clin Chem*, 1999. **45**(10):1789–1796.
20. Labugger, R., et al., Extensive troponin I and T modification detected in serum from patients with acute myocardial infarction. *Circulation*, 2000. **102**(11):1221–1226.
21. Shi, Q., et al., Degradation of cardiac troponin I in serum complicates comparisons of cardiac troponin I assays. *Clin Chem*, 1999. **45**(7):1018–1025.
22. Bohlmeyer, T.J., A.H. Wu, and M.B. Perryman, Evaluation of laboratory tests as a guide to diagnosis and therapy of myositis. *Rheum Dis Clin North Am*, 1994. **20**(4):845–856.
23. Larca, L.J., J.T. Coppola, and S. Honig, Creatine kinase MB isoenzyme in dermatomyositis: a noncardiac source. *Ann Intern Med*, 1981. **94**(3):341–343.
24. Young, A., Plasma creatine kinase after the marathon–a diagnostic dilemma. *Br J Sports Med*, 1984. **18**(4):269–272.
25. Eggers, K.M., et al., Diagnostic value of serial measurement of cardiac markers in patients with chest pain: limited value of adding myoglobin to troponin I for exclusion of myocardial infarction. *Am Heart J*, 2004. **148**(4):574–581.
26. Thygesen, K., et al., Universal definition of myocardial infarction. *Eur Heart J*, 2007. **28**(20):2525–2538.
27. Iwanaga, Y., et al., B-type natriuretic peptide strongly reflects diastolic wall stress in patients with chronic heart failure: comparison between systolic and diastolic heart failure. *J Am Coll Cardiol*, 2006. **47**(4):742–748.
28. Maisel, A., et al., State of the art: using natriuretic peptide levels in clinical practice. *Eur J Heart Fail*, 2008. **10**(9):824–839.
29. Clerico, A., et al., Clinical relevance of biological variation: the lesson of brain natriuretic peptide (BNP) and NT-proBNP assay. *Clin Chem Lab Med*, 2006. **44**(4):366–378.
30. Rosseneu, M., et al., Some considerations of methodology and standardization of apolipoprotein B immunoassays. *Clin Chem*, 1983. **29**(3):427–433.

31. Dati, F., et al., First WHO/IFCC international reference reagent for lipoprotein(a) for immunoassay–Lp(a) SRM 2B. *Clin Chem Lab Med*, 2004. **42**(6):670–676.

32. Werno, A.M., and D.R. Murdoch, Medical microbiology: laboratory diagnosis of invasive pneumococcal disease. *Clin Infect Dis*, 2008. **46**(6):926–932.

33. Mandell, L.A., et al., Infectious Diseases Society of America/American Thoracic Society consensus guidelines on the management of community-acquired pneumonia in adults. *Clin Infect Dis*, 2007. **44**(Suppl 2): S27–72.

34. Smith, M.D., et al., Rapid diagnosis of bacteremic pneumococcal infections in adults by using the Binax NOW Streptococcus pneumoniae urinary antigen test: a prospective, controlled clinical evaluation. *J Clin Microbiol*, 2003. **41**(7):2810–2813.

35. Helbig, J.H., et al., Clinical utility of urinary antigen detection for diagnosis of community-acquired, travel-associated, and nosocomial Legionnaires' disease. *J Clin Microbiol*, 2003. **41**(2):838–840.

36. Daxboeck, F., R. Krause, and C. Wenisch, Laboratory diagnosis of Mycoplasma pneumoniae infection. *Clin Microbiol Infect*, 2003. **9**(4):263–273.

37. Singhi, S.C., et al., Evaluation of polymerase chain reaction (PCR) for diagnosing Haemophilus influenzae b meningitis. *Ann Trop Paediatr*, 2002. **22**(4):347–353.

38. Gaydos, C.A., et al., Diagnostic utility of PCR-enzyme immunoassay, culture, and serology for detection of Chlamydia pneumoniae in symptomatic and asymptomatic patients. *J Clin Microbiol*, 1994. **32**(4): 903–905.

39. Agarwal, R., Allergic bronchopulmonary aspergillosis. *Chest*, 2009. **135**(3):805–826.

40. Goss, C.H., and F. Ratjen, Update in cystic fibrosis 2012. *Am J Respir Crit Care Med*, 2013. **187**(9):915–919.

41. Wells, J., et al., A decision-tree approach to cost comparison of newborn screening strategies for cystic fibrosis. *Pediatrics*, 2012. **129**(2):e339–347.

42. Stein, P.D., et al., D-dimer for the exclusion of acute venous thrombosis and pulmonary embolism: a systematic review. *Ann Intern Med*, 2004. **140**(8):589–602.

43. Pietropaolo, M., and G.S. Eisenbarth, Autoantibodies in human diabetes. *Curr Dir Autoimmun*, 2001. **4**:252–282.

44. Verge, C.F., et al., Prediction of type I diabetes in first-degree relatives using a combination of insulin, GAD, and ICA512bdc/IA-2 autoantibodies. *Diabetes*, 1996. **45**(7):926–933.
45. Umehara, A., et al., A novel ultra-sensitive enzyme immunoassay for soluble human insulin receptor ectodomain and its measurement in urine from healthy subjects and patients with diabetes mellitus. *Clin Biochem*, 2009. **42**(13–14):1468–1475.
46. Ross, D.S., L.J. Ardisson, and M.J. Meskell, Measurement of thyrotropin in clinical and subclinical hyperthyroidism using a new chemiluminescent assay. *J Clin Endocrinol Metab*, 1989. **69**(3):684–688.
47. Ekins, R., The free hormone hypothesis and measurement of free hormones. *Clin Chem*, 1992. **38**(7):1289–1293.
48. Michalek, K., et al., TSH receptor autoantibodies. *Autoimmun Rev*, 2009. **9**(2):113–116.
49. Montwill, J., D. Igoe, and T.J. McKenna, The overnight dexamethasone test is the procedure of choice in screening for Cushing's syndrome. *Steroids*, 1994. **59**(5):296–298.
50. Streeten, D.H., et al., The diagnosis of hypercortisolism. Biochemical criteria differentiating patients from lean and obese normal subjects and from females on oral contraceptives. *J Clin Endocrinol Metab*, 1969. **29**(9):1191–1211.
51. Aletaha, D., et al., 2010 Rheumatoid arthritis classification criteria: an American College of Rheumatology/European League Against Rheumatism collaborative initiative. *Arthritis Rheum*, 2010. **62**(9):2569–2581.
52. Shmerling, R.H., and T.L. Delbanco, The rheumatoid factor: an analysis of clinical utility. *Am J Med*, 1991. **91**(5):528–534.
53. Eberhardt, K.B., et al., Disease activity and joint damage progression in early rheumatoid arthritis: relation to IgG, IgA, and IgM rheumatoid factor. *Ann Rheum Dis*, 1990. **49**(11):906–909.
54. Lee, D.M., and P.H. Schur, Clinical utility of the anti-CCP assay in patients with rheumatic diseases. *Ann Rheum Dis*, 2003. **62**(9):870–874.
55. Whiting, P.F., et al., Systematic review: accuracy of anti-citrullinated peptide antibodies for diagnosing rheumatoid arthritis. *Ann Intern Med*, 2010. **152**(7):456–464; W155–66.
56. Harley, J.B., Autoantibodies are central to the diagnosis and clinical manifestations of lupus. *J Rheumatol*, 1994. **21**(7):1183–1185.
57. Liu, C.C., S. Manzi, and J.M. Ahearn, Biomarkers for systemic lupus erythematosus: a review and perspective. *Curr Opin Rheumatol*, 2005. **17**(5):543–549.

58. Walker, J.G., and M.J. Fritzler, Update on autoantibodies in systemic sclerosis. *Curr Opin Rheumatol*, 2007. **19**(6):580–591.
59. Ramos-Casals, M., A.G. Tzioufas, and J. Font, Primary Sjogren's syndrome: new clinical and therapeutic concepts. *Ann Rheum Dis*, 2005. **64**(3):347–354.
60. Tan, E.M., et al., A critical evaluation of enzyme immunoassays for detection of antinuclear autoantibodies of defined specificities. I. Precision, sensitivity, and specificity. *Arthritis Rheum*, 1999. **42**(3):455–464.
61. Hagen, E.C., et al., Diagnostic value of standardized assays for anti-neutrophil cytoplasmic antibodies in idiopathic systemic vasculitis. EC/BCR Project for ANCA Assay Standardization. *Kidney Int*, 1998. **53**(3):743–753.
62. Drake, L.A., et al., Guidelines of care for dermatomyositis. American Academy of Dermatology. *J Am Acad Dermatol*, 1996. **34**(5 Pt 1):824–829.
63. Hector, S., et al., A reverse-ELISA for the detection of TRIM28/KAP1 serum autoantibodies in colorectal cancer patients. *Acta Oncol*, 2012. **51**(3):394–396.
64. Fiorentino, D., and L. Casciola-Rosen, Autoantibodies to transcription intermediary factor 1 in dermatomyositis shed insight into the cancer-myositis connection. *Arthritis Rheum*, 2012. **64**(2):346–349.
65. Love, L.A., et al., A new approach to the classification of idiopathic inflammatory myopathy: myositis-specific autoantibodies define useful homogeneous patient groups. *Medicine (Baltimore)*, 1991. **70**(6):360–374.
66. Perkins, G.L., et al., Serum tumor markers. *Am Fam Physician*, 2003. **68**(6):1075–1082.
67. Wu, J.T., Serum alpha-fetoprotein and its lectin reactivity in liver diseases: a review. *Ann Clin Lab Sci*, 1990. **20**(2):98–105.
68. Gupta, S., S. Bent, and J. Kohlwes, Test characteristics of alpha-fetoprotein for detecting hepatocellular carcinoma in patients with hepatitis C. A systematic review and critical analysis. *Ann Intern Med*, 2003. **139**(1):46–50.
69. Gilligan, T.D., et al., American Society of Clinical Oncology Clinical Practice Guideline on uses of serum tumor markers in adult males with germ cell tumors. *J Clin Oncol*, 2010. **28**(20):3388–3404.
70. Oesterling, J.E., et al., Serum prostate-specific antigen in a community-based population of healthy men. Establishment of age-specific reference ranges. *JAMA*, 1993. **270**(7):860–864.

71. Morgan, T.O., et al., Age-specific reference ranges for prostate-specific antigen in black men. *N Engl J Med*, 1996. **335**(5):304–310.

72. Wolf, A.M., et al., American Cancer Society guideline for the early detection of prostate cancer: update 2010. *CA Cancer J Clin*, 2010. **60**(2):70–98.

73. Polascik, T.J., J.E. Oesterling, and A.W. Partin, Prostate specific antigen: a decade of discovery–what we have learned and where we are going. *J Urol*, 1999. **162**(2):293–306.

74. Gilgunn, S., et al., Aberrant PSA glycosylation-a sweet predictor of prostate cancer. *Nat Rev Urol*, 2013. **10**(2):99–107.

75. Carlson, K.J., S.J. Skates, and D.E. Singer, Screening for ovarian cancer. *Ann Intern Med*, 1994. **121**(2):124–132.

76. Jacobs, I.J., et al., Risk of diagnosis of ovarian cancer after raised serum CA 125 concentration: a prospective cohort study. *BMJ*, 1996. **313**(7069):1355–1358.

77. Skates, S.J., et al., Calculation of the risk of ovarian cancer from serial CA-125 values for preclinical detection in postmenopausal women. *J Clin Oncol*, 2003. **21**(10 Suppl):206s–210s.

78. Harris, L., et al., American Society of Clinical Oncology 2007 update of recommendations for the use of tumor markers in breast cancer. *J Clin Oncol*, 2007. **25**(33):5287–5312.

79. Steinberg, W., The clinical utility of the CA 19-9 tumor-associated antigen. *Am J Gastroenterol*, 1990. **85**(4):350–355.

80. Cwik, G., et al., Cancer antigens 19-9 and 125 in the differential diagnosis of pancreatic mass lesions. *Arch Surg*, 2006. **141**(10):968–973; discussion 974.

81. Fletcher, R.H., Carcinoembryonic antigen. *Ann Intern Med*, 1986. **104**(1):66–73.

82. Locker, G.Y., et al., ASCO 2006 update of recommendations for the use of tumor markers in gastrointestinal cancer. *J Clin Oncol*, 2006. **24**(33):5313–5327.

83. Goldstein, M.J., and E.P. Mitchell, Carcinoembryonic antigen in the staging and follow-up of patients with colorectal cancer. *Cancer Invest*, 2005. **23**(4):338–351.

84. Muller, C.Y., and L.A. Cole, The quagmire of hCG and hCG testing in gynecologic oncology. *Gynecol Oncol*, 2009. **112**(3):663–672.

85. Cole, L.A., Immunoassay of human chorionic gonadotropin, its free subunits, and metabolites. *Clin Chem*, 1997. **43**(12):2233–2243.

86. Dalmau, J., H.S. Gultekin, and J.B. Posner, Paraneoplastic neurologic syndromes: pathogenesis and physiopathology. *Brain Pathol*, 1999. **9**(2):275–284.

87. Rudnicki, S.A., and J. Dalmau, Paraneoplastic syndromes of the spinal cord, nerve, and muscle. *Muscle Nerve*, 2000. **23**(12):1800–1818.

88. Pittock, S.J., T.J. Kryzer, and V.A. Lennon, Paraneoplastic antibodies coexist and predict cancer, not neurological syndrome. *Ann Neurol*, 2004. **56**(5):715–719.

89. Kijanka, G., et al., Human IgG antibody profiles differentiate between symptomatic patients with and without colorectal cancer. *Gut*, 2010. **59**(1):69–78.

90. O'Reilly, J.A., et al., Diagnostic potential of zinc finger protein-specific autoantibodies and associated linear B-cell epitopes in colorectal cancer. *PLoS One*, 2015. **10**(4):e0123469.

Chapter 7

Immunoassay-Based Detection of Infectious and Parasitic Diseases

Paul J. Conroy

Department of Biochemistry and Molecular Biology, Faculty of Medicine, Nursing and Health Science, Monash University, Melbourne, VIC 3800, Australia

paul.conroy@monash.edu

In the 'decade of the vaccine' infectious and parasitic diseases still represent a significant healthcare and socio-economic burden on modern society. Like many such diseases their prevalence is much higher in poorer resource areas. Significantly, the ability to detect causative agents in the environment and in patients is vital to aid intervention, thus preventing contagion. Many causative agents of infectious disease currently reside on a number of international government 'watch-lists' as biological agents for terrorism. This too strengthens the case for the rapid detection of infectious disease agents in individuals and the environment. In this chapter, the challenges in producing antibodies against indicators of infectious diseases will be discussed and current assay technologies for their detection outlined, highlighting their strengths and limitations. A future prospective will outline how the field of microfluidic 'point-of-care' devices can offer an attractive and low-cost solution for

Immunoassays: Development, Applications and Future Trends
Edited by Richard O'Kennedy and Caroline Murphy

ISBN 978-981-4669-97-9 (Hardcover), 978-1-315-20654-7 (eBook)
www.panstanford.com

the detection infectious diseases and their causative agents in the regions that require them the most.

7.1 Introduction

Over the last number of decades, substantial improvements in public health have resulted in lower incidences of communicable diseases. However, this progress is not distributed evenly between the developed and the developing world. Worldwide, 5.7 million people died from infectious and parasitic disease in 2015, of which 1.45 million were children (<5 years old). The lack of facilities and services taken for granted in the Western world means that 50% of these deaths occurred in the African region. This is in stark contrast to Europe and the Americas combined totallying 6.5% of all deaths attributed to infectious and parasitic disease (Fig. 7.1) [1].

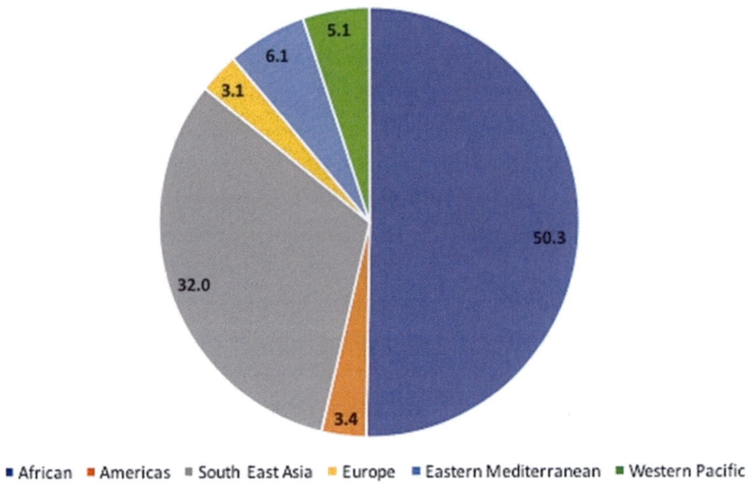

Figure 7.1 Infectious and parasitic disease as a percentage of all deaths grouped by World Health Organization (WHO) regions. Clearly, poorer resource regions, such as the African region, have a significantly higher percentage of deaths related to infectious and parasitic disease. The data presented was compiled from reports by the World Health Organization [1].

Infectious disease, although typically initiated in localised areas, can rapidly spread, a fact exacerbated by the ease at which people can be transported across the globe [2]. Despite a reduction in new tuberculosis (TB) cases and a decrease in deaths due to malaria, outbreaks such as encephalitis in India (2,300 infected, 400 dead [3]) remind us that infectious diseases are still a major healthcare concern. Figure 7.2 illustrates the particularly high prevalence and incidence of these diseases in developing countries (Africa and Southeast Asia) over the developed 'West'. The lack of technologies to efficiently identify such diseases is exacerbated by poor sanitation, poor access to safe water and additional transmission routes (e.g. the mosquito) coupled with socio-economic and political instability [4]. The ability to detect such infectious agents is critical to preventing their spread, and for the purposes of this book chapter, a focus on the world's leading infectious disease, human immunodeficiency virus (HIV), a related re-emerging one (TB) and a vaccine-treatable yet neglected disease (malaria) serves to highlight the significant advances in immunoassay-based testing. In addition, examples addressing the issue of bioterrorism detection and increased influenza infection rates are highlighted.

Pathogen-induced diseases in man are capable of rapid, prolonged or latent infection and can cause significant morbidity and mortality. The diagnosis of such conditions is challenging due to the numerous routes of infection by a very broad range of contagious elements [4]. Pathogen classification includes prions, viruses, bacteria, fungi and protozoa. Such diseases can be divided into several disease groups; respiratory infections, sexually transmitted infections (STI), and food-, water- and vector-borne and vaccine-preventable diseases (Table 7.1).

7.2 Current Technologies for the Detection of Infectious Diseases in Humans

At present, approaches to diagnose infections include laboratory-based examination of patient samples (e.g. biopsy or disease-associated fluids), serological testing, molecular-based testing

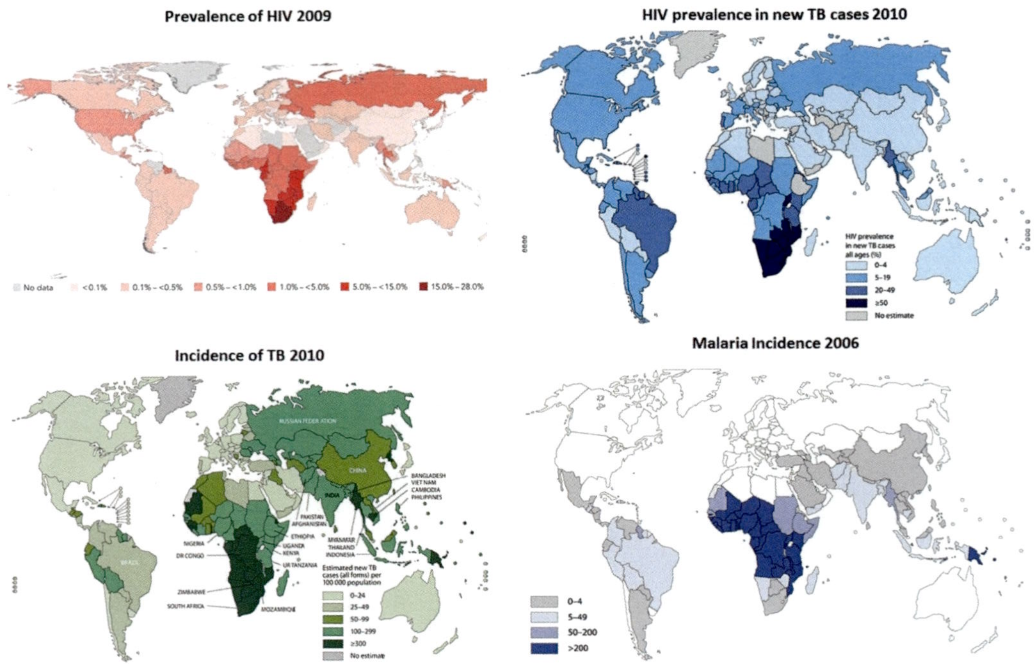

Figure 7.2 Worldwide prevalence of major infectious diseases. HIV (% adult population), TB (per 100,000) and malaria (per 1,000) represent some of the most significant disease burdens across the globe. Notably, the incidence of HIV in TB patients (%) is of considerable concern to already immune-compromised individuals, particularly in the light of drug-resistant forms of TB. This figure was prepared from statistical maps available from the WHO and the Joint United Nations Program on HIV/AIDS (UNAIDS) [5].

Table 7.1 Selected examples of infectious and parasitic diseases

Disease	Causative agent	Bioterrorism [6]
Respiratory infection		
Tuberculosis	*Mycobacterium tuberculosis*	
Influenza	*Orthomyxoviridae* family	
Legionnaires	*Legionella pneumophila*	
Sexually transmitted infection (STI)		
Hepatitis C	Hepatitis C virus	
Hepatitis B	Hepatitis B virus	
AIDs	Human immunodeficiency virus (HIV)	
Chlamydia	*Chlamydia trachomatis*	
Food- and water-borne infection		
Yersiniosis	*Yersinia enterocolitica*	
Anthrax	*Bacillus anthracis*	Y
Cholera	*Vibrio cholerae*	
Hepatitis A	Hepatitis A virus	
Listeriosis	*Listeria monocytogenes*	
Botulism	*Clostridium botulinum*	Y
Brucellosis	*Brucella* genus	
Vector-borne infection		
Malaria	*Plasmodium* genus	
Plague	*Yersinia pestis*	Y
Q Fever	*Coxiella burnetii*	Y
Severe acute respiratory syndrome (SARS)	*SARS coronavirus*	Y
Vaccine-preventable infection		
Meningococcal disease	*Neisseria meningitidis*	
Measles	Measles virus	
Diphtheria	*Corynebacterium diphtheriae*	
Pertussis	*Bordetella pertussis*	
Rabies	Rabies virus	

and immunoassays. Immunoassay-based detection of infectious agents is the most widely used and successful approach for both specific antigen and host-produced antibody analyses [7]. To be of value for low-resource communities, the current technologies are required to be or are moving towards more appropriate methodologies.

7.2.1 Appropriate Technologies

The global health statistics forum has reported that a TB diagnostic test with >85% sensitivity and >97% specificity could save 400 million lives annually [8], while a >95% sensitivity and >95% specificity malarial test could prevent >100 million deaths in children [9]. Therefore, appropriate technologies for improved diagnostics have the potential to lead to a dramatic reduction in disability-adjusted life years and mortality [10].

Point-of-care (POC) tests are those carried out at the primary care facility where the results are available in a short space of time, providing rapid diagnosis. Typically, these tests are based on lateral flow immunoassays which are cheap to produce, easy to carry out and often require no ancillary equipment. Increasingly novel microfluidic technology has the potential to propel such POC devices into the realm of effective, rapid and quantitative results for low-resource areas. However, to impact disease burden, these devices must conform to the characteristics of an ideal test. The 'ASSURED' principle (see Box 7.1) is used to guide diagnostic test development for low-resource areas. This further reinforces the need to adopt diagnostic approaches in developing tests for infectious diseases which are deliverable and usable by those who require them [11, 12].

Box 7.1 ASSURED: Characteristics of an ideal diagnostic test [13] for developing countries

Affordable to those at highest risk of infection
Sensitive
Specific
User-friendly
Rapid and Robust
Equipment-free
Deliverable to those who require it

Immunoassay-based POC has real potential to meet the needs of infectious disease diagnosis by building on the successful application of immuno-chromatographic systems, such as the iconic home pregnancy test kit and glucose monitoring systems. Technologies based on disposable cassettes, which accept a sample, perform some pre-analytical steps (e.g. clearing of the sample from its matrix), introduce the sample to the test zone where a result can be reported by a hand-held reader, have huge potential in lower-resource communities [14]. In such communities, guaranteed electricity supply, adequate operator training and centralised laboratory testing are often non-existent. Lower-resource areas are typically not targeted as markets for diagnostic platforms by multinational companies. However, organisations such as the Bill and Melinda Gates Foundation and entities such as the Program for Appropriate Technology in Health (PATH) and European and Developing Countries Clinical Trials Partnership (EDCTP) have championed the development of diagnostic tests for low-resource areas, and many of the in-place immunoassay systems for several diseases result from PATH-driven developments.

7.2.2 Human Immunodeficiency Virus (HIV)

HIV is an RNA-based virus which targets cells of the immune system. Undiagnosed HIV infection progresses to acquired immune deficiency syndrome (AIDS) without treatment and is a fatal disease. The eradication of AIDS is made all the more challenging due to the high mutation rate of the virus. The AIDS epidemic, although showing a reduction in the number of infected individuals (~25%), continues to affect over 36.7 million people. Since the start of the AIDS epidemic 35 million people have died from AIDS releated illnesses [5, 15]. A number of HIV tests currently in existence have seen successful application to the diagnosis and management of HIV which is largely driven by the private sector to answer the demands of control programs and blood banks [13]. The current gold standard test for HIV is the enzyme immunoassay (EIA), and in 2010 the fourth-generation device from Abbot (Architect HIV Ag/Ab Combo Assay) received FDA approval, followed in 2011 by BioRad (GS HIV Combo Ag/Ab EIA) [15]. In both cases, the devices detect both HIV antibodies (IgG and IgM) and the HIV antigen (p24), allowing earlier diagnosis of infection. However, both are designed for use in clinical laboratory settings rather than in low-resource settings or even at POC. The earliest possible detection of HIV involves RNA-based tests which are disadvantageous for low-resource settings, due to long processing times and requirements for electricity and trained staff

[2]. Currently there are eight FDA-approved rapid test kits for HIV 1 or HIV 1 and 2 detection [15], of which the most recent (INSTI™ HIV-1 Antibody Test Kit, 2010) device is approved for use in POC settings by trained personnel largely as a result of the fact that such devices are covered by the Clinical Laboratory Improvement Amendments (CLIA) waiver, permitting more widespread use.

7.2.3 Tuberculosis

Mycobacterium tuberculosis (MTB) is the causative agent of tuberculosis (TB) and presents in the lung (pulmonary) or elsewhere as extra-pulmonary TB. Rapid transmission of TB is possible through coughing and the disease can remain latent until an environmental trigger, which impairs the immune system, can reactivate the disease. TB is a significant problem for HIV-infected individuals, and the UNAIDS 2010 report suggests the need for a dual-screening program to deal with such dual epidemics [5]. TB affects approximately 8.6 million people and is the cause of 1.26 million deaths (2012-combined HIV-positive and HIV-negative deaths) [16]. The most commonly used test for TB diagnosis is sputum smear microscopy. TB cultures are more sensitive, but they require class 3 facilities. Progress in TB care and control is described as 'constrained by old technologies', but recent investments have led to the development of a suitable laboratory-based nucleic acid amplification system (Xpert MTB/RIF) capable of identifying both TB and drug-resistant infections. Immunoassay technology may yet have a significant role to play in the diagnosis and control of TB, as POC-based detection is predicated to be of significant value, particularly in low-resource settings [17]. Rapid methodologies to monitor the disease will be of substantial commercial interest in light of a number of phase II/III drugs and vaccines in development [16]. Key research areas identified include biomarker discovery for diagnostic targeting and developing POC-orientated tools for diagnosis [18]. While culture and molecular methods are the gold-standard approaches, microscopy is still widely employed in low-resource areas. Immunological methods most commonly associated with TB diagnosis rely on detecting circulating serum antibodies to antigens from MTB [19] and circulating MTB antigen detection. The serological diagnosis of TB by detection of antibodies to MTB antigens is an attractive approach for low-resource settings. Distinguishing latent TB has been the goal of such tests for several years. However, lack of suitable antigens (in children especially) combined with low sensitivity and specificity of antibodies, in cases further complicated by HIV co-infection, have limited the currently available commercial tests [17, 20, 21]. Such is the variability that the WHO issued a negative policy for TB serodiagnosis, recommending it not be used for the diagnosis of pulmonary or extra-pulmonary TB [16]. However, serodiagnosis may have adjunctive value in the diagnosis of TB in HIV co-infected individuals and it is suggested that antibody reactivity may be identifying a true serological response for MTB where the prognostic value has yet to be understood [22]. Urine-based TB diagnosis by detection of MTB antigens has yielded a promising urinalysis candidate, liboarabinomannan (LAM), which appears to be suited for HIV-associated TB diagnostics. Several initial studies, using commercial kits, demonstrated variable sensitivity but high specificity. Sensitivity could be improved by employing superior reagents or novel platforms, including, for example, use of standardised poly- or monoclonal or recombinant antibodies [20]. Enhanced antigen detection using LAM in an ELISA format has recently demonstrated improved sensitivity over sputum smear microscopy [23, 24]. Additionally, a LFIA-based 'dip-stick' assay for LAM with similar sensitivity and sensitivity to ELISA (in low T-cell count HIV patients) is under evaluation for POC settings [24]. TB diagnostics has proven to be a significant challenge and numerous bottlenecks have resulted in a slower development of diagnostic tests compared to other infectious diseases [2].

7.2.4 Malaria

In 2010, of the 216 million new cases of malaria, 81% occurred in the Africa region. In the same year, 81% of the total deaths were children [25], although recently the death figures were reported to be underestimated by a factor of 2 [26]. In 2015, of the 214 million new cases of malaria world-wide, 438,000 people died, of which 80% of these were children [1]. In the continuum of malarial infection, most researchers believe that an effective malarial vaccine will target a number of crucial molecular epitopes in more than one stage of the parasitic lifecycle [19, 27]. There are three stages of the malaria parasites' life cycle: pre-erythrocytic (liver), erythrocytic (blood stage) and transmission. The multi-stage nature of infection offers viable opportunities for diagnostics. As for TB, microscopy is the gold standard for malarial detection; however, lateral flow-based tests have been successfully applied to the diagnosis of malarial infection particularly in improving parasite detection in endemic regions [28]. The current assays apply classical sandwich formats with either poly- (more sensitive but less specific) or monoclonal (more specific but less sensitive) antibodies [29]. Current rapid tests for malaria detect several antigens, including histidine-rich protein 2 (HRP2, *P. falciparum*), plasmodium acetate dehydrogenase (*P. falciparum* and *P. vivax*) and plasmodium aldolase (all malaria species) [28]. HRP2-based tests are highly specific for *P. falciparum*, but are less sensitive to low-density parasitaemia. Significant challenges for POC-based malarial devices are firstly the detection of low levels of parasitic infection (<100–200 parasites μL^{-1}) for which PCR is still the mainstay, but unsuited for poorer resource areas and, secondly, the identification of infections with similar symptoms to prevent the high mortality rates associated with mistreated patients [10]. With variability in sensitivity dipping below the required 90% level, concerns for misdiagnosis arise. This becomes important for malaria management as overuse of anti-malarial therapies leads to drug-resistant forms of the parasite [2, 29]. The WHO has undertaken an extensive evaluation of the performance of rapid diagnostic tests (RDT) over the last number of years. The recent tests showed an increase in sensitivity of such tests at low density parasitemia and all were aimed at detecting the HRP2 antigen [30]. These reports provide guidance on procurement of such tests with a particular emphasis on application in low-resource areas.

7.2.5 Rapidly Spreading Infectious Agents

Biological agents as weapons present a significant threat to public health. An ideal agent is readily aerosolised, infective and communicable [31]. Table 7.1 contains several agents, which are currently listed on bioterrorism watch lists, of which *Bacillus anthracis* is considered to have potentially severe effects in terms of casualties and associated disruption, if released. Global outbreaks of infectious agents, including those on bioterror watch lists and influenza, have the propensity to rapidly spread across the world. In addition, clinical identification of such infections may not be immediate as symptoms take several days to present and clinicians may not be aware of suspicious cases until the numbers of patients reaches unusual levels [32]. Important devices are in development for *B. anthracis* detection in the air and other transmission sources but are outside the scope of rapid tests for humans. However, for such bioterror agents environmental monitoring is critical to prevent contagion. For human infection, the FDA approved immunological assay is the Red Line Alert™ (TetracoreR). This rapid test allows for confirmation of *B. anthracis* cultured from patient samples. Serological diagnosis is also of value and typically detects the bacterial protective antigen (PA) of *B. anthracis.* Immunetics® quick ELISA Anthrax-PA kit™ is FDA approved for use in patient diagnostics without centralised laboratory testing for qualitative or semi-quantitate diagnosis by detection of infection-elicited IgG/IgM antibodies.

The rapid detection of influenza is critical due to recent incidences of seasonal and avian influenza outbreaks. Although sporadic infection of humans with avian flu can occur, concerns reside around the ability of the virus to adapt and transmit more readily as demonstrated by the H1N1 outbreak in 2009. For these reasons, monitoring of influenza and the virology associated with the infection is crucial for controlling pandemic spread. A number of rapid influenza diagnostic tests exist and typically detect influenza A and B in nasal passage samples. Many of these kits have CLIA waivers permitting their POC use and the assay times are typically in the order of 10–15 minutes. These tests target viral nucleoproteins using monoclonal antibodies and employ many labels permitting visual detection or more complex yes/no reader systems. The most recently approved system from BD® (Veritor System™ for Rapid Detection of Flu A + B) is an immunochromatographic test (ICT) with a portable reader detecting influenza A+B without distinguishing between A subtypes. Alere's® Clearview Exact™ Influenza A + B delivers simple qualitative results in LFIA format with specificities and sensitivities for influenza A of 98.5% and 81.7%, respectively. Again, the test does not distinguish subtypes of influenza and is an example of another presumptive test to direct clinicians to order further testing. In the case of presumptive positive tests PCR is the mainstay for sub-type confirmation. In combination, rapid immunological identification kits assist in clinical decision making before employing more complex methodologies/kits for subtype categorisation. However, many kits do not provide adequate early diagnosis due to limitations in sensitivity (50–70%) and specificities (90–95%) in comparison to culture techniques [33].

The value of combining both specific antigen recognition and antibody presence (IgM/IgG) for improving the sensitivity of presumptive tests is of significance. A comparison of Bio-Rad® NS1 Ag Strip and Standard Diagnostics® Dengue Duo™ (NS1/IgM/IgG) lateral flow rapid tests demonstrated up to 21.3% improvement in sensitivity with no compromise in specificity in a dengue-endemic region [34]. In this case the assay can detect the antigen in an early stage of infection (days 1–9, where day 0 is onset of fever) and revert to IgG/IgM detection (days 3–4) when the antigen positive rate decreases (post days 8/9). Additionally, the infection can be identified as a primary or a re-occurrence. Combining serodiagnosis with specific antigen detection in the same format has obvious value for specific detection of infectious diseases. However, such approaches require extensive evaluation in large cohorts in both endemic and other regions to assess their true specificity.

7.3 Challenges in Detecting Infectious and Parasitic Diseases

In response to improving the sensitivities of POC-based assays, several novel disease biomarkers, reagents (antibodies), functionalisation strategies (labels, etc.), platforms and transducers are under investigation. This section outlines the novel approaches taken and the challenges associated with migration of such research from the confines of the pristine laboratory into the 'real-world' of infectious disease monitoring.

7.3.1 Current Research into New Platform Development

Table 7.2 highlights some novel antibody-based approaches to infectious disease detection deployed on several platforms in

Table 7.2 Assays in research for detecting infectious diseases

Analyte	Assay format	Platform	LOD[a]	Ref.
Tuberculosis				
38 kDa antigen	Direct (serological)	RIfS	ND	[35]
Ag231	Sandwich (Biotin SPEC)	Enzyme CV	1.0 ng mL^{-1}	[36]
55 kDa antigen	Direct	Dot-ELISA	ND	[37]
Multiple kDa antigen	Direct (serological)	MAPIA	ND	[38]
A60	Direct (serological)	Rapid Filtering Cartridge	ND	[39]
LAM	FLISA	Glass slides	10^{-14}M	[40]
HIV				
p24 antigen	Direct (Label-less)	EIS	6.4 pg mL^{-1}	[41]
Ad5 capsid	Direct (Label-less)	EIS	10^3 particles mL^{-1}	[42]
p24 antigen	Direct (Label-less)	Amperometric	ND	[43]
gp36	Direct (serological)	EMPAS	100 μg mL^{-1}	[44]
Malaria				
Plasmodium spp.	Sandwich (PCR product)	NALIFA	3 parasites mL^{-1}	[45]
Plasmodium HRP-2	Direct (Label-less)	QCM	12 ng mL^{-1}	[46]
	Sandwich (IgM/IgG-HRP)	Magneto-ELISA Magneto-sensor	0.35 ng mL^{-1} 0.36 ng mL^{-1}	[47]
	Sandwich	Amperometric	8 ng mL^{-1}	[48]
Plasmodium falciparum	Agglutination	Laser light-scattering	ND	[49]
Anthrax				
Bacillus anthracis	Direct (Label-less)	QCM	10^3 spores mL^{-1}	[50]
	Fluorescent Sandwich	FO	10^5 spores mg^{-1}	[51]
	Direct (Label-less)	PEMC	38 spores L^{-1}	[52]
	Fluorescent Sandwich	Waveguide	10^3 spores mL^{-1}	[53]
	Direct (Label-less)	Magnetoelastic	10^3 spores mL^{-1}	[54]

(*Contd.*)

Table 7.2 (*Continued*)

Analyte	Assay format	Platform	LOD[a]	Ref.
Influenza				
A	Direct (Label-less)	QCM	4 particles mL^{-1}	[55]
H5N1	Direct (RBC amplification)	EIS	10^3 EID_{50} mL^{-1}	[56]
A	Direct (Label-less)	EIS	8 ng mL^{-1}	[57]
Avian H5N1	Sandwich	QCM (Magnetic nanoparticles)	0.0128 HA unit	[58]
Avian	Sandwich (DNA-probe)	Immuno-PCR	10^{-4} EID_{50} mL^{-1}	[59]
A	Aggregation	DLS	<100 $TCID_{50}$ mL^{-1}	[33]
Hepatitis				
A and C	Direct (Label-less)	MEMS cantilever	0.1 ng mL^{-1}	[60]
B	Direct (Label-less)	Potentiometric	1.9 ng mL^{-1}	[61]
	Fluorescent sandwich	LFIA (nanocrystals)	50 pg mL^{-1}	[62]
	Direct (Label-less)	Amperometric	40 pg mL^{-1}	[63]
B and alpha-fetoprotein	Direct (Label-less	µ Piezoelectric	100 pg mL^{-1}	[64]
Tularemia				
Francisella tularensis	Direct (serological)	Piezoelectric	ND	[65]
Plague				
F1 capsule protein	Sandwich (Magnetic particles)	Immunosensor	2.5 ng mL^{-1}	[66]
	Sandwich (Up-converting phosphor particles)	LFIA	10^4 CFU mL^{-1}	[67]

[a]ND, Not determined; CV, cyclic voltammetry; DLS, dynamic light scattering; EID_{50}, 50% egg infective dose; EIS, electrochemical impedance spectroscopy; EMPAS, electromagnetic piezoelectric acoustic sensor; FO, fiber optic; LFIA, lateral flow immunoassay; MAPIA, multi-antigen print immunoassay; MEMS, micro-electromechanical systems, NALIFA, nucleic acid LIFA; PEMC, piezoelectric-excited millimeter-sized cantilever; QCM, quartz crystal microbalance; RIfS, reflectometric interference spectroscopy; SPEC, screen-printed carbon electrode; $TCID_{50}$, median tissue culture infective dose.

numerous assay formats. Despite demonstrating the value of novel transduction platforms some of the published literature suffers from sub-optimal assay design or sub-optimal real-sample analysis. Biosensor-based platforms are required to be compatible with sample environments where they are required to be of high sensitivity, robustness and have lower limits of detection. Additionally, such approaches must be suitable for disease monitoring in, low-resource areas. Although the technologies address current technical challenges in the area of infectious and parasitic disease diagnostics, there are challenges that must be faced when developing highly-specific antibodies for incorporation into immunological tests.

7.3.2 Current Antibodies for Infectious Disease Agents

Antibodies are ideal biorecognition elements due to their exquisite specificities and strong affinities for their cognate antigens. In the continuum of infectious and parasitic diseases, immunological tests rely on the development of specific antibodies capable of detecting the analyte in a multitude of matrices. Owing to the varied nature of the causative agents of such infections, antibody generation against viruses, bacteria and fungi presents a significant challenge. However, due to the diverse nature of the causative agents and their transmission routes no one generic approach to specific antibody generation can be applied, rather, tailored approaches combining diagnostic marker discovery and rationalised antibody generation. Using a knowledge-driven and focused approach to raise antibodies against key markers or epitopes maximises the odds of developing highly-specific biorecognition elements for incorporation into immunoassays.

The identification of influenza A subtypes within rapid diagnostic testing (RDT) is a limitation of the currently approved tests and a topic of consideration for improving the diagnostic sensitivity of current systems. Accordingly, significant interest in approaches to achieve sub-type classification has ensued. In this case, improved antibody reagents have the potential to improve sup-type recognition. Linke and co-workers developed a panel of monoclonal antibodies, which were specific for various influenza A subtypes, suggesting conserved epitopes, and the H5 subtype.

The authors correctly state that no mAb alone was sufficient for detection of several isolates of the H5N1 virus, but a battery of monoclonal antibody combinations was applied to specific clades of influenza A. Such an approach applies to improving current assays by detection of differing epitopes on the virus combined with conserved regions with sub-nanogram limits of detection (0.1 ng mL^{-1} per 0.005 HA) [68]. Similarly, Miyagawa and co-workers combined their developed mAb pairings into three tests with a commercial influenza A-specific LFIA. This increased the tests capacity to identify influenza A and to further differentiate H5 subtype [69]. Masalova and co-workers demonstrated mAbs with broad specificity for pandemic H1N1, typing avian influenza and subclade identification of highly pathogenic H5N1 [70]. Mizuike and co-workers investigated antibodies raised against pandemic H1N1 (H1N1 pdm), which do not react with seasonal variants of the influenza virus. Using this approach in combination with confirmatory RT-PCR, sensitivities of 85.5% and specificities of up to 100% were achieved [71]. Such approaches, demonstrate the substantial effort that is undertaken assessing the multiple strain and sub-clade reactivity of the mAbs in various formats applicable to improving the specificity and sensitivity of RDTs for pathogenic and seasonal influenza. Such approaches identify new clade-specific epitopes, conserved viral epitopes and permit monitoring of antigenic variation for possible effective prevention of large-scale outbreaks.

For malaria detection, an RDT [72] differentiating the Plasmodium species, live versus dead infection and the sexual stage of the parasitemia would be of benefit for diagnosis and crucially the guidance of the intervention to be taken. The main challenge appears to be in the area of low-level parasitemia. Examination of the stages of the life-cycle for infection identifies many critical targets including the HRP2 protein (*P. falciparum)*, parasite lactate dehydrogenase (pLDH, pan-*plasmodium* spp.) and Plasmodium aldolase (pan spp.). Therefore, differentiation between *P. falciparum* from other species is not a straightforward exercise. Piper and co-workers presented a thorough and rigorous empirical approach to ascertaining how combinations of existing pLDH antibodies perform in numerous combinations for *P. falciparum*, pan-specific and differential diagnosis of malarial parasites in an interesting detailed study. It is suggested from crystal structure studies that the difference in reactivity is likely to be associated with small differences in the pLDH surface where subtle amino acid changes are responsible for species specificity [73]. Additionally, the authors examined the effect of conjugation to gold colloids, but the antibody affinities were not assessed and perhaps could be attributed to the sensitivity differences upon conjugation or attributed to diffusion rate changes. The comprehensive evaluation of 'best assay pairings' for RDT formats in conjunction with the development of specific pairings to identify (i) pan-specific malarial infection, (ii) specifically *P. falciparum* and (iii) differentiation of all four human malarial parasites (*P. vivax, P. malaria and P. ovale*), was successfully applied to improving malarial diagnosis using the suggested diagnostic approach (algorithm) for pLDH [73].

7.4 Future Trends

The currently approved tests for many parasitic diseases are acknowledged to be limited by specificity, or sensitivity or requirements for ancillary components and trained personnel. The issues of specificity are currently being addressed by rigorous approaches to rational antibody development for specific antigen detection. The development of such antibodies with extremely high affinities impacts upon the assay sensitivity; however, the greatest contribution to sensitivity may in fact come from improved assay platforms and components. This too can impact on the requirements for centralised laboratory testing with trained personnel which in low-resource settings are not available.

7.4.1 Rapid Assay Development: Antibodies

Several factors will affect the quality of any analytical test. Irrespective of format, the specificity of the test is paramount and in the immunoassay arena is dependent on the specific interaction between the antibody and the target antigen. The numerous routes to the generation of specific antibodies are outlined in Fig. 7.3.

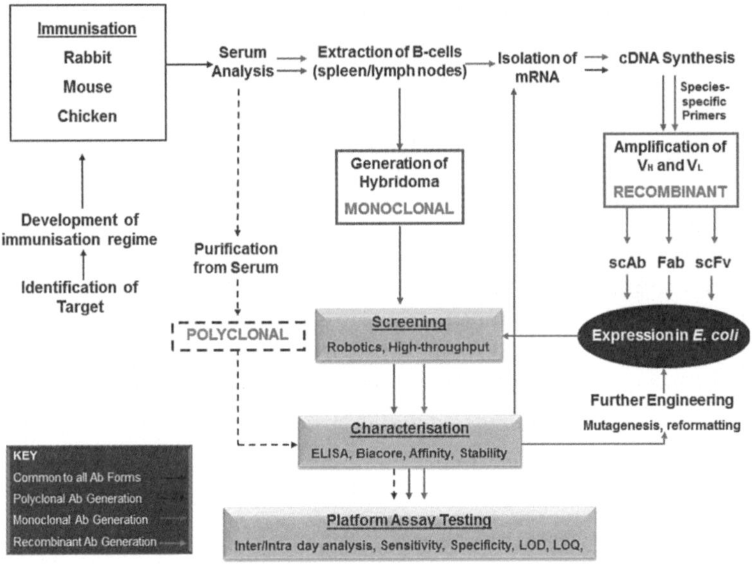

Figure 7.3 Overview of antibody generation routes. From the identification of the target biomarkers, key steps in the development of superior biorecognition elements for diagnostic assay development are outlined. Reproduced with permission from Conroy et al. [74].

The use polyclonal reagents is compromised by the broad specificities generated, the requirement for numerous laboratory animals and batch-to-batch variation. Monoclonal antibody generation is a route to generation of specific antibodies, which is countered by reduced sensitivity, in comparison to the broad coverage of polyclonal antibodies. Classically, such reagents exhibit low nanomolar affinity due to the concept of the affinity ceiling [75]. These limitations can be addressed by recombinant antibody technologies which have allowed the development of extremely high affinity–specific reagents by a number of display technologies [76]. Coupled with advanced approaches for reformatting, these recombinant antibodies can be of considerable importance to diagnostic applications. The development of recombinant antibody-based diagnostic tests is anticipated to come to the fore in the near future. To address cross-reactivity, a knowledge driven approach based upon detailed target evaluation can minimise, or if required maximise target cross-reactivity. The use of alternative hosts for antibody generation, such as chickens, can also assist in reducing false positives due to complement elements and human anti-mouse antibody (HAMA) crosslinking [77]. Thus the quality of the reagents generated will impact significantly on both the sensitivity and specificity of the designed assay. The sample matrix and its preparation combined with the signal detection methodology applied will have a dramatic effect on the sensitivity and several of the approaches outlined in Table 7.2 show sophisticated methodologies to improve assays for infectious disease.

7.4.2 Rapid Assay Development: Microfluidics and Nanotechnology and Their Relevance to Infectious Disease Detection

Microfluidic approaches are powerful methodologies to address the current limitations of RDT. Microfluidic systems are trending towards platforms that are essentially a 'lab-on-a-chip' and are of potentially major benefit for low resource settings. This subject is discussed in depth in Chapter 5 of this book. Such systems integrate the assay steps within a sophisticated network of channels, mixers and zones, at the micro scale, which allow the test to be carried out with minimal operator training and input. The area of minimally or non-instrumented microfluidic devices is very nicely reviewed by Weigl and co-workers [78]. The authors address the major developments required for such devices in the areas of novel alternatives to pumping, mixing and valving, separation of the analyte from the matrix, separation of the sample, concentration and detection. The ability to integrate numerous sample manipulation steps autonomously has advantages for improving the reliability of the RDT. The cost per device [79] is of considerable importance, especially in poorly developed countries where fabrication techniques are moving towards polymer microfabrication to reduce the associated costs [80]. In addition to these novel microfluidic devices, the ability to multiplex assays is of interest for the evaluation of a number of biomarkers of a disease or an number of biomarkers for multiple diseases in a single test [10]. For some diseases, the geographical location or pathogenic drift could introduce potential limitations for these devices, however, the ability to examine multiple pathogens, reduce costs and the incorporation of controls, sub-typing and drug resistance testing would be of significant benefit for infectious disease diagnosis in low resource settings [14]. The use of nanostructures such as gold nanoparticles, supermagnetic nanoparticles and quantum dots (QDots) is of interest as novel methodologies for detection. QDots, for example, are convenient as they require only one excitation light and are amenable to barcode-type multiplex assays.

Tang and co-workers demonstrated an ELISA-like approach for using nanoparticles in sensitive detection of anthrax toxins from infected mouse sera. This Europium nanoparticle plate-based immunoassay (ENIA) detected anthrax PA in a sandwich assay of mono- and polyclonal antibodies, which was 100-fold more sensitive than the same assay in ELISA format [81]. The authors demonstrated nanotechnology-assisted rapid testing for anthrax infection, although not on a microfluidic platform. The convergence of nanotechnology and microfluidics was demonstrated by Sia and co-workers, who developed a novel approach to HIV diagnostics by adopting a portable, low-cost approach well suited for low-resource settings. The device used polydimethylsiloxane (PDMS)-based soft lithography to generate the microfluidic surface and a combination of gold colloid and silver film opacity with a simple semiconductor laser-diode for HIV (gp41) serodiagnosis [82]. A barcode-type approach for the simultaneous detection of hepatitis B and C and HIV was developed by Klostrancec and co-workers which integrated a multiplex assay on a microfluidic platform [83]. In this assay, specific antigens were coated onto the QDot (HBsAg, HCV NSP4 and HIV-gp41) and incubated with human serum spiked with cognate antibodies and detected by anti-species AlexaFluor-488-labelled antibodies. When introduced into the microfluidics architecture, the electrokinetic force transported the QDot sandwich to a laser, where the fluorescent signal was detected. The demonstrated convergence of microfluidics and nanotechnology achieved assay times of approximately 1 hour and sensitivities far greater than the FDA-approved equivalent. Kim and co-workers developed a bio-barcode amplification approach for HIV-1 diagnosis in patient sera samples, using a nanoparticle-based sandwich immunoassay followed by

RT-PCR or chip-based scanometric detection methodologies [84]. The latter approach, requiring no enzymatic amplification cycle steps, could have potential application for POC and the devised system was superior to ELISA in terms of sensitivity, with an assay range of 0.1 pg mL^{-1} to 10 ng mL^{-1} p24 Gag. Targeting the capsid p24 antigen Tang and co-workers developed a similar bio-barcode assay and an ENIA for HIV-1 diagnostics with LODs of 0.1 pg mL^{-1} and 0.5 pg mL^{-1}, respectively [85]. The ENIA simplified the assay and reduced the assay time but still outperformed the ELISA LOD (10–15 pg mL^{-1}) and is suggested as a more viable alternative for low-resource settings. Myyryläinen and co-workers illustrated a dual time-resolved immunofluorescent assay for HIV-1 and HBV using lanthanide tracers measured by time-resolved fluorescence (TRF) in human samples [86]. The assay exploits the inherent fluorescence of the lanthanide tracers, which are longer lived than for QDs; however, the cross-talk between the tracers is an issue and could be dealt with by spatially resolving the multiplex assay.

Stephens and co-workers demonstrate an instrumental microfluidic immunoassay concept using the malaria antigen *Pf*HRP2 and gold colloid conjugated antibody. The developed assay took advantage of stabilising the reagents by anhydrous storage and demonstrated retained reactivity after storage at elevated temperatures [87]. The assay was sensitive to sub-nanomolar concentrations of the antigen in assay times of ~9 minutes. The authors highlighted the requirement to balance reduced assay times and flow rates to ensure sensitivity. This publication sought to address the issues surrounding reagent storage and stability with particular emphasis on lack of 'cold supply chain' capabilities. Integrating a number of micro-mixers and micro–pumps into a microfluidic cartridge, Lee and co-workers developed a sensitive assay for the detection of dengue virus by serodiagnosis using magnetic particles and dengue virus antigen by quantitation of human IgG and IgM, achieving a LOD of 21 pg in 30 minutes [88], and while nanotechnologies are powerful avenues of approach for diagnostics their biocompatibility and toxicity are of considerable concern, in addition to insolubility in biologically-relevant buffers. The shelf-life of QDots is important as photo bleaching and oxidation contribute to instability, while gold nanoparticles require well-characterised methodologies to control shape, size and prevent aggregation [89]. Such systems applicability to minimally and non-instrumented devices is also of concern particularly given the urgent need for improved sensitive diagnostics in low resource settings. The integration of such devices with mobile phone technology is of considerable interest given that 5.1 billion of the world's 6.8 billion people have such devices, which would allow global monitoring of infectious disease progression and spread.

7.5 Conclusion

For the last 20 years immunoassays have been exemplified by the ELISA and a litany of publications demonstrate immunoassay on a wide range of platforms, transducers surfaces and devices. Searching 'immunoassay and diagnostic' in PubMed (www.pubmed.com) yields over 8000 references which stretch back to 1963. The application of the immunoassay to diagnostics for global health and particularity for low-resource areas has identified numerous technologies and approaches in the laboratory. However, application of many of these approaches outside the controlled conditions of laboratory will render them impractical for impacting on low-resource areas. The immunoassay has a massive role to play in future rapid diagnostic tests in either stand-alone and/or integrated multiplexed devices. Current research aspires to support those aims, and ultimately, some of these emerging technologies appropriate for POC-based diagnostics will make an impact on global health and contribute to the diagnosis, management and potential eradication of infectious disease. For this to become a reality the balance of complexity, sensitivity, specificity, cost, reliability and user friendly nature of the technologies must be achieved. Exciting advances in the area of microfluidics, nanotechnology and biomarker discovery, coupled with integration with communications technology, have the potential to contribute significantly to controlling infectious diseases. In tandem, provision of significant financial supports and engagement of multinational companies are absolutely required to develop live-saving devices.

Suggested key papers

Antibody generation: References 73–75.
Microfluidics: References 14 and 77.
Nanotechnologies for infectious disease: References 4, 6, 11 and 82.

References

1. WHO. Cause specific mortality. Health Statistics and Informatics Department, World Health Organization, Geneva, Switzerland, 2015.
2. Hauck, T.S., Giri, S., Gao, Y., and Chan, W.C. Nanotechnology diagnostics for infectious diseases prevalent in developing countries. *Adv Drug Deliv Rev*, 2010; **62**:438–448.
3. Biswas, S. India encephalitis outbreak kills 400, mainly children. BBC, http://www.bbc.co.uk/news/world-south-asia-15269441, 2011.
4. Kaittanis, C., Santra, S., and Perez, J.M. Emerging nanotechnology-based strategies for the identification of microbial pathogenesis. *Adv Drug Deliv Rev*, 2010; **62**:408–423.
5. UNAIDS. http://www.unaids.org/globalreport/. 2011.
6. CDC. Bioterrorism agents. Centers for Disease Control and Prevention, https://emergency.cdc.gov/agent/agentlist.asp, 2015.
7. Andreotti, P.E., Ludwig, G.V., Peruski, A.H., Tuite, J.J., Morse, S.S., and Peruski, L.F., Jr. Immunoassay of infectious agents. *Biotechniques*, 2003; **35**:850–859.
8. Keeler, E., Perkins, M.D., Small, P., et al. Reducing the global burden of tuberculosis: the contribution of improved diagnostics. *Nature*, 2006; **444**(Suppl 1):49–57.
9. Rafael, M.E., Taylor, T., Magill, A., Lim, Y.W., Girosi, F., and Allan, R. Reducing the burden of childhood malaria in Africa: the role of improved diagnostics. *Nature*, 2006; **444**(Suppl 1):39–48.
10. Yager, P., Domingo, G.J., and Gerdes, J. Point-of-care diagnostics for global health. *Annu Rev Biomed Eng*, 2008; **10**:107–144.
11. Pang, T., and Peeling, R.W. Diagnostic tests for infectious diseases in the developing world: two sides of the coin. *Trans R Soc Trop Med Hyg*, 2007; **101**:856–857.
12. Peeling, R. Bringing diagnostics to developing countries: an interview with Rosanna Peeling. *Expert Rev Mol Diagn*, 2015; **15**:1107–1110.

13. Mabey, D., Peeling, R.W., Ustianowski, A., and Perkins, M.D. Diagnostics for the developing world. *Nat Rev Microbiol*, 2004; **2**:231–240.
14. Yager, P., Edwards, T., Fu, E., et al. Microfluidic diagnostic technologies for global public health. *Nature*, 2006; **442**:412–418.
15. FDA. http://www.fda.gov/ForConsumers/ByAudience/ForPatientAdvocates/HIVandAIDSActivities/ucm117922.htm. 2010.
16. WHO. Global tuberculosis control 2011. Health Statistics and Informatics Department, World Health Organization, Geneva, Switzerland, 2011.
17. Chegou, N.N., Hoek, K.G., Kriel, M., Warren, R.M., Victor, T.C., and Walzl, G. Tuberculosis assays: past, present and future. *Expert Rev Anti Infect Ther*, 2011; **9**:457–469.
18. WHO_Stop_TB_Partnership. An international roadmap for tuberculosis research. Health Statistics and Informatics Department, World Health Organization, Geneva, Switzerland, 2011.
19. Palma-Nicolas, J.P., and Bocanegra-Garcia, V. Innovative strategies to diagnose and monitor tuberculosis patients. *Arch Bronconeumol*, 2007; **43**:225–232.
20. Achkar, J.M., Lawn, S.D., Moosa, M.Y., Wright, C.A., and Kasprowicz, V.O. Adjunctive tests for diagnosis of tuberculosis: serology, ELISPOT for site-specific lymphocytes, urinary lipoarabinomannan, string test, and fine needle aspiration. *J Infect Dis*, 2011; **204**(Suppl 4):S1130–1141.
21. Ivanyi, J. Serodiagnosis of tuberculosis: due to shift track. *Tuberculosis (Edinb)*, 2011.
22. Achkar, J.M., Jenny-Avital, E., Yu, X., et al. Antibodies against immunodominant antigens of *Mycobacterium tuberculosis* in subjects with suspected tuberculosis in the United States compared by HIV status. *Clin Vaccine Immunol*, 2010; **17**:384–392.
23. Dheda, K., Davids, V., Lenders, L., et al. Clinical utility of a commercial LAM-ELISA assay for TB diagnosis in HIV-infected patients using urine and sputum samples. *PLoS One*, 2010; **5**:e9848.
24. Lawn, S.D., and Wood, R. Tuberculosis in antiretroviral treatment services in resource-limited settings: addressing the challenges of screening and diagnosis. *J Infect Dis*, 2011; **204**(Suppl 4):S1159–1167.
25. WHO. World malaria report 2011. Health Statistics and Informatics Department, World Health Organization, Geneva, Switzerland, 2011.
26. Murray, C.J.L., Rosenfeld, L.C., Lim, S.S., et al. Global malaria mortality between 1980 and 2010: a systematic analysis. *Lancet*, 2012; **379**:413–431.

27. Hearty, S., Conroy, P.J., Ayyar, B.V., Byrne, B., and O'Kennedy, R. Surface plasmon resonance for vaccine design and efficacy studies: recent applications and future trends. *Expert Rev Vaccines*, 2010; **9**:645–664.

28. McMorrow, M.L., Aidoo, M., and Kachur, S.P. Malaria rapid diagnostic tests in elimination settings-can they find the last parasite? *Clin Microbiol Infect*, 2011; **17**:1624–1631.

29. Murray, C.K., Gasser, R.A., Jr., Magill, A.J., and Miller, R.S. Update on rapid diagnostic testing for malaria. *Clin Microbiol Rev*, 2008; **21**:97–110.

30. WHO. Rapid diagnostic tests. Health Statistics and Informatics Department, World Health Organization, Geneva, Switzerland, 2015.

31. Peruski, L.F., Jr., and Peruski, A.H. Rapid diagnostic assays in the genomic biology era: detection and identification of infectious disease and biological weapon agents. *Biotechniques*, 2003; **35**:840–846.

32. Petrenko, V.A., and Sorokulova, I.B. Detection of biological threats. A challenge for directed molecular evolution. *J Microbiol Methods*, 2004; **58**:147–168.

33. Driskell, J.D., Jones, C.A., Tompkins, S.M., and Tripp, R.A. One-step assay for detecting influenza virus using dynamic light scattering and gold nanoparticles. *Analyst*, 2011; **136**:3083–3090.

34. Tricou, V., Vu, H.T., Quynh, N.V., et al. Comparison of two dengue NS1 rapid tests for sensitivity, specificity and relationship to viraemia and antibody responses. *BMC Infect Dis*, 2010; **10**:142.

35. Nagel, T., Ehrentreich-Forster, E., Singh, M., et al. Direct detection of tuberculosis infection in blood serum using three optical label-free approaches. *Sens Actuators B*, 2008; **129**:934–940.

36. Diaz-Gonzalez, M., Gonzalez-Garcia, M.B., and Costa-Garcia, A. Immunosensor for *Mycobacterium tuberculosis* on screen-printed carbon electrodes. *Biosens Bioelectron*, 2005; **20**:2035–2043.

37. Attallah, A.M., Osman, S., Saad, A., et al. Application of a circulating antigen detection immunoassay for laboratory diagnosis of extra-pulmonary and pulmonary tuberculosis. *Clin Chim Acta*, 2005; **356**:58–66.

38. Lyashchenko, K.P., Singh, M., Colangeli, R., and Gennaro, M.L. A multi-antigen print immunoassay for the development of serological diagnosis of infectious diseases. *J Immunol Methods*, 2000; **242**:91–100.

39. Yari, S., Hadizadeh Tasbiti, A., Fateh, A., et al. Purification of modified mycobacterial A60 antigen by affinity chromatography and its use for rapid diagnostic tuberculosis infection. *J Microbiol Methods*, 2011; **87**:184–188.

40. Schmidt, R., Jacak, J., Schirwitz, C., et al. Single-molecule detection on a protein-array assay platform for the exposure of a tuberculosis antigen. *J Proteome Res*, 2011; **10**:1316–1322.
41. Kheiri, F., Sabzi, R.E., Jannatdoust, E., Shojaeefar, E., and Sedghi, H. A novel amperometric immunosensor based on acetone-extracted propolis for the detection of the HIV-1 p24 antigen. *Biosens Bioelectron*, 2011; **26**:4457–4463.
42. Caygill, R.L., Hodges, C.S., Holmes, J.L., Higson, S.P., Blair, G.E., and Millner, P.A. Novel impedimetric immunosensor for the detection and quantitation of Adenovirus using reduced antibody fragments immobilized onto a conducting copolymer surface. *Biosens Bioelectron*, 2012; **32**(1):104–110.
43. Gan, N., Luo, N.-X., Li, T.-H., Zheng, L., and Ni, M.-J. A non-enzyme amperometric immunosensor for rapid determination of human immunodeficiency virus p24 based on magnetism controlled carbon nanotubes modified printed electrode. *Chin J Anal Chem*, 2010; **38**:1556–1562.
44. Sheikh, S., Blaszykowski, C., and Thompson, M. Label-free detection of HIV-2 antibodies in serum with an ultra-high frequency acoustic wave sensor. *Talanta*, 2011; **85**:816–819.
45. Mens, P.F., van Amerongen, A., Sawa, P., Kager, P.A., and Schallig, H.D. Molecular diagnosis of malaria in the field: development of a novel 1-step nucleic acid lateral flow immunoassay for the detection of all 4 human Plasmodium spp. and its evaluation in Mbita, Kenya. *Diagn Microbiol Infect Dis*, 2008; **61**:421–427.
46. Sharma, M.K., Rao, V.K., Merwyn, S., Agarwal, G.S., Upadhyay, S., and Vijayaraghavan, R. A novel piezoelectric immunosensor for the detection of malarial *Plasmodium falciparum* histidine rich protein-2 antigen. *Talanta*, 2011; **85**:1812–1817.
47. Castilho Mde, S., Laube, T., Yamanaka, H., Alegret, S., and Pividori, M.I. Magneto immunoassays for *Plasmodium falciparum* histidine-rich protein 2 related to malaria based on magnetic nanoparticles. *Anal Chem*, 2011; **83**:5570–5577.
48. Sharma, M.K., Rao, V.K., Agarwal, G.S., et al. Highly sensitive amperometric immunosensor for detection of *Plasmodium falciparum* histidine-rich protein 2 in serum of humans with malaria: comparison with a commercial kit. *J Clin Microbiol*, 2008; **46**:3759–3765.
49. Mya, M.M., Saxena, R.K., Roy, A., and Roy, K.B. Design and development of an immunosensor for the detection of malaria in field conditions. *Parasitol Res*, 2003; **89**:371–374.

50. Hao, R., Wang, D., Zhang, X., et al. Rapid detection of *Bacillus anthracis* using monoclonal antibody functionalized QCM sensor. *Biosens Bioelectron*, 2009; **24**:1330–1335.

51. Tims, T.B., and Lim, D.V. Rapid detection of *Bacillus anthracis* spores directly from powders with an evanescent wave fiber-optic biosensor. *J Microbiol Methods*, 2004; **59**:127–130.

52. Campbell, G.A., Delesdernier, D., and Mutharasan, R. Detection of airborne *Bacillus anthracis* spores by an integrated system of an air sampler and a cantilever immunosensor. *Sens Actuators B*, 2007; **127**:376–382.

53. Hang, J., Sundaram, A.K., Zhu, P., et al. Development of a rapid and sensitive immunoassay for detection and subsequent recovery of *Bacillus anthracis* spores in environmental samples. *J Immunol Methods*, 2008; **73**:242–246.

54. Shen, W., Lakshmanan, R.S., Mathison, L.C., Petrenko, V.A., and Chin, B.A. Phage coated magnetoelastic micro-biosensors for real-time detection of *Bacillus anthracis* spores. *Sens Actuators B*, 2009; **137**:501–506.

55. Owen, T.W., Al-Kaysi, R.O., Bardeen, C.J., and Cheng Q. Microgravimetric immunosensor for direct detection of aerosolized influenza A virus particles. *Sens Actuators B*, 2007; **126**:691–699.

56. Wang, R., Wang, Y., Lassiter, K., et al. Interdigitated array microelectrode based impedance immunosensor for detection of avian influenza virus H5N1. *Talanta*, 2009; **79**:159–164.

57. Hassen, W.M., Duplan, V., Frost, E., and Dubowski, J.J. Quantitation of influenza A virus in the presence of extraneous protein using electrochemical impedance spectroscopy. *Electrochim Acta*, 2011; **56**:8325–8328.

58. Li, D., Wang, J., Wang, R., et al. A nanobeads amplified QCM immunosensor for the detection of avian influenza virus H5N1. *Biosens Bioelectron*, 2011; **26**:4146–4154.

59. Deng, M., Long, L., Xiao, X., et al. Immuno-PCR for one step detection of H5N1 avian influenza virus and Newcastle disease virus using magnetic gold particles as carriers. *Vet Immunol Immunopathol*, 2011; **141**:183–189.

60. Timurdogan, E., Alaca, B.E., Kavakli, I.H., and Urey, H. MEMS biosensor for detection of Hepatitis A and C viruses in serum. *Biosens Bioelectron*, 2011; **28**:189–194.

61. Tang, D., Yuan, R., Chai, Y., Zhong, X., Liu, Y., and Dai, J. Electrochemical detection of hepatitis B surface antigen using colloidal gold

nanoparticles modified by a sol-gel network interface. *Clin Biochem*, 2006; **39**:309–314.

62. Shen, H., Yuan, H., Niu, J.Z., et al. Phosphine-free synthesis of high-quality reverse type-I ZnSe/CdSe core with CdS/Cd(x)Zn(1 - x)S/ZnS multishell nanocrystals and their application for detection of human hepatitis B surface antigen. *Nanotechnology*, 2011; **22**:375602.
63. Qiu, J.D., Huang, H., and Liang, R.P. Biocompatible and label-free amperometric immunosensor for hepatitis B surface antigen using a sensing film composed of poly(allylamine)-branched ferrocene and gold nanoparticles. *Microchim Acta*, 2011; **174**:97–105.
64. Xu, T., Miao, J., Wang, Z., Yu, L., and Li, C.M. Micro-piezoelectric immunoassay chip for simultaneous detection of Hepatitis B virus and α-fetoprotein. *Sens Actuators B*, 2011; **151**:370–376.
65. Pohanka, M., Pavlis, O., and Skladal, P. Diagnosis of tularemia using piezoelectric biosensor technology. *Talanta*, 2007; **71**:981–985.
66. Meyer, M.H., Stehr, M., Bhuju, S., et al. Magnetic biosensor for the detection of *Yersinia pestis*. *J Microbiol Methods*, 2007; **68**:218–224.
67. Yan, Z., Zhou, L., Zhao, Y., et al. Rapid quantitative detection of *Yersinia pestis* by lateral-flow immunoassay and up-converting phosphor technology-based biosensor. *Sens Actuators B*, 2006; **119**:656–663.
68. Linke, S., Neubauer, K., Dorner, M.B., Dorner, B.G., Pauli, G., and Schweiger, B. Generation and characterisation of monoclonal antibodies against influenza virus A, subtype H5N1. *J Virol Methods*, 2011; **175**:85–94.
69. Miyagawa, E., Kogaki, H., Uchida, Y., et al. Development of a novel rapid immunochromatographic test specific for the H5 influenza virus. *J Virol Methods*, 2011; **173**:213–219.
70. Masalova, O.V., Klimova, R.R., Chichev, E.V., et al. Development of monoclonal antibodies to highly pathogenic avian influenza H5N1 virus and their application to diagnostics, prophylaxis, and therapy. *Acta Virol*, 2011; **55**:3–14.
71. Mizuike, R., Sasaki, T., Baba, K., et al. Development of two types of rapid diagnostic test kits to detect the hemagglutinin or nucleoprotein of the swine-origin pandemic influenza A virus H1N1. *Clin Vaccine Immunol*, 2011; **18**:494–499.
72. Bell, D., Wongsrichanalai, C., and Barnwell, J.W. Ensuring quality and access for malaria diagnosis: how can it be achieved? *Nat Rev Microbiol*, 2006; **4**:S7–20.

73. Piper, R.C., Buchanan, I., Choi, Y.H., and Makler, M.T. Opportunities for improving pLDH-based malaria diagnostic tests. *Malar J*, 2011; **10**:213.
74. Conroy, P.J., Hearty, S., Leonard, P., and O'Kennedy, R.J. Antibody production, design and use for biosensor-based applications. *Semin Cell Dev Biol*, 2009; **20**:10–26.
75. Hearty, S., and O'Kennedy, R. Exploiting recombinant antibodies in point-of-care (POC) diagnostics: the combinatorial advantage. *Bioeng Bugs*, 2011; **2**:182–186.
76. Hoogenboom, H.R. Selecting and screening recombinant antibody libraries. *Nat Biotechnol*, 2005; **23**:1105–1116.
77. Greunke, K., Braren, I., Alpers, I., et al. Recombinant IgY for improvement of immunoglobulin-based analytical applications. *Clin Biochem*, 2008; **41**:1237–1244.
78. Weigl, B., Domingo, G., Labarre, P., and Gerlach, J. Towards non- and minimally instrumented, microfluidics-based diagnostic devices. *Lab Chip*, 2008; **8**:1999–2014.
79. Antia, M., Herricks, T., and Rathod, P.K. Microfluidic approaches to malaria pathogenesis. *Cell Microbiol*, 2008; **10**:1968–1974.
80. Mairhofer, J., Roppert, K., and Ertl, P. Microfluidic systems for pathogen sensing: a review. *Sensors*, 2009; **9**:4804–4823.
81. Tang, S., Moayeri, M., Chen, Z., et al. Detection of anthrax toxin by an ultrasensitive immunoassay using Europium nanoparticles. *Clin Vaccine Immunol*, 2009; **16**:408–413.
82. Sia, S.K., Linder, V., Parviz, B.A., Siegel, A., and Whitesides, G.M. An integrated approach to a portable and low-cost immunoassay for resource-poor settings. *Angew Chem Int Ed*, 2004; **43**:498–502.
83. Azzazy, H.M., and Mansour, M.M. In vitro diagnostic prospects of nanoparticles. *Clin Chim Acta*, 2009; **403**:1–8.
84. Kim, E.Y., Stanton, J., Korber, B.T., et al. Detection of HIV-1 p24 Gag in plasma by a nanoparticle-based bio-barcode-amplification method. *Nanomedicine (Lond)*, 2008; **3**:293–303.
85. Tang, S., and Hewlett, I. Nanoparticle-based immunoassays for sensitive and early detection of HIV-1 capsid (p24) antigen. *J Infect Dis*, 2010; **201**(Suppl 1):S59–64.
86. Myyrylainen, T., Talha, S.M., Swaminathan, S., et al. Simultaneous detection of Human Immunodeficiency Virus 1 and Hepatitis B virus infections using a dual-label time-resolved fluorometric assay. *J Nanobiotechnol*, 2010; **8**:27.

87. Stevens, D.Y., Petri, C.R., Osborn, J.L., Spicar-Mihalic, P., McKenzie, K.G., and Yager, P. Enabling a microfluidic immunoassay for the developing world by integration of on-card dry reagent storage. *Lab Chip*, 2008; **8**:2038–2045.
88. Lee, Y.F., Lien, K.Y., Lei, H.Y., and Lee, G.B. An integrated microfluidic system for rapid diagnosis of dengue virus infection. *Biosens Bioelectron*, 2009; **25**:745–752.
89. Ray, S., Reddy, P.J., Choudhary, S., Raghu, D., and Srivastava, S. Emerging nanoproteomics approaches for disease biomarker detection: a current perspective. *J Proteomics*, 2011; **74**:2660–2681.

Chapter 8

Detection of Food, Agricultural and Aquatic Contaminants

Marie Le Berre,[a*] Caroline Viguier,[b*] Caroline Murphy,[b] and Niamh Gilmartin[b,c*]

[a] *National Centre for Biomedical Engineering Science, National University of Ireland, University Road, Galway, Ireland*

[b] *School of Biotechnology and Biomedical Diagnostics Institute, National Centre for Sensor Research, Dublin City University, Collins Avenue, Dublin 9, Ireland*

[c] *School of Biological Sciences, Dublin Institute of Technology, Kevin Street, Dublin 8, Ireland*

niamh.gilmartin@dit.ie

The Food and Agriculture Organisation of the United Nations (FAO) predicts that food production will need to increase by 70% by 2050 in order to meet the demands of the projected growth in population. This projected increase and the constant risk posed from contaminants puts greater pressure on the food industry to provide safe food to the consumer and to meet the demands for food production. Intensive farming and food production have been linked to increased agricultural and environmental contaminants including chemicals, industrial waste and to naturally occurring

*These authors contributed equally to this work.

Immunoassays: Development, Applications and Future Trends
Edited by Richard O'Kennedy and Caroline Murphy

ISBN 978-981-4669-97-9 (Hardcover), 978-1-315-20654-7 (eBook)
www.panstanford.com

components such as toxins, bacteria and viruses. If released into the environment, these contaminants can affect livestock, fish or shellfish and travel through the food chain to humans. There are well-established regulations; e.g. (EC) No. 1881/2006 sets maximum levels for certain contaminants in foodstuffs to protect public health. Similarly, monitoring programmes involving detection of contaminants have been established in order to avoid the large costs of contamination, clean-up in the environment and associated health costs [1]. Immunoassay-based tests are now very widely used by producers, food processors, regulatory authorities and consumers. While a comprehensive discussion of the current detection of all contaminants is beyond the scope of this chapter, particular emphasis will be placed on the use of immunoassays for the detection of contaminants in food, agriculture and in aquatic environments.

8.1 Immunoassays Used in the Detection of Contaminants in Food

8.1.1 Foodborne Pathogens

The four main bacterial pathogens responsible for the highest levels of foodborne illnesses are Salmonella, Campylobacter, Shiga toxin/verotoxin-producing *Escherichia coli* (STEC/VTEC) and *Listeria monocytogenes.* Since 2010 the cases of campylobacteriosis and STEC/VTEC *E. coli* are increasing annually, while outbreaks of listeriosis and salmonellosis are continuing on a global scale, thus highlighting the need to monitor foodborne pathogens throughout the food chain, including production, processing and distribution to the point of sale. Pathogens may be present in low numbers in a sample, thus making detection difficult. The permitted limits of microbes (Table 8.1) in food are governed by commission regulation (EC) No. 2073/2005. Culture methods remain the gold standard for detection and they are the primary methods cited in the legislation for the determination of foodborne pathogens. A comparison of enzyme-linked immunosorbent assay (ELISA), polymerase chain reaction (PCR) and lateral-flow immunoprecipitation technologies

Table 8.1 Permitted limits of major foodborne pathogens (adapted from McGrath et al. 2012 [3])

Pathogen	Acceptable limits in food
Salmonella	Absent within a set weight of food during shelf life
E. coli (STEC/VTEC)	50 CFU g^{-1} minced meat during processing (value set for *E. coli*) 1000 CFU g^{-1} ready-to-eat fruit and vegetables (value set for *E. coli*)
L. monocytogenes	100 CFU g^{-1} in ready-to-eat foods during their shelf life or <1 cell in 25 g of food before the food has left the control of the producer
Campylobacter	To date, no criteria have been established in legislation for Campylobacter spp. in foodstuffs

CFU: colony-forming units.

to conventional culture methodology for the detection of Salmonella, Campylobacter, Listeria, and *E. coli* O157:H7 in processed meat showed agreement ranging from 80% to 100% depending on the pathogen detected and the method used [2]. Immunoassays, however, offer significant advantages over culture-based methods as they are rapid, easy to use and capable of detecting viable but non-culturable pathogens.

In pathogen detection, a 'sandwich-type' assay format is most commonly used. This format involves the capture of a pathogen in a sample through the use of an immobilised antibody and detection using a labelled antibody. Several different immunoassays, including ELISA, fluorescence-linked immunosorbent assay (FLISA) and lateral flow immunoassays, have been developed over the years for the detection of a wide variety of food pathogens (Table 8.2) with varying sensitivities. The presence of pathogens in food is detected using electrochemical (potentiometric, amperometric and conductometric), optical (absorbance, fluorescence, luminescence, refractive index and surface-plasmon resonance) mass, thermal and magnetic methods. (The principles of these methods are discussed elsewhere in this book in Chapters 1, 10 and 12). For example, two different detection technologies for *L. monocytogenes* resulted in similar sensitivities. Davis et al. [4] demonstrated detection of 10^2

Table 8.2 Examples of the determination of food pathogens using immunoassays

Pathogen	Technique	Detection method	Detection limit CFU mL^{-1}	Ref.
S. typhimurium	FLISA (Quantum dots)	Fluorescence	1.95×10^3	[9]
	Copper enhanced gold nanoparticles	Electrochemical	98.9	[10]
	FLISA (magnetic nanoparticle and quantum dots)	Fluorescence	10^3	[11]
	Localised surface plasmon resonance (SPR)	Optical	10^2	[12]
Campylobacter	Voltammetry with multi-walled carbon nanotubes	Electrochemical	400	[13]
	Indirect ELISA	Optical	10^4–10^6	[14]
L. monocytogenes	ELISA	Optical	1–10	[15]
	Surface plasmon resonance	Optical	10^5	[16]
E. coli O157:H7	Flow cytometer (Ruβpy-doped silica NPs)	Fluorescence	1	[17]
	FLISA (magnetic nanoparticle and quantum dots)	Fluorescence	10^3	[11]
	Surface plasmon resonance	Optical	10^7	[18]
	Piezoelectric-excited millimetre-sized cantilever	Electrochemical	1	[19]

CFU g^{-1} using disposable screen-printed carbon electrode (SPCE) strips with commercial anti-*L. monocytogenes* antibodies in about 1 hour. Whereas a similar level of *L. monocytogenes* was detected in milk using a mass-based piezoelectric cantilever biosensor and a commercial polyclonal anti-*L. monocytogenes* antibody in 1 hour [5].

The use of nanomaterials has proven invaluable in signal amplification in immunoassays, resulting in detection of a single cell in some cases. For example, Wang and colleagues [6] formed a sandwich complex using Salmonella species-specific antibodies and antibody-coated gold nanoparticles (AuNPs). Silver was then deposited around the AuNPs resulting in signal amplification of the chemiluminescence-based assay and a detection limit of 5 CFU mL^{-1}. Using a similar but enhanced AuNP approach Cao and co-workers demonstrated 'on-slide' detection of the foodborne pathogen, *Campylobacter jejuni*. This simple and cost-effective detection format resulted in a strong colour intensity that can easily be detected by the unaided eye or measured by an inexpensive flatbed scanner [7]. The ultimate goal of an immunoassay for the detection of pathogens is the detection of a single cell. Using nanoparticles, the capture of a single Salmonella bacterium was observed when a gold/silica heterostructured nanorod scaffold was functionalised with anti-Salmonella antibodies [8].

While ultra-sensitive detection of a pathogen is desirable, significant development in multiplex nanoparticle-based immunodetection of pathogens in food was observed in recent years [20]. The use of quantum dots (QDs) rather than traditional dyes results in brighter fluorescence intensities for longer and signal amplification has resulted in lower detection thresholds. For example, Zhao et al. [17] used fluorescent nanoparticles conjugated to anti-*E. coli* O157 antibodies for the detection of *E. coli* O157 in ground beef. The fluorescence of the nanoparticles was amplified 1000-fold, and as a result, a single *E. coli* O157 cell was detectable. Use of QDs allowed simultaneous detection of several biomarkers due to their broad Stokes shift, which permits the simultaneous excitation of many different QDs at a single excitation wavelength. Using QDs, Zhao and colleagues detected three foodborne pathogenic bacteria, *S. typhimurium*, *Shigella flexneri*, and *E. coli* O157:H7, to a detection limit of 10^3 CFU mL^{-1} in milk and apple juice [11]. An equivalent detection limit was demonstrated with the use of AuNPs for the multiplexed detection of *S. typhimurium* and *Staphylococcus aureus* using silica-coated magnetic probes functionalised with pathogen-specific antibodies for capture, followed by detection using pathogen-specific surface-enhanced Raman scattering probes [21]. The low detection capability (10^3 CFU mL^{-1}) demonstrated by these studies in complex food matrices (milk, apple juice, spinach solution and peanut butter) proffers great potential for cost-effective, rapid multiplex immunoassays. Typical ELISA assays consist of several different steps, namely, blocking, washing, incubation of primary and, possibly, secondary antibodies, substrate development and reading. These can take several hours to complete and, understandably, this may be problematic in instances where rapid detection is a requisite. Hence, more rapid immunoassay-based platforms may be used as alternatives for pathogen detection.

Lateral flow immunoassays (LFIA) offer a rapid (10–20 min) point-of-need, i.e. outside-the-laboratory immunoassay for the detection of pathogens such as Salmonella, Campylobacter, Listeria, and *E. coli* O157:H7. When LFIA was compared to culture methods, however, a higher number of false-positive results were observed [2]. Despite this and the need for pre-enrichment, the speed and simplicity of these methods resulted in the development of commercial LFIA-based tests (Singlepath®, Duopath®, RapidChek®) for the preliminary screening for pathogen contamination in foods. The reported limit of detection of bacteria using such strips ranges from 10^4 to 10^7 CFU mL^{-1} without an enrichment step [22].

A field-portable colorimetric lateral flow immunoassay using immunoliposomes encapsulating methylene blue dye and tagged with anti-Salmonella antibodies showed a detection limit of 1.6×10^3 CFU with heat-killed *Salmonella typhimurium* [23]. Pre-concentration steps were used to increase the sensitivity of immunoassays and a lateral flow chromatographic enzyme immunoassay together with a magnetic concentration step was demonstrated to detect 10^2 CFU mL^{-1} *L. monocytogenes* in spiked milk within 2 hours [24]. Nucleic acid lateral flow immunoassay (NALFIA) is a method combining a molecular biological principle of detection with an immunochemical principle of visualisation.

Blazkova et al. [25] combined polymerase chain reaction (PCR) and lateral flow immunoassay for detecting the amplified products for Listeria spp. and *L. monocytogenes*. This method was successfully used for identification of *L. monocytogenes* and strains of Listeria spp. in 20 different food matrices and was in concordance with the International Organisation for Standardisation (ISO) method.

While the improvement and enhancement of existing immunoassay detection is ongoing, new technologies are also in development. For example Chai et al. [26] demonstrated in a 'proof-of-principle' study a method for the detection of bacterial pathogens on fresh food surfaces in real-time and in situ using a phage-coated magnetoelastic biosensor for detecting Salmonella. Further advancements in technology, rapidity and multiplex detection of food pathogens will be a huge advantage to the food industry.

8.1.2 Foodborne Toxins

Often it is both the presence of the pathogen and the presence of an associated toxin that cause the adverse effects to human health. An example of this was the outbreak of *E. coli* serotype O104:H4 and its associated Shiga-like toxin in Germany in 2011 in which a total of 3602 cases were reported and 47 people died [27]. In addition to *E. coli* vero- and Shiga-toxins, staphylococcal enterotoxins, botulinum neurotoxins and the plant toxin ricin have also been implicated in food-related health concerns. Detection of both ricin and botulinum toxins has caused increased interest due to the threat of their use in a terrorist attack on drinking water.

Shiga toxin-producing *E. coli* (STEC) strains can sometimes secrete levels of toxins that cannot be detected using traditional cell cytotoxicity or immunological assays. Zhang and colleagues [28] demonstrated a sensitive immuno-PCR assay for the detection of Shiga toxin and its variants by combining antibody capture using a Shiga-specific biotinylated antibody and a biotinylated DNA fragment for amplification of the signal. The immuno-PCR assay detected 10 pg mL^{-1} of Shiga toxin, compared to 1 ng mL^{-1} of Stx2 detected by a commercial enzyme immunoassay (EIA). A competitive assay was used by Harteveld and co-workers [29] for the detection of 0.1 μg mL^{-1} of Staphylococcal enterotoxin B

(SEB) through the development of a competition assay. Samples containing SEB were preincubated with an anti-SEB polyclonal antibody and subsequently passed over the sensor surface containing immobilised toxin. The SEB present in the sample prevented the antibody binding to the surface, thus reducing the signal and indicating the presence of SEB in the sample. Conversely, Rowe-Taitt and colleagues [30] used a sandwich-type assay format in their fluorescence-based array biosensor which was capable of detecting 20 ng mL^{-1} SEB. This work used specific biotinylated polyclonal and monoclonal antibodies captured on a neutravidin-coated surface for the multiplex detection of SEB and *Clostridium botulinum* toxins A (40 ng mL^{-1}) and B (200 ng mL^{-1}) and *Vibrio cholera* toxins (1.6 ng mL^{-1}). A similar approach was demonstrated by Pauly and coworkers [31] with the simultaneous detection of ricin, abrin, botulinum neurotoxin A and SEB, in baby food, milk, yoghurt, iced coffee and carrot juice. This assay used toxin-specific antibody-tagged magnetic beads to isolate the toxin from the matrix and the detection of low ng L^{-1} quantities was achieved using fluorescently labelled secondary antibodies.

8.2 Immunoassays in the Agricultural Environment

Livestock production is increasing significantly as a consequence of the rise in the human population, leading to a higher need for food products and the removal of the 'cap' on milk production in Europe in 2015. A study predicts that worldwide meat production and consumption will increase from 233 million tonnes (in year 2000) to 300 million tonnes (in year 2020), dairy production from 568 to 700 million tonnes and egg production will increase by 30% [32].

8.2.1 Immunoassays in Animal Feedstuffs

The use of antibiotics as feed additives is one of the most effective management tools available to meat/cattle producers [33].

Added in low doses to the feed of farm animals, they improve growth performance. Although most veterinary drugs used in animal production are not harmful to human health, antibiotic residues have the potential to cause the development of antibiotic-resistant strains and allergic reactions. Hence, the EC has imposed maximum residue limits (MRL) for drug residues in food detailed in EC Directives No. 470/2009 and 37/2010 (Table 8.3). In these regulations the use of physicochemical analysis methods such as mass spectrometry are specified. However, as these methods can be expensive time-consuming and require specially trained personnel, the use of rapid cost-effective screening approaches such as immunoassays are increasing in popularity.

Table 8.3 Maximum residue limits (MRL) ng g^{-1} from common drug residues (adapted from Meng et al. [34])

	Veterinary drugs	**MRL (ng g^{-1})**
Antibiotics	Penicillins	4–30
	Tetracyclines	100
	Cephalosporins	100–200
	Polymyxin	50
	Macrolides	40–200
	Aminoglycosides	100–200
Antibacterials	Sulphonamides	100
	Quinolones	50–100
	Diamino pyrimidine derivatives	50
	Nitrofurans	0
	Nitromidazole	0
Anthelmintics	Avermectins	15–40
Growth promoter	Beta-2 sympathomimetic agents	0–0.01
	Steroid hormones	
Sedatives	Chlorpromazine	0

Due to the small size of these drugs and their residues most immunoassays used for their detection are competitive in format. For example, Cooper et al. [35] used a novel carboxyphenyl semicarbazide (SEM) derivative to raise a polyclonal antibody to SEM, the marker residue for the banned nitrofuran veterinary antibiotic nitrofurazone (NFZ). This antibody was incorporated into a direct competitive ELISA format for the detection of SEM in chicken muscle with a detection capability of 0.25 g kg^{-1}, thus satisfying the EU minimum required performance limit of 1 g kg^{-1} for nitrofurans. Samples containing SEM at 0.5–5.0 g kg^{-1} by LC–MS/MS, all screened positive by this ELISA, indicating the utility of this assay in screening samples for the presence of drug residues. A recombinant antibody developed against halofuginone (an antiprotozoal drug used in poultry) was also used in a competitive assay format and showed a limit of detection of 80 pg mL^{-1} well below the MRL of 1 ng mL^{-1} [36].

Polyclonal antibodies are used extensively in immunoassays for the detection of drug residues as they offer the advantage of containing a mixture of antibodies, which can bind to different epitopes on the same compound. A polyclonal antibody was used in a competitive format for the screening of sulphonamide residues in pig muscle and milk [37]. This dipstick ELISA assay had a detection limit of 1–10 μg L^{-1} in buffer for seven sulphonamides and the results correlated well to a validated high-performance liquid chromatographic (HPLC) method. With an assay time of 15 minutes, this test offers simple, rapid and cost-effective 'on-site' screening to detect sulphonamides in pig muscle or milk. Similarly, Zacco et al. [38] developed a novel electrochemical immunosensing strategy for the detection of sulphonamide antibiotics in milk based on magnetic beads coated with class-specific anti-sulphonamide antibodies and a sulphonamide-peroxidase as tracer. While Conzuelo et al. [39] developed a disposable amperometric immunosensor, based on the use of a selective capture antibody and screen-printed carbon electrodes (SPCEs), for the specific detection and quantification of sulphonamide residues in milk. Detection of a number of sulphonimides is more efficient than a single immunoassay for each sulphonimide. The development of such a generic assay for sulphonimides, although it appears reasonably straightforward due to the general similarity in structures, is still proving difficult [40]. Commercial immunoassays for the detection of drug residues such a receptor-based assay dipstick format (Twin sensorBT) for the rapid detection of β-lactams and tetracyclines in raw milk and the Rapid One Step Assay (ROSA®) tests for β-lactams, tetracyclines, enrofloxacin and sulphadimethoxine/sulphamethazine of Charm

Sciences Inc. (Lawrence, MA, USA) are extensively used for milk analysis.

The multiplex detection of drug residues from different classes is extremely beneficial due to the large number of veterinary residues potentially present in a food sample. A flow-based surface plasmon resonance (SPR) assay for the detection of seven compounds (neomycin, gentamicin, kanamycin, and streptomycin, sulphamethazine, chloramphenicol, enrofloxacin), from four different residue classes aminoglycosides, sulphonamides, fenicols and fluoroquinolones using a single sensor chip was developed [41]. The assays for neomycin, kanamycin, streptomycin, enrofloxacin, and sulphamethazine were significantly sensitive for detection in milk at the MRL levels established by the European Union. This represents a powerful screening tool indicative of future developments in the area of drug residue detection.

Natural and synthetic hormones have been widely used in animal husbandry as they can help to increase the growth, feed conversion efficiency and carcass leanness of cattle. They include naturally-occurring steroids such as 17beta-oestradiol, progesterone and testosterone, and their synthetic counterparts zeranol, melengestrol acetate and trenbolone acetate. Although hormonal implants are widely used in countries such as the USA and Australia, the consumption of products containing growth-enhancing drugs and steroids for farm-raised meat animals has been banned by the EU since 1988. Analytical techniques help to achieve the effective surveillance of their prohibited use and immunoassays have been successfully developed for on-site use. For instance, Zhang proposed an immunochromatographic lateral flow for the detection of clenbuterol, a synthesized β-adrenergic agonist (used to treat bronchial obstructions in human medicine but has also been used illegally for promoting animal growth with increased accretion of skeletal muscle mass and decreased accretion of body fat ratio in many species, including cattle, sheep, swine, poultry and man), in swine urine [42]. Huo and colleagues developed a colloidal gold–based lateral-flow assay for the detection of medroxyprogesterone acetate residue. The detection limit was 5 $\mu g\ kg^{-1}$ in standard solutions and 10 $\mu g\ kg^{-1}$ in spiked swine urine and liver samples [43]. The assay time for test was less than 5 min and is suitable for field use. Huo also reported a similar assay for detecting hexoestrol residues in swine urine and liver [44].

8.2.2 Immunoassays for Agricultural Veterinary Infections

Animal diseases are a significant factor in reducing livestock productivity and infectious diseases can have significant economic consequences costing the UK economy over £230 million every year. The use of immunological assays may contribute to improving animal disease control, stimulating food production and enhancing livestock trade. The use of such assays can potentially also avoid serious disease out-breaks and help to determine the prevalence and incidence of infectious diseases within a geographical zone to monitor the efficiency of vaccination programs. The assays involved can either test for the presence of the disease causative agents or for the host's immunological responses to them.

For instance, bovine mastitis, an inflammation of the mammary gland in cows, is a burden for the dairy industry worldwide as it lowers milk yield, reduces milk quality and increases production costs. Economically, bovine mastitis costs around US$2 billion every year to the dairy industry in the United States alone and has been identified as one of the most economically relevant diseases in Ireland by Animal Health Ireland [33, 45]. There is an increased interest in using biomarkers present in milk for mastitis detection. Immunoassays are now available to detect such inflammation-related markers at the different stages of mastitis. For instance, serum amyloid A and haptoglobin are hepatically produced, but they can also be found in the udder of the animal [46, 47]. Both haptoglobin and serum amyloid A have antibacterial functions and thus could be used for the detection of infected animals [48]. Haptoglobin concentrations were reported to increase significantly in plasma and in milk during mastitis and, thus, it could be a possible marker for diagnosis [49]. An assay developed by Hiss had a detection limit of 0.07 mg mL^{-1} in both milk and serum [46], while with the commercially available solid phase-sandwich ELISA (Tridelta Phase TM range serum amyloid A kit, Tridelta Development Ltd, Co. Wicklow, Ireland), Szczubial and his coworkers [50] could detect concentrations of serum amyloid A of up to 322.26 mg mL^{-1} in mastitis milk compared with normal levels of 11.67 mg mL^{-1}.

The early detection of diseases such as bovine tuberculosis and foot-and-mouth disease is critical for the meat industry. Cui et al. [51] developed a rapid and sensitive impedance-based immunosensing method for the detection of antibodies produced due to tuberculosis infection with a limit of detection of 10 ng mL^{-1}. However, distinguishing infected animals from vaccinated animals is a challenge. Whelan et al. [52] reported the performance of a novel multiplex serological test with sera collected from skin-tested animals with bovine tuberculosis, TB-free animals, and cattle vaccinated with *Mycobacterium bovis* BCG. The results showed the test to have a sensitivity range of 77.0–86.5% and thus this assay is suitable for distinguishing vaccinated from infected animals. A similar approach was shown by Gao and colleagues [53] to differentiate infected from vaccinated animals with foot-and-mouth disease virus. An indirect ELISA was developed based on the recombinant 8BF protein and the sensitivity of the assay was 96.8% and the specificities for naive and vaccinated cattle were 99.8% and 99.0%, respectively.

8.2.3 Immunoassays Used to Assist in the Management of Reproduction in Animals

The reproductive management of a herd is of major importance particularly in the dairy industry, where heat detection and time of insemination are vital. In addition, late recognition of unsuccessful insemination can lead to important economic losses due to lower annual milk yields, a lower birth level and the additional cost of extended dry periods. In order to be efficient and profitable, dairy reproductive management requires routine heat detection, which ensures properly timed artificial insemination. Failure to detect the heat of the animal can result in low level of fertility. Currently up to half of oestrus events fail to be detected in the USA and 15% of the animals inseminated are not in heat [54]. Thus, the major application of immunoassays in livestock reproduction involves the measurement of reproductive hormone levels in blood and milk samples.

Progesterone levels fluctuate and accurately reflect the different stages of the oestrous cycle. It is minimal on the day of oestrus, but within two days, secretion increases. Its level reaches its peak on the tenth day after oestrus and remains stable for three to four days until the next oestrus on day 21 [54]. The success of an insemination can be detected if the progesterone concentration remains high between day 18 and day 21. Therefore, monitoring progesterone levels in the animals is a challenging task. It requires development of rapid and sensitive analytical method able to detect and identify appropriate levels of progesterone in complex biological samples (milk and plasma).

Simersky [55] reported the development of an ELISA to estimate the level of progesterone in milk samples using highly specific polyclonal antibodies against 11α-hydroxyprogesterone-hemisuccinate and a conjugate of 11α-hydroxyprogesterone-hemisuccinate with horseradish peroxidase. The test is simple, can be used in 'on-farm' conditions and can be applied in time to facilitate re-insemination in the current oestrus cycle, and hence, one does not wait 28 days to detect a failed or successful insemination. A highly sensitive magnetic nanoparticle enzyme immunoassay of progesterone was established by Ivanova and Godjevargova [56] with a limit of detection of 0.04 ng mL^{-1}.

Immunoassay-based techniques for progesterone detection can be difficult to automate, but a few examples have been reported. Delwiche [57] proposed a biosensor for 'on-line' measurement of progesterone based on the measurement of progesterone in milk at follicular phase concentrations in 'real time'. The assay design involves an anti-progesterone antibody coated on small discs of nitrocellulose membrane inserted in the reaction chamber prior to performance of the assay. The sensor uses computerised micropumps and valves and has a 1 mL sample size requirement. The system could execute a measurement cycle in 10 min and detect progesterone levels between 2 and 10 ng mL^{-1}.

It is clear that immunoassays with improved sensitivity and simple operation are already superseding the traditional enzyme-linked immunosorbent assay for a wide range of applications in agriculture, including determination of contaminants in animal feed, disease diagnosis and veterinary reproduction management.

8.3 Immunoassays in Aquatic Environments

8.3.1 Detection of Marine Toxins

Marine toxins, such as phycotoxins, are naturally occurring contaminants made up of a variety of toxins from different groups of phytoplanktons. Poisoning that results from the ingestion of shellfish contaminated with toxin is classified according to the associated symptoms: neurotoxic shellfish poisoning (NSP), paralytic shellfish poisoning (PSP), amnesic shellfish poisoning (ASP), diarrhetic shellfish poisoning (DSP), and azaspiracid poisoning (AZP). Phycotoxins are also classified according to their chemical properties, for example lipophilic toxins (e.g. okadaic acid (OA), dinophysis toxins, yessotoxins (YTZ), azaspiracid (AZA), pectenotoxins [58] and ciguatera fish poisoning (CFP)) and hydrophilic toxins (e.g. palytoxin, domoic acid (DA) and saxitoxin (STX)) (Table 8.4).

Marine toxins have been monitored for over 20 years in many countries worldwide [59] and much of the testing still relies on the mouse bioassay (MBA), although this is no longer permissible in the EU. Hence, there is a very real need for the development of alternative rapid and effective analytical methods. A description of all methods for the detection of marine toxins is beyond the remit of this chapter; however, they have been extensively reviewed [60–62].

In the early 1990s, Shestowsky et al. [63] described the development of monoclonal anti-okadaic acid (OA) antibodies and anti-idiotypic antibodies, which were both used for the commercial assay provided by Rougier Bio-Tech®. Another commercial kit, DSP-Check® ELISA (SCETI Laboratories, Tokyo, Japan), with a sensitivity of 10 ng mL^{-1}, used an enzyme-conjugated anti-OA monoclonal antibody and has been used widely for research. Its high sensitivity meant it could be used to monitor phytoplankton as an early warning system. Imai et al. [64] demonstrated that OA could be detected in seawater two weeks prior to contamination

Table 8.4 Information on some important marine algal-toxins, their causative species and toxic occurrences

Toxin analogues and size	Chemical properties	Poisoning	Causative genus	Causative species	Location	Regulatory limit in shellfish	Ref.
Azaspiracid (AZA) (20 different analogues exist) thought to be more toxic than OA. (MW > 600 Da)	Nitrogen containing lipophilic polyether	Azaspiracid Shellfish poisoning (AZP)	*Azadinium*	*spinosum, obesum* sp. nov.	Ireland, England, Norway, France, Galacia, NW Portugal, Canada, North West Africa, Denmark and Japan.	AZA1-3 max limit in shellfish 0.16 mg kg^{-1} shellfish meat.	[76–85]
Okadaic Acid (OA) (MW 805 Da) and dinophysis toxins (DTX) (MW > 600 Da)	Lipophilic polyether	Diarrheic shellfish poisoning (DSP)	*Dinophysis* *Prorocentrum*	*acuminate, acuta, rotunda* (and more) *lima*	UK, Ireland, Denmark, Sweden, Norway, France, Spain, Italy, Portugal, The Nederlands, Belguim, Canada, Chile, Japan, Australia and Morocco.	160 μg OA equivalents* kg^{-1} shellfish meat (EU 2008, EFSA reduced OA equivalents to 45 μg OA eq kg^{-1})	[86–91]
Domoic acid (DA) (MW < 500 Da)	Hydrophilic	Amnesic Shellfish Poisoning (ASP)	*Pseudo-nitzschia*	*australis, pungens, multiseries* (and many more)	Canada, UK, Spain, Ireland and Portugal	20 mg kg^{-1}	[79, 92–97]

Saxitoxin (STX) and analogues, (MW < 500 Da)	Hydrophilic	Paralytic shellfish poisoning (PSP)	*Alexandrium*	*catanella, angustitabulatum fundyense, tamarense* (and many more)	USA, EU, Japan, Chile and S. Africa.	0.8 mg kg^{-1} shellfish meat	[79, 98, 99]
			Gymnodinium	*catenatum*			
			Pyrodinium	*bahamense*			
			Aphanizomenon	*flosaquae*	Germany and France		

OA equivalents* expressed as sum of okadaic acid, dinophysis toxins and pectenotoxins.

being detected in shellfish. Sheep polyclonal antibodies against domoic acid (DA) were used in an ELISA that was developed by Garthwaite et al. [65]. The assay could detect DA in seawater at concentrations that were undetectable by HPLC and thus could potentially be useful for early warning of toxin contamination. The method, originally developed by AgResearch (New Zealand), was further optimised by Biosense® Laboratories and approved by the Association of Official Analytical Chemists (AOAC) [66] for quantitation of DA and as an alternative method for monitoring ASP (Commission regulation (EC) No. 1244/2007 of 24 October 2007 amending regulation (EC) No. 2074/2005). Garthwaite et al. [67] presented an integrated ELISA screening system for ASP, DSP, NSP and PSP, to identify contaminated shellfish samples. Suspected positive samples were confirmed by methods approved by international regulatory authorities. Recently, Garet et al. [68] confirmed the possibility of using ELISAs as alternative screening methods for the detection of ASP and PSP, using the Biosense® ELISA for detection of DA and the Ridascreen Fast PSP Test (R-Biopharm AG, Darmstadt, Germany).

The development of lateral flow immunoassays (LFA) for use as screening tools for marine toxins has been demonstrated for the detection of DSP [69], ASP [70] and PSP [71]. The LFA for the detection of PSP was accepted as a screening tool at the Interstate Shellfish Sanitation Conference in 2003. These rapid lateral flow immunochromatographic test kits have been shown to be as efficient as the mouse bioassay (MBA) as a method of screening and are commercially available (www.jellett.ca/www.neogen.com).

Many studies using immunobiosensors have been described for the detection of marine toxins [1, 60]. For instance, Kreuzer et al. [72] developed an immunosensor for the detection of OA and DA, using screen-printed electrodes as the working surface and anti-OA monoclonal and anti-DA polyclonal antibodies as the biological recognition elements. The assays showed a sensitivity of 32 ng mL^{-1} for OA (defined by the ED-50) and limit of detection of 2 ng mL^{-1} for DA. Similarly, Tang et al. [73] produced a disposable immunosensor for OA using a commercial monoclonal antibody, with a limit of detection of 2 ng mL^{-1}. Micheli et al. [74] also developed a disposable immunosensor for DA, with a detection limit of 5 ng

mL^{-1}. Tang et al. [75] also described preliminary studies on the development of a quartz crystal microbalance (QCM) immunosensor for the detection of OA. These assays were still in the preliminary stages of development as no data were given on sample analyses and improvements were needed for high-throughput analysis.

8.3.2 Detection of Freshwater Algal Toxins

Other types of natural occurring contaminants are cyanotoxins, produced by cyanobacteria (Table 8.5). Cyanotoxins are the main toxins associated with fresh-water contamination [100]. The largest group of cyanotoxins are microcystins (MC), which comprise approximately 80 heptapeptide and pentapeptide analogues. Owing to their association with human intoxication and casualties, the World Health Organisation (WHO) has set an acceptable limit of 1 μg L^{-1} of microcystin in drinking water [101]. Antibodies with broad cross-reactivity to the microcystin analogues are a pre-requisite for assay development to monitor their levels.

A sensitive microchip-based ELISA with low sample volume was developed by Pyo and Hahn [102], with a minimum detection level of 0.025 μg L^{-1}. Likewise, a monoclonal antibody from Khreich et al. [103] showed a broad specificity for the microcystin analogues and its application in ELISA resulted in a very sensitive assay (1 fmol of microcystin per mL, WHO threshold 1 pmol mL^{-1}), allowing dilution of samples and hence reduction of matrix effect, and a reproducible assay. A novel immuno-sensing format for the detection of free microcystin-LR to limit of detection of 0.19 ng mL^{-1} was developed using antibody-based optical-planar waveguide platform [104]. This assay can be carried out in less than 20 minutes, uses inexpensive cartridges and low sample volumes. An alternative method of toxin detection is to detect the presence of the cyanobacteria that produce the toxins. Blanco et al. [105] have produced a antibody array (CYANOCHIP) which can detect 17 different strains of cyanobacteria to a level of 100 CFU mL^{-1}.

Commercial ELISA kits are also available from Abraxis LLC, Pennsylvania, USA, Wako Chemicals, Osaka, Japan, EnviroLogix Inc., Portland, ME, USA or Strategic Diagnostics Inc., Newark, DE, USA. Two of these commercial kits (Abraxis LLC and EnviroLogix)

Table 8.5 Information on important freshwater algal-toxins, their causative species and toxic occurrences

Toxin and analogue size	Chemical properties	Poisoning	Causative genus	Causative species	Location	Regulatory limit in drinking water	Ref.
Microcystin (MC) and analogues. (MW 1 KDa)	Hydrophilic, cyclic heptapeptides and pentapeptides	Hepatotoxic	*Microcystis*	*aeruginosa*	Ubiquitous in temperate regions of the world	1 μg L^{-1} in drinking water	[114–117]
			Anabaena	(exact species not fully identified)	Baltic sea		
			Oscillatoria	*aghardii*	Finnish lakes		
			Nodularia	*spumigena*	Western Australia		
Anatoxin, homoanatoxin-a (MW 280 Da)	Hydrophilic, alkaloid	Neurotoxic	*Anabaena*	–	USA, Africa, Asia and Europe and Baltic sea.	Various reports from 1 μg L^{-1} to 61 μg L^{-1} in drinking water	[118–125]
			Aphanizomenon	*issatschenkoi*	North Eastern Germany		
			Planktothrix	*rubescens*	Northern Italy		
Cylindrospermopsin (CYN) (MW 415 Da)	Cytotoxic alkaloid	Cytotoxic, dermatotoxic, genotoxic and hepatotoxic	*Cylindrospermopsis*	*raciborskii*	Australia	1 μg L^{-1} in drinking water	[126–129]

were used in a feasibility study [106]. This group presented a detailed protocol and validation of an integrated multi-method laboratory system for the detection of microcystins and analogues in different aquatic matrices, using kit assays along with a protein phosphatase inhibition (PPI) assay as a screening method, with confirmation of the positive samples on HPLC/PDA and LC-MS/MS. Both assays tested using toxin spiked fresh water samples showed good cross-reactivity to the microcystin analogues and fulfilled the requirements set by the WHO.

'On-site' detection of toxins is highly desirable. A lateral flow immunoassay (LFA) application was described by Kim et al. [107] using an 'in-house' produced monoclonal antibody-based monitoring system that utilised a 'hand-held' fluorescence scanner, making the assay very useful for 'on-site' detection. Two different assay formats were evaluated: antibody immobilised and antigen immobilised, the latter producing better reproducibility and sensitivity. An LFA developed by Khreich et al. [108] using fluorescent liposome-labelled monoclonal antibodies could detect MC levels as low as 0.06 ng mL^{-1}, also using a handheld commercial fluorometer from ESE (US).

A four-channel SPR sensor platform was developed at the Institute of Photonics and Electronics (Prague) and was used for the detection of MC using commercial antibodies (AbKem Iberia S.L., Vigo, Spain). The assay allowed the analysis of 4 samples simultaneously on the instrument's four different flow channels. The assay fulfilled all WHO requirements: sensitivity (0.67 μg L^{-1}) and cross-reactivity to analogues (>85%) [109]. An automated portable array biosensor using Leopard Array Biosensor (Hanson Technologies, USA), a commercial version of the NRL Array Biosensor prototype, that could analyse up to 6 samples at a time and was suitable for on-site testing, has also been described [110].

Although predominately considered a marine toxin, saxitoxin can also be produced by cyanobacteria in fresh water. The multiplex detection of freshwater toxins microcystin, saxitoxin and other major cyanotoxins, was demonstrated by Zhang et al. [111]. In less than 25 minutes, multiple samples for these three cyanotoxins could be analysed in a simple microfluidic chip that has the potential to be fully automated. Similarly, a novel multiplex microarray was developed for the detection of five toxins: domoic acid (DA), okadaic acid (OA, and analogues), saxitoxin (STX, and analogues), cylindrospermopsin (CYN) and microcystins (MC, and analogues) [112]. Detection limits for the 15 min assay were 0.37, 0.44, 0.05, 0.08, and 0.40 ng mL^{-1} for DA, OA, STX, CYN, and MC, respectively. Due to the rapid, easy-to-use and highly sensitive features of this assay it could potentially be used as a screening tool for the aforementioned toxins in water.

Capitalising on the sensitivity of antibodies for the detection of toxins allows multiplex detection of toxins coupled with rapid, easy-to-use assays. One of the major challenges as articulated by Yakes et al. [113] is the development of suitable antibodies which can detect the range of toxins and analogues and can be effectively utilised to develop rapid assays for toxin detection in water. These challenges are now being addressed.

8.4 Conclusion

The need for rapid detection of food contaminants, either directly in the food we eat or indirectly in the marine or agriculture environment providing the food, has resulted in the development of highly sensitive immunoassays. Improvements in technology lead to rapid sample preparation, the removal of matrix-associated inhibitors and the detection of food contaminants below the maximum limits set in legislation. The development of rapid, simple and inexpensive assays has potential for screening for contaminants. However, in order for the food industry to routinely use immunoassays, further development is required to make systems that are universal (e.g. applicable to multiple food types and contaminants) and portable.

The production of food that is safe to consume is vital to the continued growth of the food sector and as a result it becomes an absolute necessity to provide companies with techniques that allow them to monitor contamination in industrial food-producing plants in a fast, safe and efficient manner. Promising immunoassay developments coupled with advances in microfluidics and miniaturised devices could make portable, rapid, sensitive, easy-to-use diagnostic tools for in situ food contaminant detection a reality. As a consequence, 'farm-to-fork' monitoring of food for contaminants will reduce the number of foodborne incidents, thus increasing consumer confidence in the quality and safety of food thereby strengthening the competiveness of the industry.

Useful Information

European Food Safety Authority http://www.efsa.europa.eu/

US Food and Drug Administration http://www.fda.gov/

Eurosurveillance http://www.eurosurveillance.org/

EU Legislation

Regulations (EEC) No. 315/93 and (EC) No 1881/2006 sets maximum levels for certain contaminants in foodstuffs.

Commission regulation (EC) No. 2073/2005 sets limits for microbes and recommended detection methods.

Commission Regulation (EC) 1126/2007 and Commission Regulation (EU) 165/2010 set maximum residues limits (MRL) for mycotoxins in food.

Commission regulation (EC) No. 470/2009 and EU No. 37/2010 sets maximum residues limits (MRL) for drug residues in food.

References

1. Byrne, B., et al., Antibody-based sensors: principles, problems and potential for detection of pathogens and associated toxins. *Sensors (Basel)*, 2009. **9**(6):4407–4445.
2. Bohaychuk, V.M., et al., Evaluation of detection methods for screening meat and poultry products for the presence of foodborne pathogens. *J Food Prot*, 2005. **68**(12):2637–2647.
3. McGrath, T.F., et al., Development of a rapid low cost fluorescent biosensor for the detection of food contaminants. *Biosens Bioelectron*, 2013. **41**:96–102.

4. Davis, D., et al., Gold Nanoparticle-modified carbon electrode biosensor for the detection of *Listeria monocytogenes*. *Ind Biotech*, 2013. **9**(1):31–36.
5. Sharma, H. and R. Mutharasan, Rapid and sensitive immunodetection of *Listeria monocytogenes* in milk using a novel piezoelectric cantilever sensor. *Biosens Bioelectron*, 2013. **45**:158–162.
6. Wang, Z., et al., Ultrasensitive chemiluminescent immunoassay of Salmonella with silver enhancement of nanogold labels. *Luminescence*, 2011. **26**(2):136–141.
7. Cao, C., et al., Dual enlargement of gold nanoparticles: from mechanism to scanometric detection of pathogenic bacteria. *Small*, 2011. **7**(12):1701–1708.
8. Fu, J., et al., An Au/Si hetero-nanorod-based biosensor for Salmonella detection. *Nanotechnology*, 2008. **19**(15):155502.
9. Lee, Y.C., et al., Chicken single-chain variable fragments against the SARS-CoV spike protein. *J Virol Methods*, 2007. **146**(1–2):104–111.
10. Dungchai, W., et al., *Salmonella typhi* determination using voltammetric amplification of nanoparticles: a highly sensitive strategy for metalloimmunoassay based on a copper-enhanced gold label. *Talanta*, 2008. **77**(2):727–732.
11. Zhao, Y., et al., Simultaneous detection of multifood-borne pathogenic bacteria based on functionalized quantum dots coupled with immunomagnetic separation in food samples. *J Agric Food Chem*, 2009. **57**(2):517–524.
12. Marinakos, S.M., S. Chen, and A. Chilkoti, Plasmonic detection of a model analyte in serum by a gold nanorod sensor. *Anal Chem*, 2007. **79**(14):5278–5283.
13. Viswanathan, S., C. Rani, and J.A. Ho, Electrochemical immunosensor for multiplexed detection of food-borne pathogens using nanocrystal bioconjugates and MWCNT screen-printed electrode. *Talanta*, 2012. **94**:315–319.
14. Hochel, I., et al., Detection of Campylobacter species in foods by indirect competitive ELISA using hen and rabbit antibodies. *Food Agric Immunol*, 2007. **18**(3–4):151–167.
15. Kim, S.H., et al., Development of a sandwich ELISA for the detection of Listeria spp. using specific flagella antibodies. *J Vet Sci*, 2005. **6**(1):41–46.

16. Leonard, P., et al., A generic approach for the detection of whole *Listeria monocytogenes* cells in contaminated samples using surface plasmon resonance. *Biosens Bioelectron*, 2004. **19**(10):1331–1335.
17. Zhao, X., et al., A rapid bioassay for single bacterial cell quantitation using bioconjugated nanoparticles. *Proc Natl Acad Sci U S A*, 2004. **101**(42):15027–15032.
18. Meeusen, C.A., E.C. Alocilja, and W.N. Osburn, Detection of *E. coli* O157:H7 using a miniaturized surface plasmon resonance biosensor. *Trans Am Soc Agric Eng*, 2005. **48**(6):2409–2416.
19. Campbell, G.A. and R. Mutharasan, A method of measuring *Escherichia coli* O157:H7 at 1 cell/mL in 1 liter sample using antibody functionalized piezoelectric-excited millimeter-sized cantilever sensor. *Environ Sci Technol*, 2007. **41**(5):1668–1674.
20. Gilmartin, N. and R. O'Kennedy, Nanobiotechnologies for the detection and reduction of pathogens. *Enzyme Microb Technol*, 2012. **50**(2):87–95.
21. Wang, Y., S. Ravindranath, and J. Irudayaraj, Separation and detection of multiple pathogens in a food matrix by magnetic SERS nanoprobes. *Anal Bioanal Chem*, 2011. **399**(3):1271–1278.
22. Hossain, S.M., et al., Multiplexed paper test strip for quantitative bacterial detection. *Anal Bioanal Chem*, 2012. **403**(6):1567–1576.
23. Ho, J.A., et al., Liposome-based immunostrip for the rapid detection of Salmonella. *Anal Bioanal Chem*, 2008. **391**(2):479–485.
24. Cho, I.H. and J. Irudayaraj, In-situ immuno-gold nanoparticle network ELISA biosensors for pathogen detection. *Int J Food Microbiol*, 2013. **164**(1):70–75.
25. Blažková, M., et al., Development of a nucleic acid lateral flow immunoassay for simultaneous detection of Listeria spp. and *Listeria monocytogenes* in food. *Eur Food Res Technol*, 2009. **229**(6):867–874.
26. Chai, Y., et al., A surface-scanning coil detector for real-time, in-situ detection of bacteria on fresh food surfaces. *Biosens Bioelectron*, 2013. **50**:311–317.
27. EHEC/HUS O104:H4 The outbreak is considered to be over. Press release from Robert Koch-Institute, 2001.
28. Zhang, W., et al., New immuno-PCR assay for detection of low concentrations of Shiga toxin 2 and its variants. *J Clin Microbiol*, 2008. **46**(4):1292–1297.

29. Harteveld, J.L., M.S. Nieuwenhuizen, and E.R. Wils, Detection of staphylococcal enterotoxin B employing a piezoelectric crystal immunosensor. *Biosens Bioelectron*, 1997. **12**(7):661–667.
30. Rowe-Taitt, C.A., et al., Array biosensor for detection of biohazards. *Biosens Bioelectron*, 2000. **14**(10–11):785–794.
31. Pauly, D., et al., Simultaneous quantification of five bacterial and plant toxins from complex matrices using a multiplexed fluorescent magnetic suspension assay. *Analyst*, 2009. **134**(10):2028–2039.
32. Delgado, C., et al., Livestock to 2020: The Next Food Revolution. Food Agriculture and Discussion Paper No. 28. International Food Policy Research Institute, Food and Agriculture Organization, International Livestock Research Institute, 1999.
33. Geary, U., et al., Estimating the effect of mastitis on the profitability of Irish dairy farms. *J Dairy Sci*, 2012. **95**(7):3662–3673.
34. Meng, M. and R. Xi, Review: current development of immunoassay for analyzing veterinary drug residue in foods and food products. *Anal Lett*, 2011. **44**(15):2543–2558.
35. Cooper, K.M., et al., Enzyme immunoassay for semicarbazide–the nitrofuran metabolite and food contaminant. *Anal Chim Acta*, 2007. **592**(1):64–71.
36. Fitzgerald, J., et al., Light-chain shuffling from an antigen-biased phage pool allows 185-fold improvement of an anti-halofuginone single-chain variable fragment. *Anal Biochem*, 2011. **410**(1):27–33.
37. Zhang, H., Y. Zhang, and S. Wang, Development of flow-through and dipstick immunoassays for screening of sulfonamide residues. *J Immunol Methods*, 2008. **337**(1):1–6.
38. Zacco, E., et al., Electrochemical magneto immunosensing of antibiotic residues in milk. *Biosens Bioelectron*, 2007. **22**(9–10):2184–2191.
39. Conzuelo, F., et al., Disposable and integrated amperometric immunosensor for direct determination of sulfonamide antibiotics in milk. *Biosens Bioelectron*, 2012. **36**(1):81–88.
40. Zhang, H. and S. Wang, Review on enzyme-linked immunosorbent assays for sulfonamide residues in edible animal products. *J Immunol Methods*, 2009. **350**(1–2):1–13.
41. Rebe Raz, S., et al., Label-free and multiplex detection of antibiotic residues in milk using imaging surface plasmon resonance-based immunosensor. *Anal Chem*, 2009. **81**(18):7743–7749.

42. Zhang, G.P., et al., Development of an immunochromatographic lateral flow test strip for detection of beta-adrenergic agonist Clenbuterol residues. *J Immunol Methods*, 2006. **312**(1–2):27–33.

43. Huo, T.M., et al., Development of colloidal gold-based immunochromatographic assay for the rapid detection of medroxyprogesterone acetate residues. *Food Agric Immunol*, 2006. **17**(3–4):183–190.

44. Huo, T.M., et al., Immumochromatographic assay for determination of hexoestrol residues. *Eur Food Res Technol*, 2007. **225**(5–6):743–747.

45. Viguier, C., et al., Mastitis detection: current trends and future perspectives. *Trends Biotechnol*, 2009. **27**(8):486–493.

46. Hiss, S., et al., Haptoglobin concentrations in blood and milk after endotoxin challenge and quantification of mammary Hp mRNA expression. *J Dairy Sci*, 2004. **87**(11):3778–3784.

47. McDonald, T.L., et al., Elevated extrahepatic expression and secretion of mammary-associated serum amyloid A 3 (M-SAA3) into colostrum. *Vet Immunol Immunopathol*, 2001. **83**(3–4):203–211.

48. Eckersall, P.D. and R. Bell, Acute phase proteins: Biomarkers of infection and inflammation in veterinary medicine. *Vet J*, 2010. **185**(1):23–27.

49. Åkerstedt, M., et al., Relationship between haptoglobin and serum amyloid A in milk and milk quality. *Int Dairy J*, 2008. **18**(6):669–674.

50. Szczubial, M., et al., Concentration of serum amyloid A and ceruloplasmin activity in milk from cows with subclinical mastitis caused by different, pathogens. *Pol J Vet Sci*, 2012. **15**(2):291–296.

51. Cui, H., et al., An AC electrokinetic impedance immunosensor for rapid detection of tuberculosis. *Analyst*, 2013. **138**(23):7188–7196.

52. Whelan, C., et al., Performance of the enferplex TB assay with cattle in Great Britain and assessment of its suitability as a test to distinguish infected and vaccinated animals. *Clin Vaccine Immunol*, 2010. **17**(5):813–817.

53. Gao, M.C., et al., An ELISA based on the repeated foot-and-mouth disease virus 3B epitope peptide can distinguish infected and vaccinated cattle. *Appl Microbiol Biotechnol*, 2012. **93**(3):1271–1279.

54. O'Connor, M., *Heat Detection and Timing of Insemination for Cattle*. College of Agricultural Sciences and Cooperative Extension: Penn State University. Vol. 402, 1993.

55. Simersky, R., et al., Development of an ELISA-based kit for the on-farm determination of progesterone in milk. *Verinarni Medicina*, 2007. **52**:19–28.

56. Ivanova, T. and T. Godjevargova, Sensitive progesterone determination using a magnetic particle-based enzyme-linked immunosorbent assay. *Anal Lett*, 2014. **48**(5):843–860.
57. Delwiche, M., et al., Improved biosensor for measurement of progesterone in bovine milk. *Trans Am Soc Agric Eng*, 2001. **44**(6):1997–2002.
58. Hess, P., Requirements for screening and confirmatory methods for the detection and quantification of marine biotoxins in end-product and official control. *Anal Bioanal Chem*, 2010. **397**(5):1683–1694.
59. Humbert, J.F., Advances in the detection of phycotoxins and cyanotoxins. *Anal Bioanal Chem*, 2010. **397**(5):1653–1654.
60. Campas, M., B. Prieto-Simon, and J.L. Marty, Biosensors to detect marine toxins: assessing seafood safety. *Talanta*, 2007. **72**(3):884–895.
61. Vilarino, N., et al., Biological methods for marine toxin detection. *Anal Bioanal Chem*, 2010. **397**(5):1673–1681.
62. Campbell, K., et al., A European perspective on progress in moving away from the mouse bioassay for marine-toxin analysis. *Trends Anal Chem*, 2011. **30**(2):239–253.
63. Shestowsky, W.S., M.A. Quilliam, and H.M. Sikorska, An idiotypic-anti-idiotypic competitive immunoassay for quantitation of okadaic acid. *Toxicon*, 1992. **30**(11):1441–1418.
64. Imai, I., et al., Monitoring of DSP toxins in small-sized plankton fraction of seawater collected in Mutsu Bay, Japan, by ELISA method: relation with toxin contamination of scallop. *Mar Pollut Bull*, 2003. **47**(1–6):114–117.
65. Garthwaite, I., et al., Polyclonal antibodies to domoic acid, and their use in immunoassays for domoic acid in sea water and shellfish. *Nat Toxins*, 1998. **6**(3–4):93–104.
66. Horwitz, W., ed. Domoic acid in mussels, liquid chromatographic method. Official Methods of Analysis of AOAC International, AOAC International: Gaithersburg, Maryland, USA, 2000.
67. Garthwaite, I., et al., Integrated enzyme-linked immunosorbent assay screening system for amnesic, neurotoxic, diarrhetic, and paralytic shellfish poisoning toxins found in New Zealand. *J AOAC Int*, 2001. **84**(5):1643–1648.
68. Garet, E., et al., Comparative evaluation of enzyme-linked immunoassay and reference methods for the detection of shellfish hydrophilic toxins in several presentations of seafood. *J Agric Food Chem*, 2010. **58**(3):1410–1415.

69. Laycock, M.V., et al., First report of a new rapid assay for diarrhetic shellfish poisoning toxins. *Harmful Algae*, 2006. **5**:74–78.
70. Jellett, J.F., M.V. Laycock, and M.A. Quilliam, Developments in rapid test kit for toxin testing (PSP, ASP and DSP). *Proc 6th Irish Shellfish Safety Scientific Workshop*, 2006. **23**:77–81.
71. Laycock, M.V., M.A. Donovan, and D.J. Easy, Sensitivity of lateral flow tests to mixtures of saxitoxins and applications to shellfish and phytoplankton monitoring. *Toxicon*, 2010. **55**(2–3):597–605.
72. Kreuzer, M.P., et al., Novel electrochemical immunosensors for seafood toxin analysis. *Toxicon*, 2002. **40**(9):1267–1274.
73. Tang, A., et al., Immunosensor for the determination of okadaic acid based on screen-printed electrode. *Int J Environ Anal Chem*, 2003. **83**(7–8):663–670.
74. Micheli, L., et al., Disposable immunosensor for the determination of domoic acid in shellfish. *Biosens Bioelectron*, 2004. **20**(2):190–196.
75. Tang, A.X.J., et al., Immunosensor for okadaic acid using quartz crystal microbalance. *Anal Chim Acta*, 2002. **471**(1):33–40.
76. Regel, E., Regulation (EC) No 853/2004 of the European Parliment and of the Council of 29 April 2004 laying down specific hygiene rules for food of animal origin, O.J.E. Commun., Editor 2004: OJ L 139.
77. Tillmann, U., et al., Azadinium spinosum gen. et sp. nov. (Dinophyceae) identified as a primary producer of azaspiracid toxins. *Eur J Phycol*, 2009. **44**:63–79.
78. Ryan, M., et al., Azaspiracids: Assessment and management of biotoxins risks in bivalve molluscs, in *Food and Agricultural Organization of the United Nations* 2011, Rome.
79. Gerssen, A., et al., Marine toxins: chemistry, toxicity, occurrence and detection, with special reference to the Dutch situation. *Toxins (Basel)*, 2010. **2**(4):878–904.
80. Marine biotoxins in shellfish - Azaspiracid group, *European Food Safety Authority: The EFSA Journal*, 2008. **723**:1–52.
81. Amzil, Z., et al., First report on azaspiracid and yessotoxin groups detection in French shellfish. *Toxicon*, 2008. **52**(1):39–48.
82. Vale, P., R. Bire, and P. Hess, Confirmation by LC-MS/MS of azaspiracids in shellfish from the Portuguese north-western coast. *Toxicon*, 2008. **51**(8):1449–1456.
83. Taleb, H., et al., First detection of azaspiracids in mussels in north west Africa. *J Shellfish Res*, 2006. **25**:1067–1070.

84. Krock, B., U. Tillmann, and A. Cembella. Isolation and toxin composition of the azaspiracid-producing dinoflagellate *Azadinium spinosum* from the Danish west coast, in *Oral presentation at the 7th Intl. Conf. Molluscan Shellfish Safety,* 2009. Nantes, France.
85. Ueoka, R., et al., Isolation of azaspiracid-2 from a marine sponge Echinoclathria sp. as a potent cytotoxin. *Toxicon*, 2009. **53**(6):680–684.
86. Garcia, C., et al., Metabolic transformation of dinophysistoxin-3 into dinophysistoxin-1 causes human intoxication by consumption of O-acyl-derivatives dinophysistoxins contaminated shellfish. *J Toxicol Sci*, 2005. **30**(4):287–296.
87. Scoging, A. and M. Bahl, Diarrhetic shellfish poisoning in the UK. *Lancet*, 1998. **352**(9122):117.
88. Elgarch, A., et al., Detection of diarrheic shellfish poisoning and azaspiracid toxins in Moroccan mussels: comparison of the LC-MS method with the commercial immunoassay kit. *Mar Drugs*, 2008. **6**(4):587–594.
89. Vilarino, N., et al., Innovative detection methods for aquatic algal toxins and their presence in the food chain. *Anal Bioanal Chem*, 2013. **405**(24):7719–7732.
90. Sassolas, A., et al., Detection of the marine toxin okadaic acid: assessing seafood safety. *Talanta*, 2013. **105**:306–316.
91. Prego-Faraldo, M.V., et al., Okadaic acid meet and greet: an insight into detection methods, response strategies and genotoxic effects in marine invertebrates. *Mar Drugs*, 2013. **11**(8):2829–2845.
92. Perl, T.M., et al., An outbreak of toxic encephalopathy caused by eating mussels contaminated with domoic acid. *N Engl J Med*, 1990. **322**(25):1775–1780.
93. Campbell, D.A., et al., Amnesic shellfish poisoning in the king scallop, *Pecten maximus*, from the west coast of Scotland. *J Shellfish Res*, 2001. **20**:75–84.
94. Blanco, J., et al., Effect of phytoplankton containing paralytic shellfish and amnesic shellfish toxins on the culture of the king scallop, *Pecten maximus* in Malaga (SE Spain). *Aquat Living Resour*, 2006. **19**:267–273.
95. James, K.J., et al., Amnesic shellfish poisoning toxins in bivalve molluscs in Ireland. *Toxicon*, 2005. **46**(8):852–858.
96. Vale, P. and M.A. Sampayo, Domoic acid in Portuguese shellfish and fish. *Toxicon*, 2001. **39**(6):893–904.
97. Horowitz, W., ed. *AOAC Official Method of Analysis*. International AOAC2000: AOAC International, Gaithersburg.

98. Etheridge, S.M., Paralytic shellfish poisoning: seafood safety and human health perspectives. *Toxicon*, 2010. **56**(2):108–122.

99. Wiese, M., et al., Neurotoxic alkaloids: saxitoxin and its analogs. *Mar Drugs*, 2010. **8**(7):2185–2211.

100. Neilan, B.A., et al., Environmental conditions that influence toxin biosynthesis in cyanobacteria. *Environ Microbiol*, 2013. **15**(5):1239–1253.

101. World Health Organization (WHO), Cyanobacterial Toxins: microcystin-LR in drinking water, background document for development of WHO guidelines for drinking-water quality. 2003, World Health Organization, Geneva: Addendum to Vol. 2 Health criteria and other supporting information.

102. Pyo, D. and J.H. Hahn, Determination of trace amount of cyanobacterial toxin in water by microchip based enzyme-linked immunosorbent assay. *J Immunoassay Immunochem*, 2009. **30**(1):97–105.

103. Khreich, N., et al., A highly sensitive competitive enzyme immunoassay of broad specificity quantifying microcystins and nodularins in water samples. *Toxicon*, 2009. **53**(5):551–559.

104. Murphy, C., et al., Detection of the cyanobacterial toxin, microcystin-LR, using a novel recombinant antibody-based optical-planar waveguide platform. *Biosens Bioelectron*, 2015. **67**:708–714.

105. Blanco, Y., et al., CYANOCHIP: an antibody microarray for high-taxonomical-resolution cyanobacterial monitoring. *Environ Sci Technol*, 2015. **49**(3):1611–1620.

106. Triantis, T., et al., Development of an integrated laboratory system for the monitoring of cyanotoxins in surface and drinking waters. *Toxicon*, 2010. **55**(5):979–989.

107. Kim, Y.M., et al., Development of an ultrarapid one-step fluorescence immunochromatographic assay system for the quantification of microcystins. *Environ Sci Technol*, 2003. **37**(9):1899–1904.

108. Khreich, N., et al., A fluorescent immunochromatographic test using immunoliposomes for detecting microcystins and nodularins. *Anal Bioanal Chem*, 2010. **397**(5):1733–1742.

109. Herranz, S., et al., An SPR biosensor for the detection of microcystins in drinking water. *Anal Bioanal Chem*, 2010. **398**(6):2625–2634.

110. Herranz, S., M.D. Marazuela, and M.C. Moreno-Bondi, Automated portable array biosensor for multisample microcystin analysis in freshwater samples. *Biosens Bioelectron*, 2012. **33**(1):50–55.

111. Zhang, J., et al., Rapid detection of algal toxins by microfluidic immunoassay. *Lab Chip*, 2011. **11**(20):3516–3522.
112. McNamee, S.E., et al., Development of a planar waveguide microarray for the monitoring and early detection of five harmful algal toxins in water and cultures. *Environ Sci Technol*, 2014. **48**(22):13340–13349.
113. Yakes, B.J., S.M. Prezioso, and S.L. DeGrasse, Developing improved immunoassays for paralytic shellfish toxins: the need for multiple, superior antibodies. *Talanta*, 2012. **99**:668–676.
114. Bell, S.G. and G.A. Codd, Cyanobacterial toxins and human health. *Rev Med Microbiol*, 1994. **5**:256–264.
115. Halinen, K., et al., Direct evidence for production of microcystins by Anabaena strains from the Baltic sea. *Appl Environ Microbiol*, 2007. **73**(20):6543–6550.
116. Luukkainen, R., et al., Isolation and identification of eight microcystins from thirteen *Oscillatoria agardhii* strains and structure of a new microcystin. *Appl Environ Microbiol*, 1993. **59**(7):2204–2209.
117. Falconer, I.R., A. Choice, and W. Hosja, Toxicity of edible mussels (Mytilus edulis) growing naturally in an estuary during a water bloom of the blue-green alga *Nodularia spumigena*. *Environ Toxicol Water Qual*, 1992. **7**(2):119–123.
118. Osswald, J., et al., Toxicology and detection methods of the alkaloid neurotoxin produced by cyanobacteria, anatoxin-a. *Environ Int*, 2007. **33**(8):1070–1089.
119. Ballot, A., et al., Cyanobacterial toxins in Lake Baringo, Kenya. *Limnologica*, 2003. **33**(1):2–9.
120. Namikoshi, M., et al., Simultaneous production of homoanatoxin-a, anatoxin-a, and a new non-toxic 4-hydroxyhomoanatoxin-a by the cyanobacterium *Raphidiopsis mediterranea* Skuja. *Toxicon*, 2003. **42**(5):533–538.
121. Carrasco, D., et al., Anatoxin-a occurrence and potential cyanobacterial anatoxin-a producers in Spanish reservoirs. *J Phycol*, 2007. **43**(6):1120–1125.
122. Gugger, M., et al., First report in a river in France of the benthic cyanobacterium *Phormidium favosum* producing anatoxin-a associated with dog neurotoxicosis. *Toxicon*, 2005. **45**(7):919–928.
123. Codd, G.A., Eutrophication, blooms and toxins of cyanobacteria (blue-green algae), and health. In A.Z. Keller and H.C. Wilson, eds. Proceedings of the Fourth Disaster Prevention and Limitation Conference. The

changing face of Europe: Disasters, pollution and the environment. Vol. 14. 1992, University of Bradford: Aquatic problems. pp. 33–62.

124. van Apeldoorn, M.E., et al., Toxins of cyanobacteria. *Mol Nutr Food Res*, 2007. **51**(1):7–60.

125. Ballot, A., et al., First report of anatoxin-a-producing cyanobacterium *Aphanizomenon issatschenkoi* in northeastern Germany. *Toxicon*, 2010. **56**(6):964–971.

126. de la Cruz, A.A., et al., A review on cylindrospermopsin: the global occurrence, detection, toxicity and degradation of a potent cyanotoxin. *Environ Sci Processes Impacts*, 2013. **15**(11):1979–2003.

127. Hawkins, P.R., et al., Severe hepatotoxicity caused by the tropical cyanobacterium (blue-green alga) *Cylindrospermopsis raciborskii* (Woloszynska) Seenaya and Subba Raju isolated from a domestic water supply reservoir. *Appl Environ Microbiol*, 1985. **50**:1292–1295.

128. Preussel, K., et al., First report on cylindrospermopsin producing *Aphanizomenon flos-aquae* (Cyanobacteria) isolated from two German lakes. *Toxicon*, 2006. **47**(2):156–162.

129. Brient, L., et al., First occurrence of cylindrospermopsin in freshwater in France. *Environ Toxicol*, 2009. **24**(4):415–420.

Chapter 9

Next-Generation Immunoassays

Valerie Fitzgerald and Paul Leonard
School of Biotechnology, Dublin City University, Glasnevin, Collins Avenue, Dublin 9, Ireland
valerie.fitzgerald4@mail.dcu.ie

The immunoassay has advanced tremendously since its introduction in 1959 [1]. These advances are driven by the need for sensitive, specific, rapid and robust detection systems while reducing costs and removing the need for highly skilled operators. Advances in immunoassay efficiency tend to focus predominantly in two areas: the first is improvement of the bio-recognition element (i.e. antibody) and the second focuses on enhancement of the detection platform. The purpose of this chapter is to detail advances in each of these areas as well as providing a focus on future directions for immunoassay.

9.1 History of the Immunoassay

The impact of the development of the immunoassay is clearly evidenced by the number used as standard methodologies in quality assessment, medical testing, diagnostics as well as a plethora of other laboratory settings [2]. It is therefore surprising that its evolution only began less than 60 years ago, when the

Immunoassays: Development, Applications and Future Trends
Edited by Richard O'Kennedy and Caroline Murphy

ISBN 978-981-4669-97-9 (Hardcover), 978-1-315-20654-7 (eBook)
www.panstanford.com

first immunoassay, a radioimmunoassay for the measurement of endogenous plasma insulin, was described by Berson and Yalow [1]. This work, for which Yalow received the Nobel Prize in 1977, led to the introduction of thousands of novel immunoassays over the next five decades.

While the first immunoassay described the use of a radioisotope for labelling, the technical and safety implications involved led to the development of alternative labels such as enzymes and fluorophores. The loss of sensitivity involved in the switch from radioimmunoassay was not overcome until 1976, when the use of chemiluminescence labelling was described [3]. Indeed the majority of commercial automated immunoassay analysers now make use of chemiluminescence because the analytical sensitivity is equal to or exceeds that of radiolabels [4].

Another scientific discovery, which greatly influenced the proliferation of immunoassay techniques was that of monoclonal antibody production. In 1975, Kohler and Milstein described the process of fusing a mouse myeloma cell with a B lymphocyte isolated from the spleen of a mouse that had been immunised with an antigen of interest [5]. This in vitro synthesis of specific monoclonal antibodies circumvented the limitations imposed when using polyclonal antibodies, namely limited source material. In addition, the availability of large volumes of antibody allowed for the development of non-competitive sandwich immunoassays, which are now a mainstay for automated immunoassays [4].

9.2 Evolution of the Immunoassay

Traditional style immunoassays based on the 96-well microtitre plate format are commonplace in analytical laboratories and, with the introduction of robotics in recent years, have become more and more automated thus increasing assay throughput. An example of such a robotic system, used in our laboratory, is shown in Fig. 9.1.

Indeed the majority of clinical analysers found in hospital laboratories are practically 'self-contained labs' with accurate, precise and highly reproducible programmed-liquid-handling, sample addition and washing steps. However, besides cost, the size limitation

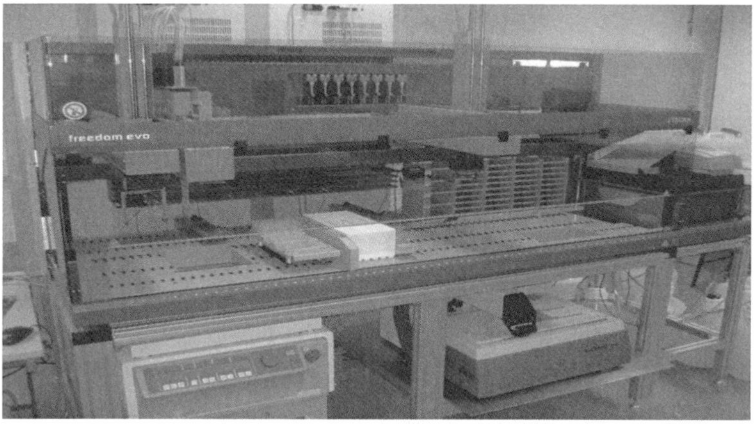

Figure 9.1 High-throughput robotic antibody screening system. The major component of this system is the Tecan freedom EVO 200 liquid handling workstation. This workstation contains a work table, three robotic arms (ecentric gripper, centric gripper and a LiHa [liquid handling arm]), one shelf and a storage rack (hotel) for storing microtiter and deep-well plates, plate holders on the worktable and a number of reagent troughs. In addition, the external pieces of equipment are shaking incubators, a centrifuge, a colony picker and waste and reagent bottles.

of these automated analysers means they are not suitable for remote applications such as point-of-care (POC) testing. This market segment has traditionally been dominated by nitrocellulose-based lateral flow assays providing a rapid user-friendly solution to a clear diagnostic need. Unfortunately, these type of tests (e.g. pregnancy tests) are usually only qualitative (pregnant/not pregnant) or at best semi-qualitative. The caveat of the ease of use and flexibility of these devices is that increased variability, and, therefore, reduced sensitivity, is often associated with their use.

Advances in microfluidics, detection strategies, antibody engineering and immunoassay readers have resulted in the development of new, 'next-generation' rapid POC diagnostics that are approaching the sensitivities of current 'gold standard' clinical analysers. This section will evaluate advances in antibody engineering, signal generation and platform design and highlight key improvements over traditional methods.

9.3 Improvements in Antibody Development

The key characteristics of antibodies, predominantly their high affinity and specificity for a binding partner, have led to their utilisation in many varied applications in diagnostic, biotechnology and biomedical fields.

The introduction of hybridoma technology in 1975 and the consequent ability to generate monoclonal antibodies (mAbs) led to a surge in antibody research and development. As a result, the field of monoclonal antibody discovery has developed into a thriving industry and has had a profound impact by providing a diverse source of therapeutic, diagnostic and research reagents. The global demand for immunoassay testing was nearly \$15.6 billion in 2011 and \$16.3 billion in 2012. This market is expected to grow to \$20.5 billion by 2017 [6] with research antibodies reaching \$2 billion in 2013 and nearly \$2.2 billion in 2014 and the market expected to reach nearly \$3 billion in 2019 [7].

Therapeutic use of mAbs has become a major part of treatments in various diseases, including transplantation, oncology, autoimmune, cardiovascular and infectious diseases. With over 40 approved mAb products and an unprecedented number of mAb-based therapeutics in clinical trials mAbs have become the fastest growing class of biological drug [8]. Initial issues resulting from immunogenicity of murine mAbs have been reduced, or removed, by the development of methods to produce chimeric, humanised and fully human antibodies [9]. The global market for antibody drugs was worth nearly \$63.4 billion in 2013. This market is expected to grow, resulting in totals near \$122.6 billion globally in 2019, according to BCC Research [10].

While these figures clearly demonstrate its success, the initial impact of monoclonal antibody technology was somewhat hindered by unwanted immune responses to murine antibodies in patients. Additional limitations include poor immunogenicity of some targets and general issues with expression of full-length antibodies, glycosylation patterns and the lack of purification tags [11]. An additional consideration when looking at the monetary outlay for these products is their effectiveness. The use of companion diagnostics could clearly be of huge benefit, if employed as standard with the roll out of any new therapeutic, to ascertain initial suitability to treatment and subsequently monitor effectiveness of the drug on each patient. Indeed drugs such as Erbitux, Herceptin, Glivex and Plavix are all seen to be highly dependent on an efficient diagnostic marketplace, and have benefitted greatly from the experience [12].

The challenge of circumventing these limitations coupled with the requirement for large quantities of high quality antibodies led to the emergence of methods for their creation, without the use of hybridoma technology. Commonly described as display methods, an array of approaches for generation of recombinant antibodies have now become commonplace in modern laboratories. The predominant processes, which include phage display, yeast display, bacterial display, ribosome display and mRNA display, are discussed below. A comparison of methods for the production of monoclonal antibodies, mentioned in this chapter, is represented in Fig. 9.2. It is important to note that while the majority of focus has been placed on the potential of antibodies as novel therapeutics the progress in the field of antibody generation, selection and manipulation has been used to great advantage in other settings. Antibodies are one of the most widely used tools in modern biochemistry, cytology and clinical chemistry as well as in the field of diagnostics [13].

9.3.1 Antibody Engineering

In recent years, the emergence of recombinant antibody display technologies has transformed the way in which we generate antibodies for the specific detection of a chosen analyte. Moreover, modifications are easily introduced in the primary antibody sequence, leading to affinity maturations, often resulting in higher affinity for binding to the antigen, generation of fusion proteins and addition of detection and purification tags. Additionally, the use of recombinant technology allows us to overcome what is termed the 'affinity ceiling' of antibodies produced in vivo and provide libraries of higher diversity than those generated in the natural immune response [14]. Display technology gives us the ability to choose those ligands which have the desired biological properties and permits us to synthesize 'tailor-made' antibodies for use in diagnosis, immunotherapy or for immunoassay development.

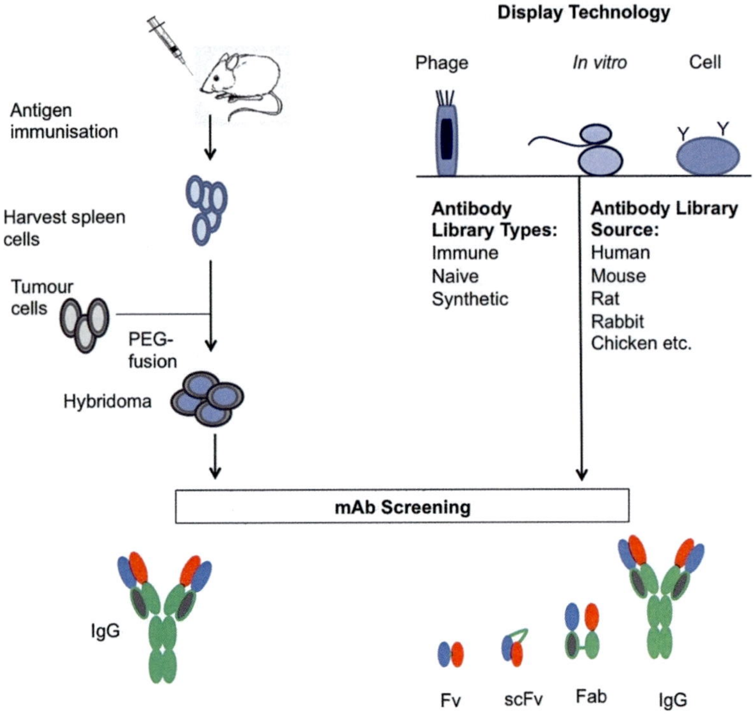

Figure 9.2 Schematic representation of the different approaches used to produce monoclonal antibodies. The traditional hybridoma technology for obtaining mouse antibodies is shown on the left. The right shows the main procedures for obtaining antibodies through display systems (phage, in vitro and cell display). With display technologies, antibodies can be developed from immune, naive or synthetic libraries and derived from different sources. There are also a number of different antibody fragments that can be produced. Image adapted from da Silva et al. [15].

9.3.1.1 Phage display

Phage display was first described in 1985, when George Smith demonstrated that a linkage between phenotype and genotype could be established in filamentous bacteriophage, which is illustrated in Fig. 9.3 [16]. Following on from this discovery, in the early 1990s several laboratories described phage display systems for antibody fragments [17, 18]. In terms of antibody generation, antibody genes are linked to the amino terminus of the phage minor coat protein

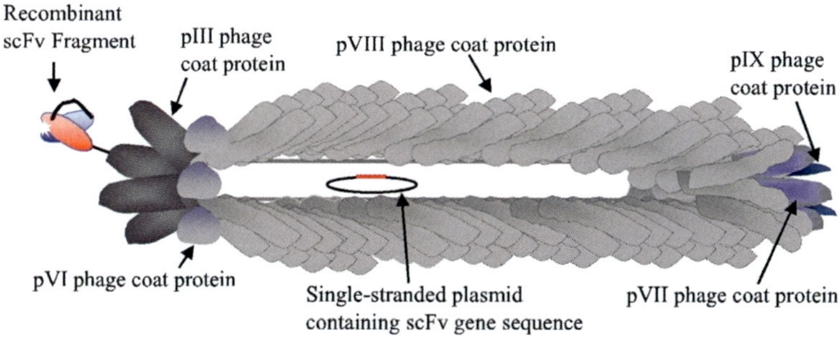

Figure 9.3 Display of a scFv on a filamentous bacteriophage particle. The location of the capsid proteins and the single chain fragment variable (scFv) are indicated by arrows. Filamentous phage particles are covered by approximately 3000 copies of the small major coat protein pVIII. A few copies of the minor coat proteins pIII and pVI are displayed at one extremity of the phage particle, while pVII and pIX proteins are located at the other extremity. The scFv is displayed as a fusion to g3p (pIII) protein at the tip of the phage. The phage particles may incorporate either pIII derived from the helper phage or from the scFv fusion protein and therefore in reality, the scFv is not fused to all pIII protein molecules, allowing the phage to retain its ability to infect bacteria.

pIII. When expressed, the encoded fusion product is incorporated into the mature phage particle during normal phage biogenesis. The resulting phage particle expresses antibody on its surface and contains the antibody encoding gene [15].

Large libraries containing millions of different antibodies can be obtained by forced cloning in *Escherichia coli*. From these repertoires, phage carrying specific antibodies can be isolated by repeated cycles of selection using the antigen of interest, which involves binding, washing, elution and amplification [19]. A more detailed description of considerations in selection processes is provided elsewhere by Conroy et al. [20].

9.3.1.2 Cell display methods

Cell display methods employ various cell systems, either prokaryotic or eukaryotic, for expression and selection of antibody fragments demonstrating desirable characteristics.

Prior to the introduction of phage display technologies, methods to display antibodies on bacterial cells had been demonstrated.

The method was hindered by the lack of an efficient screening method but with the introduction of high-speed flow cytometry technologies, namely fluorescence-activated cell sorting (FACS), its use has been reintroduced. While gram-positive bacteria (e.g. *Bacillus brevis* and *Bacillus subtilus*), which secrete proteins directly into the medium due to the lack of cell wall, have been exploited to produce and purify different antibody fragments, gram-negative bacteria (e.g. *E. coli*) are more commonly used [2]. As the expression of recombinant antibodies in the cytoplasm principally results in non-functional aggregates, most are produced in the periplasm of the bacteria using N-terminal leader sequences [2]. This was enabled by the work of Skerra and Pluckthun, who described the first expression of a functional antibody fragment in *E. coli*, and observed that directing the fragment to the oxidising environment of the periplasmic space allowed for the correct formation of disulphide bonds [21].

The expressed antibody fragment can then be isolated from the periplasmic fraction or in some cases from the culture supernatant [2]. Although bacterial display theoretically holds certain advantages over phage display (e.g. less technically demanding) a direct comparison of the methods, by Lunder et al., found that phage display tends to be more successful in identifying ligands of interest [22]. An additional disadvantage to prokaryotic expression is their inability to provide post-translational modifications such as glycosylation [13].

Using eukaryotic hosts, a more sophisticated protein secretion and folding apparatus is provided, as well as the capacity for post-translational modifications, when compared to prokaryotes. While mammalian cells are still the system of choice for the production of antibodies the disadvantages associated with their use which include a requirement for highly specialised dedicated facilities, high cost and lengthy production times mean that other systems have been investigated. Yeast, filamentous fungi, insect cells along with transgenic plants and animals have all been used in the production of recombinant antibodies [2]. Perhaps the most widely used eukaryotic display technology is yeast display. Antibody fragments are displayed on the cell surface as part of a hybrid protein that is made up of the antibody or antibody fragment and the Aga2p (agglutinin) subunit, which is covalently linked by two disulphide bonds to Aga1 (agglutinin) in the yeast cell wall [8]. The use of yeast technology combines the ease-of-culture seen with prokaryotic systems with the capacity for folding and secretion of eukaryotic systems. Other benefits of the system include rapid and quantitative screening facilitated by FACS and convenient evaluation of characteristics such as affinity without the need for soluble expression and purification of each clone of interest [23].

9.3.1.3 In vitro display technologies

The predominant technologies described as in vitro display methods are ribosome display and mRNA display. These methods are outlined in Fig. 9.4.

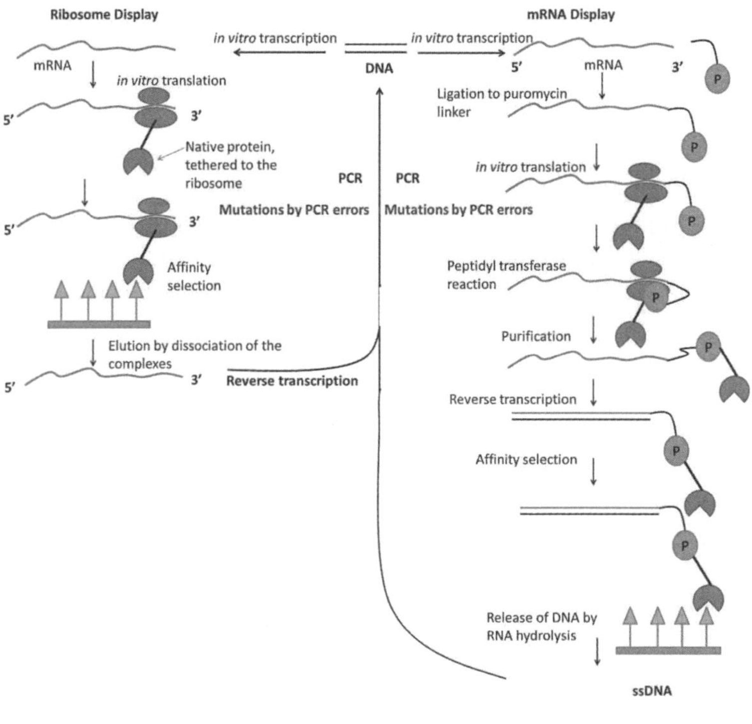

Figure 9.4 In vitro display methods. Ribosome display and mRNA display. Image amended from Lipovsek and Pluckthun [24].

During ribosome display, DNA encoding the library is transcribed in vitro. The resulting mRNA lacks a stop codon, giving rise to linked mRNA-ribosome-protein complexes during in vitro translation. These can be stabilised and directly used for selection against an antigen of interest. The mRNA incorporated in bound complexes is eluted and purified. Reverse transcription polymerase chain reaction (RT-PCR) can introduce mutations and yields a DNA pool enriched for binders that can be used for the next iteration [24].

In the case of mRNA display, covalent mRNA–protein complexes are created by ligation of a DNA linker with a small adaptor molecule, puromycin, to create the in vitro–transcribed mRNA, which lacks a stop codon. The mRNA is translated in vitro, and the ribosome stalls at the RNA-DNA junction. Puromycin then binds the ribosomal A-site and the nascent polypeptide is thereby transferred to puromycin, as if it were an aminoacyl-tRNA. The resulting covalently linked mRNA-protein complex is isolated, reverse-transcribed and used in selection procedures. The DNA strand is recovered from target-bound complexes by hydrolysing the complementary mRNA at high pH and then amplified by PCR [24].

As these methods are performed entirely in vitro, they hold two advantages over other competing technologies. The first depends on the fact that library size can be much larger (10^{12}–10^{14}) [15] as it does not depend on the transformation efficiency of competent bacteria but rather on the amount of ribosomes and different mRNA molecules present. Secondly, there is the potential to introduce random mutations after each selection round by introducing randomisation steps, using non-proofreading enzymes [25].

9.3.2 Mutagenesis Strategies

Conventional methods of antibody production such as polyclonal and hybridoma production are severely limited in their ability for improvement or modification. Reduction in maximum residue levels (MRLs) by regulatory authorities or the need to be able to detect lower biomarker levels means that immunoassays generated with these types of antibodies can often require the development of an entirely new antibody to meet the lower detection thresholds.

Recombinant antibody technology has a clear advantage over traditional antibody production in this respect. Not only can recombinant antibodies be 'tailored' through genetic modification for a particular immunoassay application, they can be 'retailored' and improved to keep up with changing detection requirements.

An excellent example of this is provided by Korpimäki and colleagues, at the University of Turku, where they converted an anti-sulphonamide mAb obtained from a hybridoma and modified its specificity to bind up to 15 sulphonamide derivatives, significantly improving the capabilities of the immunoassay [26–29]. Altering the amino acid sequence of antibodies using gene engineering allows for an improvement in characteristics such as affinity, specificity, stability and immunogenicity [30]. Mutagenesis strategies can be divided into the following categories, random mutagenesis, site-directed mutagenesis and DNA recombination.

Random mutagenesis involves the random change of any amino acid in the antibody gene sequence. Perhaps the most well known method for random mutagenesis is error-prone PCR. Error-prone PCR employs low-fidelity polymerases and/or conditions which favour mis-incorporation of nucleotides (e.g. presence of Mn^{+2}, limiting amounts of dATP and dCTP) to create libraries of random mutants [31, 32]. Alternatively a bacterial mutator strain, for example MutD5, can be used to introduce single base substitutions at high frequency compared to normal cells [31]. These strains have an impaired mismatch repair system and can have mutation frequencies in the region of 0.2–1 substitutions per 1000 nucleotides per cycle of propagation [32]. The major advantage of random mutagenesis is that it does not require any information about the antibody structure or the interacting amino acids. However, the disadvantage lies in the fact that mutant libraries often have a large proportion of functionally inactive mutants [13].

Site-directed mutagenesis, in contrast to random mutagenesis, introduces mutations at chosen positions in the antibody gene sequence. Site-directed mutagenesis can be used alongside crystallography studies to elucidate information about the active site and in this way perhaps provide an insight into antigen binding [31]. The introduction of in silico techniques adds weight to this in that it could potentially allow the simulation of mutation and its consequences at specific points. This would allow for a more rational selection of those mutations, which seem to confer positive effects on antigen–antibody binding [13].

DNA recombination, also known as antibody shuffling, somewhat mimics somatic hypermutation and as a result is thought to be more efficient than random or directed mutagenesis approaches [31]. Shuffling of antibody genes can be carried out in a number of ways. The first is chain shuffling whereby the heavy and light chains of antibodies, selected as a positive binder, from an immune library are recombined. Fitzgerald et al. describe a 185-fold increase in sensitivity of a halfuginone-specific scFv using chain shuffling and its subsequent incorporation into an immunoassay for detection in samples [33]. The second, deemed DNA shuffling, involves digestion of the antibody DNA with DNAse 1 and its subsequent reassembly and amplification by PCR. A third method called staggered extension process or StEP is also reliant on PCR and involves template switching caused by shortened extension times which shuffles portions of the parent antibody genes [31].

9.4 Improvements in Platform and Detection Methods

New antibody molecules with better affinity and specificity profiles can greatly influence next-generation assay performance. However, biorecognition elements such as antibodies are only one of the many components that need to be addressed if the boundaries of analytical detection are to be pushed to even lower levels. Improvements in reagents, platforms, signal generation and acquisition play a fundamental role in next generation immunoassay development.

9.4.1 Nanomaterials

Nanoengineered materials are fast becoming a commonly used technology for improvement in optical detection over a wide variety of applications. *Nano*, a Greek prefix, defines the smallest natural structures and the term *nanotechnology* describes the manipulation of these materials which exhibit superior electrical, chemical, mechanical or optical properties [34]. These materials have been investigated and optimised to offer tunabilities, intensities and longevities far greater than conventional labels or dyes [35].

Nanoparticles have unique chemical and physical properties that offer important possibilities for use as probes in bioanalysis. They offer several potential advantages over conventional dyes such as a low background level because they do not scatter light. As a result of the low background lower detection limits can be achieved [36]. Especially prevalent in the area of electrochemical immunoassays, a wide range of nanomaterials, which include metal nanoparticles (nanogold and nanosilver), semiconductor nanoparticles, enzyme-loaded carbon nanotubes, among others, have been used to enhance the signal generated by the antigen-antibody interaction [37].

A method exploiting carbon nanotubes (CNTs), which exhibit high surface-to-weight ratio and excellent mechanical properties, for the detection of staphylococcal enterotoxin B in foodstuffs has recently been shown to be highly sensitive and reproducible [32].

Luminescent semiconductor nanocrystals or quantum dots (QDs) possess a number of photophysical properties which offer distinct possibilities to overcome the limitations of conventional dyes. These include broad absorption spectra which would allow for excitation with a single light source, excellent photo- and chemical stability which allows for lower limits of detection and extended monitoring in assays, and narrow, symmetrical emission spectrum that is dependent on size. Ultimately these inherent properties of QDs mean that their use could allow simultaneous excitation of quantum dots with a single light source and their simultaneous resolution and visualisation as different colours [34, 38]. The prospect of multiplex QD-based immunoassays is where the greatest potential lies for these fluorophores but several disadvantages such as the difficulty and cost associated with their synthesis and functionalisation mean that their use and development have been somewhat hindered [35].

Another relatively new technology utilising ceramic nanospheres is up-converting phosphor technology (UPT). These particles, do not photo-bleach, are available in different colours and exhibit excellent signal-to-noise ratios. The UPT technology is currently being commercialised by OraSure Technologies [35].

There are numerous examples where different nanomaterials have been used in combination with each other to provide new methods for ultrasensitive detection. In one instance, a strategy to simultaneously detect three liver cancer biomarkers utilised gold nanoparticle-coated carbon nanotubes as carriers to immobilise labelled antibodies and to enhance output signals [39]. In a different example, an assay system combining chimeric nanoparticles and nickel nanohair structures allowed for controlled orientation of antibodies in the system, which in turn increased the density and ratio of antibodies to protein markers. When applied to an assay for the detection of troponin I levels in human serum samples, this unique approach resulted in a sensitivity which was seven orders of magnitude (~100,000 fold) greater than that observed in a traditional ELISA format [40].

An additional application of nanomaterials is localised surface plasmon resonance (LSPR). LSPR describes the collective resonant oscillation of conduction electrons at the surface of a metal nanoparticle under the perturbation of incident light [35]. SPR is a widely used label-free detection system for studying binding events. SPR instruments (e.g. Biacore instruments manufactured by GEHC), while exhibiting excellent specificity and reliability, are expensive and require skilled operators. The fact that LSPR does not require any instrumentation and can be performed with a white light source opens up the possibility of incorporating the exquisite sensitivity exhibited by SPR instruments into microfluidic devices for point-of-care applications [35]. A study in which the authors describe the use of LSPR with gold bipyramids to perform a single-molecule immunoassay exemplifies the potential for this technology [41].

Perhaps one of the most exciting developments in immunoassays involving nanomaterials has been the development of the biobarcode assay (BCA). In this method, magnetic microbeads are used to carry out a heterogeneous immunoassay with the detection antibody labelled with gold nanoparticles which are in turn labelled with unique 'barcode' double-stranded DNA. After the immunoassay the DNA is denatured and the resulting single-stranded DNA is used in a sandwich DNA assay or PCR-based methods [42]. This assay offers a number of advantages, including ultrahigh sensitivity, high selectivity, adaptability to multiple targets and potentially direct detection in complex samples. Since each gold nanoparticle carries hundreds of DNA strands, there is substantial signal amplification. The exquisite sensitivity of the system can be illustrated in the following example, described by Chad Mirkin and colleagues, which tested for the levels of prostate-specific antigen (PSA) in patients after surgery. The authors theorised that in order to rule out residual prostate cancer, PSA levels as low as 5 pg mL^{-1} would need to be detected. This is 20 times more sensitive than most assays currently available. The biobarcode assay developed by Mirkin and co-workers can detect PSA at concentrations as low as 330 fg mL^{-1}, thus exceeding the sensitivity required [43].

9.4.2 Nucleic Acid–Based Signal Amplification

Nucleic acid amplification methods have been employed to greatly enhance the sensitivity of traditional immunoassays by improving signal generation and, thus, assay sensitivity. Several techniques including polymerase chain reaction (PCR) and variations which include 'real-time' PCR (rt-PCR) and immuno-PCR (iPCR), nucleic acid sequence–based amplification (NASBA), self-sustained sequence replication (3SR) and strand displacement amplification (SDA), among others, are becoming widely available in laboratory settings. A number of nucleic acid amplification methods, which are particularly suitable for use in immunoassay applications, are discussed below.

9.4.2.1 Immuno-PCR

First described by Sano et al., immuno-PCR (iPCR) has become a well-established method for routine use in healthcare, medicine and immunology for detection of tumour markers, viral protein, pathogens, microorganisms and toxins, among others [44, 45]. Immuno-PCR is based on chimeric conjugates of specific antibodies and nucleic acid molecules which are used as markers to be amplified by PCR to produce a detectable signal [45]. This method can offer an increase in assay sensitivity of 1,000–10,000 fold when compared with ELISA because it utilises signal amplification by PCR [46].

In general, an iPCR system is similar to that of conventional ELISA but in place of an antibody-enzyme conjugate which converts a substrate to a detectable product an antibody conjugated to a DNA marker is employed. By inclusion of nucleotides, specific primers and polymerase, the marker is amplified to enhance the signal generated. The number of amplicons generated relates to the original amount of antigen [45]. A number of different formats have been developed and these are outlined in Fig. 9.5.

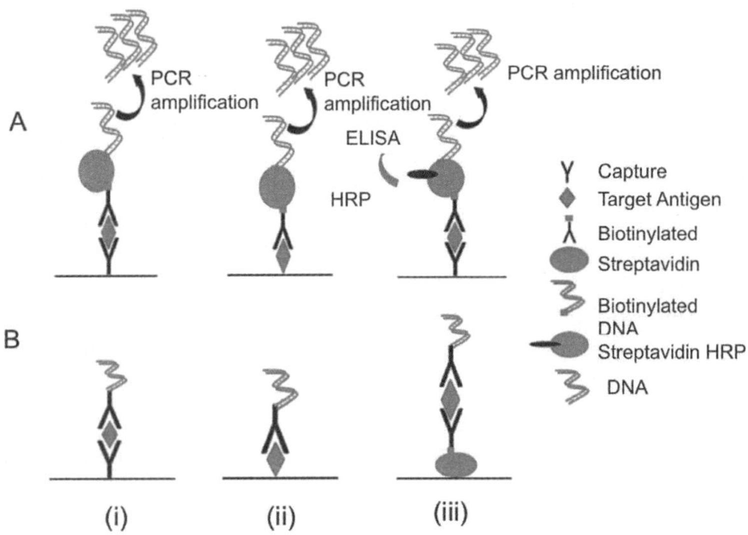

Figure 9.5 Schematic for the various formats employed in Immuno-PCR. (A) Immuno-PCR through (i) sandwich assay format, (ii) direct detection, and (iii) sandwich format allowing both iPCR and ELISA simultaneously. (B) Immuno-PCR with DNA directly conjugated to the detection antibody through (i) sandwich format, (ii) direct format, and (iii) streptavidin-coated plates with biotinylated capture antibody. Image adapted from Malou and Raoult [47].

The method has undergone huge improvements since its introduction and has been developed further into a real-time version (rt-iPCR). This rt-iPCR method provides immediate, quantified analysis of the amplified PCR product that can be used to elucidate the amount of target protein in the sample by directly monitoring fluorescent signals in the closed reaction vessel. This provides the further benefits of removing additional post-amplification analysis steps and also reduces the potential for contamination [46].

While iPCR is often hampered by the requirement for a sensitive and specific antibody to allow for successful utilisation, there are huge benefits to be availed of by the use of this technique. These include the reduced sample volume required and even the potential to use alternative sample matrices, where increased sensitivity may allow for detection where it was previously not feasible, avoiding the need for invasive procedures to obtain samples for testing [45]. However, the application of the method in point-of-care is somewhat limited by the requirement for expensive equipment.

9.4.2.2 Hybridisation chain reaction

A nucleic acid amplification method known as hybridisation chain reaction (HCR) has been described which can potentially allow for a specific, 'enzyme-free' extension using a pair of complementary, kinetically trapped hairpin oligomers [48]. More recently an adaptation of HCR, immuno-HCR for the detection of analytes secreted from single cells, has been described which offers an alternative to methods such as enzyme-linked immunosorbant spot (ELISPOT) or rolling circle amplification (RCA), which suffer limitations in time and specificity, respectively [49].

The immuno-HCR, illustrated in Fig. 9.6, utilises pairs of nucleotide-based initiators, which have been conjugated to specific antibodies, to improve the detection of chemokines or cytokines secreted from immune cells when compared with antibodies which are directly labelled with a fluorophore [49]. A 200-fold improvement in sensitivity was observed. This, coupled with the ease of integration with established practices for processing microarrays and the potential for multiplexing, makes immuno-HCR a promising isothermal, enzyme-independent method for amplification of signal from microscale spots of captured protein in sandwich immunoassays [49].

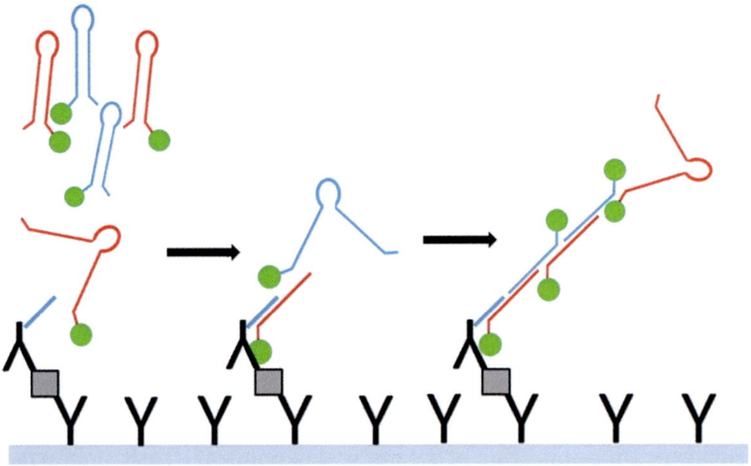

Figure 9.6 Schematic illustration of immuno-HCR. An antibody-coated glass surface captures analytes of interest. Secondary antibodies labelled with an oligonucleotide initiator are introduced and bind to the target analyte. Fluorescently labelled DNA hairpins then hybridize with their complementary oligonucleotide initiator. The fluorescence signal for each bound antibody increases with additional incorporation of hairpins bearing fluorophores during the HCR. Image amended from Choi et al. [49].

9.4.2.3 Loop-mediated isothermal amplification

Loop-mediated isothermal amplification (LAMP) is a nucleic acid amplification method which offers a rapid, accurate and cost-effective diagnostic tool for detection and identification of disease [50].

LAMP is a highly sensitive and specific one-step amplification method that amplifies a target DNA sequence under isothermal conditions. The method employs *Bst* DNA polymerase, which exhibits strand-displacement activity, and works by amplifying six distant regions in the target DNA [51]. High specificity is conferred by the fact that amplification will only occur when all six regions within a target DNA are recognised by primers [52].

There are a number of characteristics of the LAMP method that make it superior to other similar methods. Firstly, unlike other PCR-based methods, LAMP does not require high-precision thermal cycling equipment due to the use of an isothermal enzyme.

Secondly, the simplified reaction, which occurs in one tube, can be monitored and a positive reaction confirmed in a number of ways, either by turbidity or by fluorescence, without complicated or time-consuming post-amplification analysis [52]. These properties make LAMP a very attractive method for diagnosis of disease and infection in instances where sophisticated equipment and highly skilled personnel are not available. A very interesting modification of the LAMP method, described by Lee et al., outlines a reverse-transcription loop-mediated isothermal amplification–enzyme-linked immunosorbant hybridisation (RT-LAMP-ELISA) assay for the detection of *Mycobacterium tuberculosis* in patient samples. With this technique the authors detail a rapid, 'one-tube' method for detection of active tuberculosis in patients as well as the ability to differentiate *M. tuberculosis* from other *Mycobacteria* species from a single sputum sample [51].

9.4.3 Optical Detection Methods

Optical assays rely on absorbance, fluorescence or luminescence read-outs, with numerous instruments (e.g. plate readers and slide scanners) available, which allow for convenient and rapid measurement. With the ever-increasing drive to lower detection limits and increase sensitivity in existing immunoassays there has been increased development of novel detection strategies, especially in the area of fluorescence detection. One such example, of an innovative fluorescent detection method and its application, is discussed below.

Other optical detection methods based on total internal reflection, such as total internal fluorescence (TIRF), total internal reflection ellipsometry (TIRE) and the use of fibreoptics, have been described as methods for the improvement of signal detection. Supercritical angle fluorescence (SAF) has been described as an optical detection method that allows for increased sensitivity when compared to alternative detection systems. It is based on the principle, illustrated in Fig. 9.7, that incident light on a water–glass interface is refracted into angles below the critical angles, meaning that no light should enter the supercritical angles. Fluorophores bound to the glass surface can, however, emit into the supercritical

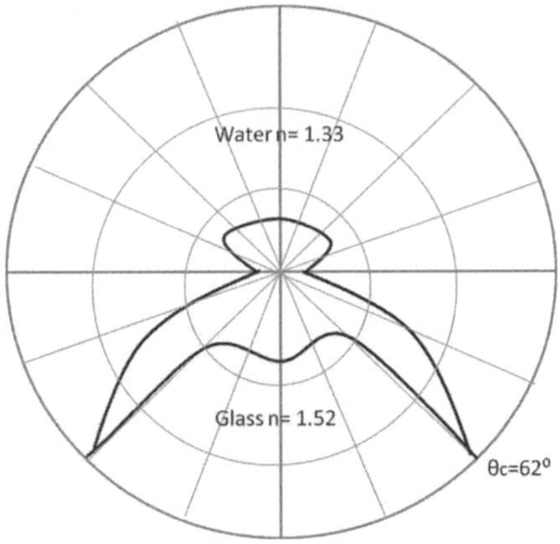

Figure 9.7 Angular distribution of the fluorescence intensity of a molecule positioned at a water–glass interface averaged over all possible emission dipole orientations. Image adapted from Kurzbuch et al. [54].

angles. By discounting light emitted into non-critical angles, only fluorophores close to the surface can be selectively detected [53]. A straightforward parabolic element can convert SAF into conveniently detectable parallel rays by 'loss-free' total internal reflection (TIR).

The combination of high collection efficiency and the ability to collect fluorescence only from molecules close to the detection surface, and not the bulk solution, provides a useful system for the sensitive readout of immunoassays [54]. The outstanding signal-to-noise ratio of the SAF technology has been used for single-molecule detection, fluorescence microscopy and fluorescence correlation spectroscopy [55]. According to Ruckstahl et al., SAF holds several advantages when compared with TIRF. The first relates to the fact that TIRF requires a very high angle illumination, whereas SAF can achieve outstanding surface confinement at any angle above the critical angle. Secondly, the ability to excite the sample at moderate surface angles allows for concurrent detection within an aqueous solution [55]. Furthermore, owing to the straightforward detection optics, it could potentially be produced by polymer injection moulding at low cost. Kurzbuch et al. describe the use of a supercritical angle fluorescence chip reader, which can provide a low-cost, highly sensitive biochip scanning system capable of application in point-of-care settings [54].

9.5 Current Immunoassay Trends

In recent years there has been an increased interest in the transfer of diagnostics from the clinical laboratory setting to the point-of-care. With driving forces such as reducing pressure on healthcare workers and the goal of faster diagnosis translating to better outcomes for patients, the development of such devices is steadily gathering pace. In this section we will focus on the area of point-of-care diagnostics and also the technologies, which allow these devices to become a reality.

9.5.1 Point-of-Care (POC) Diagnostics

The aim of point-of-care (POC) diagnostic devices is to provide an alternative to laboratory-based tests driven mainly by clinical testing needs. The rationale for their development is two-fold. Firstly, they will reduce healthcare costs by streamlining the process of diagnosis by their ability to be employed in decentralised settings such as emergency rooms, out-patient clinics, a doctor's surgery and even the home [56]. Secondly, it can improve greatly on diagnosis times and as such improve effective medical response, especially in acute care settings, where diagnostic information is critical [57].

In addition to the foreseen advantages in the developed world, the introduction of POC diagnostics has a huge potential impact in the developing world. By removing the requirement for laboratory settings and skilled operators, POC devices could be used to deliver cost-effective care in areas where it was previously not feasible [57]. To be appropriate for use as POC tests, the devices provided must be portable, require minimal user skill or involvement, make use of reagents that are stable without the need for designated storage such as a refrigerator, be cost effective to produce and operate and, most importantly, provide accurate and rapid results [58].

The quoted global market for POC testing was $13.4 billion in 2010, with an expected figure of $16.5 billion in 2016 [59].

Blood glucose testing dominates the market, largely due to the dramatic increase in diabetes cases worldwide. This is based mainly on sufferers from the Western world, but a drive by providers of these tests to reduce cost will likely see their deployment worldwide eventually [56]. The fastest-growing sector is infectious disease testing, which encompasses testing for methicillin-resistant *Staphylococcus aureus* (MRSA), flu (influenza), as well as HIV. Others which are considered to have the potential to be of significant influence on the market are coagulation monitoring, in relation to stroke, heart attack and deep vein thrombosis patients and cardiac marker testing, which is aimed at rapid diagnosis of acute coronary syndrome (ACS) and congestive heart failure (CHF). In addition, cholesterol POC testing, which has progressed to over-the-counter (OTC) testing, is likely to increase in importance driven largely by public health initiatives coupled with an ageing population and a rise in obesity and cardiovascular disorders [56].

While there has been mammoth growth in the use of diagnostic tests deployed on POC devices, there is an opinion that their use requires more ethical investigation. The question lies in whether such sensitive information (e.g. diagnosis of HIV) should be delivered in a POC setting and raises further issues of privacy, theft and medical counselling [60]. However, these reservations do not seem to be stemming the number of emerging POC devices or indeed the research and development into novel targets and platforms. It is logical to expect increased activities and advancements in the area fuelled by demand from the healthcare industry and facilitated by information technology. This is exemplified by the recent description of a cell-phone-based analysis of an immunoassay test, where the authors claim that the application would be capable of processing assay data fast enough for the results to be available to healthcare workers and patients within a single patient visit [58].

9.5.2 Microfluidics

The use of microfluidics can help to circumvent time limitations and labour requirements of traditional immunoassays. Advantages conferred by microfluidic systems are numerous. They include (i) increased surface area–to-volume ratios, which allow for improved antigen-antibody interaction; (ii) reduction in the consumption of reagents; (iii) precise liquid control, which results in improved reproducibility; and (iv) greater throughput by increased automation [42]. The focus on POC diagnostics has in turn prompted a surge in the development of 'lab-on-a-chip' devices which aim to provide a fully functional test that can incorporate sample preparation, assay execution and diagnosis without the need for additional equipment or skilled operators.

The use of microfluidic-based single-use devices could meet the demand for diagnostics with little or no instrumentation required. The demand exists predominantly in cases where the outlay for expensive instrumentation cannot be justified, where the requirement for a specific test is low-volume or sporadic. The niche markets envisioned for these devices include (i) healthcare in developing countries, (ii) home-testing in developed countries and (iii) as diagnostic or bioanalytical tools, for use in emergency settings, by first responders [61].

These lab-on-a-chip devices can potentially provide the perfect avenue for development of next-generation POC diagnostics. By taking advantage of several intrinsic characteristics of microfluidics, which include laminar flow, low consumption of costly reagents, minimal handling of hazardous materials, short reaction time required for analysis, multiple sample detection and portability, they hold huge potential for production of versatile diagnostic tests [62].

Despite their promise, only a few fully integrated systems have been described. This is most probably due to the complexity and cost of dealing with handling of real samples (e.g. whole blood) and the fluidic control of multiple reagents [63]. Additional steps required can include separation of unwanted sample components, mixing, phase extraction, analyte enrichment, analyte labelling or signal amplification and, ultimately, signal detection [61, 64]. However, there have been great strides over the past number of years in addressing the challenges associated with system integration. One such example is described by Lee et al., who reported a fully integrated lab-on-a-disc for biochemical or immunological analysis in whole blood. Utilising a novel ferro-wax valve and centrifugal microfluidics, the device allowed for simultaneous analysis of a blood chemistry panel with six analytes and an immunoassay from a whole blood sample. This technology has huge potential as a blood analyser because it uses only 350 μL of whole blood, a result can be obtained in as little as 22 minutes and it does not require highly specialised, expensive equipment [63].

Reports of such advanced fully integrated devices show the potential for development and establishment of microfluidic tests in low-resource settings for point-of-care diagnosis. Great advancements are being made in relation to these applications with particular focus being placed on analysis, which is independent of external power sources. This is exemplified in the report of the use of a hand-powered egg beater, in place of a centrifuge, to provide a means of separating plasma from a whole blood sample [65]. For a more detailed look at the advances in microfluidics, with relation to immunoassays, please refer to Chapter 5 of this book.

9.6 Commercially Available Novel Immunoassays

While many of the technological improvements discussed thus far have been reported from the academic sector, some of these improvements are being translated to commercial products. In addition, the number of new companies, new technologies and modifications to older systems and devices means that there are now an exciting range of new immunoassays. Having discussed the ways in which immunoassays are being improved upon and looking at the future directions for their development, we will now identify some examples of novel state-of-the-art immunoassay systems currently available on the market.

Singulex, Inc., has developed a single-molecule counting technology that can quantitatively measure single molecules such as proteins and metabolites directly in complex biological samples. They provide instrumentation and immunoassay kits for a range of biomarkers in the areas of inflammation and cytokines, oncology, cardiovascular disease, metabolism, neurology and toxicity. The technology uses paramagnetic microparticles (MPs) as a solid phase support for immune capture, which serves to increase surface area for detection. Coupled with instrumentation, which uses a digital counting system based on capillary flow that is capable of detecting single molecules with very little background interference, the Erenna® immunoassay system can detect even small changes in biomarker levels and, as such, can achieve exquisite sensitivity in the range of 1–3 orders of magnitude greater than traditional methods [66]. Details of these Erenna® assay kits can be found on the Singulex website (http://www.singulex.com/index.html).

The i-STAT device, provided by Abbot, is a light-weight portable cartridge technology which utilises a silicon chip with integrated microfluidics and chemically sensitive biosensor to perform standardised lab-quality bedside testing. Using only 2–3 drops of blood, a range of clinical tests, such as those for blood gases, coagulation monitoring, blood chemistries/electrolytes, haematology and cardiac markers, can be carried out. The i-STAT incorporates several quality control parameters, including monitoring sample quality and validation of reagent with each test, meaning that skilled users are not required. Additionally, Abbot have now introduced an i-STAT wireless, which means that physicians can receive immediate test information in the electronic medical record wherever they might be, enabling them to act quickly when a patient's clinical status is rapidly changing. Further information on this technology can be found at http://www.abbottpointofcare.com/Products-and-Services/iSTAT-Cartridges.aspx.

Advanced Liquid Logic (ALL) has developed methods for implementing many bioassay protocols using digital microfluidics by implementing an electrowetting effect to precisely manipulate droplets within a sealed microfluidic cartridge. Electrical signals are applied to an array of electrodes to control the size and position of each droplet. Droplets are transferred between adjacent electrodes by removing voltage from one electrode and applying it to the next one. The same processes can be used to dispense, merge or split droplets using electrical signals. Fully programmable fluid handling is thereby achieved without the use of any pumps, valves or channels.

The technology has been applied, in sub-microliter volumes with low-cost, disposable cartridges, for applications such as quantitative analysis of DNA (qPCR) and RNA (RT-qPCR), protein analysis using both enzymatic and immunoassay techniques, DNA sequencing using a sequencing-by-synthesis method, sample preparation from many different sample matrices (blood, swabs, saliva, etc.) and preparation of fragment libraries for next-generation sequencing. One of the technologies available from ALL is the LSD-100, which is an automated screening system for lysosomal storage disease in newborns. It can provide results of 5 assays on 40 dried blood spot extracts, along with 4 controls and 4 calibrators, in less than 3 hours for approximately $1 per test.

Radisens Ltd. provide a high-performance, battery-operated diagnostics platform which comprises a connected multi-fluorescent device, centrifugal microfluidic mini-disc consumables with integrated controls and calibration. With all assay and sample preparation steps integrated into the same consumable panel, they integrate over eight multiplexed immunoassay and biochemistry assays each for the management of chronic care patients suffering from diabetes, hypertension and chronic kidney disease. Each panel requires only a finger prick of the patient's blood to produce clinical results within minutes. All assay and sample preparation steps are integrated on the consumable panel, ensuring true sample-to-answer solutions. More details of their system can be sourced at http://www.radisens.com.

Perkin Elmer have developed a range of bead-based assays, including AlphaScreen® and AlphaLISA®, to study biomolecular interactions in a microplate format. The acronym 'Alpha' stands for amplified luminescent proximity homogeneous assay. The key features of these technologies are that they are non-radioactive, homogeneous proximity assays. Binding of molecules captured on the beads leads to an energy transfer from one bead to the other, ultimately producing a luminescent/fluorescent signal. The principle of the technology is illustrated in Fig. 9.8.

The assays can be designed for use in simple screening or for quantitative purposes and can be designed to replace existing immunoassays in areas such as analyte detection, antibody quantitation/characterisation, post-translational modifications, kinase assays, protease assays and more. Additional information on the technology, assay options and kits available can be found at http://www.perkinelmer.com.

Nanosphere have developed their Verigene platform based on the use of gold nanoparticles as secondary labels, which are then

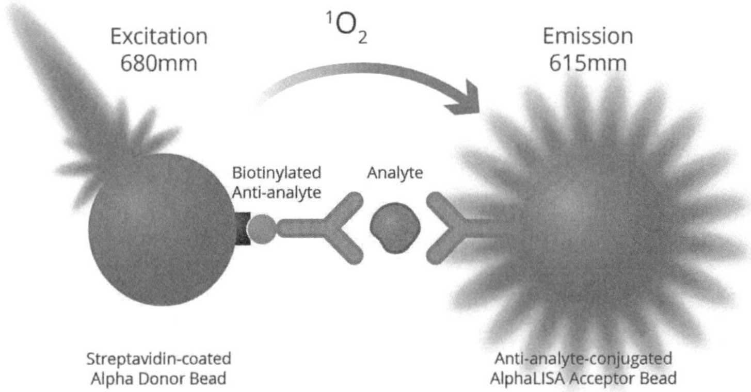

Figure 9.8 Principle of the AlphaLISA assay technology. Streptavidin-coated donor beads are used to capture a biotinylated antibody specific to a precise epitope present on the analyte. Another antibody, also specific to an epitope found on the analyte, is directly conjugated to the acceptor beads. Both the donor and acceptor beads are brought into proximity in the presence of the analyte. An AlphaLISA signal, directly proportional to the concentration of the analyte in solution, is then generated after laser excitation at 680 nm.

enlarged by catalytic silver deposition until they can be imaged using a regular slide scanner or conventional camera [30]. Depending upon the application, each nanoparticle is functionalized with either a defined number of oligonucleotides (i.e. short pieces of DNA or RNA with sequences complementary to target sequences of clinical interest) or a defined number of antibodies that are specific to a particular protein of interest (e.g. prostate-specific antigen (PSA) [67] and cardiac troponin I (cTnI)). Whole blood is dropped in a disposable cartridge which contains all required reagents for sample preparation, nanoparticle labelling and silver deposition. The processing is completely automated and results are read using a slide scanner. The complete test takes only 90 minutes. Verigene platforms are available for application in areas of infectious diseases (e.g. gram-positive and negative blood culture, enteric pathogens and for respiratory viruses such as influenza), pharmacogenetics (e.g. drug-metabolizing enzyme *CYP2C19*), cardiology (e.g. cTnI) and human genetics (e.g. the *F5* gene can be implicated in deep vein thrombosis). Additional information about the platform is available from http://www.nanosphere.us/.

9.7 Conclusion

The advent of display technologies for the production of antibody fragments has greatly extended their field of application. In addition, gene engineering has allowed for the preparation of antibodies to non-immunogenic or toxic antigens, which could not be generated using typical hybridoma technology. Coupled with this, the ability to evolve these antibodies by genetic means, to include more desirable traits (e.g. increased affinity tags for detection and purification), makes recombinant antibody production an extremely powerful tool.

There are several explanations given as to why antibodies generated by recombinant means have not superseded those produced by traditional hybridoma technology. These include the fact that the phage display platform was covered by a number of patents making it costly, the lack of knowledge about the technology and the apparent shortcomings in expertise and library availability and perceived issues with expression of the recombinant fragments [68].

There is no universal method which can reliably provide high yields of recombinant antibody and this stems from the complexity and difference in each antibody-based molecule [2]. However, the huge range of technologies currently available offer countless alternatives to hybridoma technology. Indeed it is worth mentioning that many commercial antibodies designated as 'monoclonal' are in fact reformatted recombinant antibodies [68]. The obvious advantages which include access to libraries containing billions of potential binders, the ability to sequence the generated antibody and the expiration of a number of patents surrounding several platforms in coming years will likely see an increased uptake of these technologies [68].

While it is generally accepted that fluorescence is superior to absorbance for detection, because of the increased sensitivity achieved [36], fluorescence detection methods using organic dyes also have their disadvantages. Those which commonly decrease immunoassay sensitivity include poor separation of the excitation from emission, which results in spectral overlap and hence affects the efficiency of emission signal collection, and interference from complex biological matrices [69]. There has been extensive and diverse research into methods which may help to overcome these limitations which include generation of novel fluorescence detection instruments, the employment of nanomaterials to circumvent the disadvantages of conventional organic dyes and indeed the amplification of the signal by various means [47]. These innovations, to name but a few, have allowed for the development of increasingly sensitive immunoassays.

As the areas of 3D printing [70], digital detection [71] and single cell and single molecule analysis [72] become ever more advanced we will likely see a surge in the number of novel and innovative next generation immunoassays coming to the market.

Vashist et al. provide an excellent review of some of these emerging approaches including cell phone based technologies, paper based diagnostics, lab on a chip platforms as well as discussing strategies to prolong reagent storage and shelf life of these newly developed assays chips and kits [73].

Mora et al. describes a selection of exciting, emerging technologies and approaches for the performance of next generation immunoassays which are either currently in use in the discovery or, in some cases, the regulated space. These applications involve the use of novel approaches such as single molecule array technologies, mass cytometry, reporter gene assays as well as the utilisation of novel robotics, automation and microfluidics [74].

The demand for higher content readout from immunoassay formats is increasing and as such the focus will likely be on bringing high throughput, multiplexed approaches to the fore. Immunoassays are steadily moving towards miniaturised and automated formats which can make them more accessible and more reliable for use outside of the conventional laboratory setting [75].

The immunoassay has come a long way since its first description which is impressive considering that these advancements have been made in less than 60 years. With the future firmly focused on the development of not only highly sensitive and specific tests but on their deployment in point-of-care formats, the next generation of immunoassays will most definitely provide a challenge. However, considering the vast improvements in the immunoassay, both in components used, and in the methods of detection, it is likely that these goals will be realised in the not so distant future.

References

1. Yalow, R.S., and S.A. Berson, Assay of plasma insulin in human subjects by immunological methods. *Nature*, 1959. **184**(Suppl 21):1648–1649.
2. Schirrmann, T., et al., Production systems for recombinant antibodies. *Front Biosci*, 2008. **13**:4576–4594.
3. Schroeder, H.R., et al., Competitive protein binding assay for biotin monitored by chemiluminescence. *Anal Chem*, 1976. **48**(13):1933–1937.
4. Wu, A.H., A selected history and future of immunoassay development and applications in clinical chemistry. *Clin Chim Acta*, 2006. **369**(2):119–124.
5. Kohler, G., and C. Milstein, Continuous cultures of fused cells secreting antibody of predefined specificity. *Nature*, 1975. **256**(5517):495–497.
6. Immunoassays: Technologies and Global Markets, 2013, BCC Research: http://www.bccresearch.com/pressroom/bio/immunoassays-technologies-global-markets.
7. Global Markets for Research Antibodies, 2015a, BCC Research: http://www.bccresearch.com/market-research/biotechnology/research-antibodies-global-markets-report-bio141a.html.
8. Love, K.R., et al., Microtools for single-cell analysis in biopharmaceutical development and manufacturing. *Trends Biotechnol*, 2013. **31**(5):280–286.
9. Nissim, A., and Y. Chernajovsky, Historical development of monoclonal antibody therapeutics. *Handb Exp Pharmacol*, 2008. (181):3–18.
10. Antibody Drugs: Technologies and Global Markets, 2015b, BCC Research: http://www.bccresearch.com/market-research/biotechnology/antibody-drugs-market-bio016j.html.
11. Lee, C.M.Y., et al., Selection of human antibody fragments by phage display. *Nat Protoc*, 2007. **2**(11):3001–3008.

12. Keeling, P., The impact of genetic biomarkers on drug and companion diagnostic return on investment. *Drug Discovery Today*, 2011. **16**(19–20):850–851.
13. Altshuler, E.P., D.V. Serebryanaya, and A.G. Katrukha, Generation of recombinant antibodies and means for increasing their affinity. *Biochemistry (Mosc)*, 2010. **75**(13):1584–1605.
14. Hearty, S., and R. O'Kennedy, Exploiting recombinant antibodies in point-of-care (POC) diagnostics: the combinatorial advantage. *Bioeng Bugs*, 2011. **2**(3):182–186.
15. da Silva, F.A., S. Corte-Real, and J. Goncalves, Recombinant antibodies as therapeutic agents - Pathways for modeling new biodrugs. *Biodrugs*, 2008. **22**(5):301–314.
16. Barbas, C.F., Burton, D.R., Scott, J.K., and Silverman, G.J., Phage Display: A Laboratory Manual 2001, Cold Spring Harbour, New York: Cold Spring Harbour Press.
17. McCafferty, J., et al., Phage Antibodies - Filamentous Phage Displaying Antibody Variable Domains. *Nature*, 1990. **348**(6301):552–554.
18. Barbas, C.F., et al., Assembly of combinatorial antibody libraries on phage surfaces - the gene-III site. *Proc Natl Acad Sci U S A*, 1991. **88**(18):7978–7982.
19. Hoogenboom, H.R., Overview of antibody phage-display technology and its applications. *Methods Mol Biol*, 2002. **178**: 1–37.
20. Conroy, P.J., et al., Antibody production, design and use for biosensor-based applications. *Semin Cell Dev Biol*, 2009. **20**(1):10–26.
21. Skerra, A., and A. Pluckthun, Assembly of a functional immunoglobulin Fv fragment in *Escherichia coli*. *Science*, 1988. **240**(4855):1038–1041.
22. Lunder, M., et al., Comparison of bacterial and phage display peptide libraries in search of target-binding motif. *Appl Biochem Biotechnol*, 2005. **127**(2):125–131.
23. Gai, S.A., and K.D. Wittrup, Yeast surface display for protein engineering and characterization. *Curr Opin Struct Biol*, 2007. **17**(4):467–473.
24. Lipovsek, D., and A. Pluckthun, *In vitro* protein evolution by ribosome display and mRNA display. *J Immunol Methods*, 2004. **290**(1–2):51–67.
25. Zahnd, C., P. Amstutz, and A. Pluckthun, Ribosome display: selecting and evolving proteins in vitro that specifically bind to a target. *Nat Methods*, 2007. **4**(3):269–279.
26. Korpimaki, T., et al., Improving broad specificity hapten recognition with protein engineering. *J Agric Food Chem*, 2002. **50**(15):4194–4201.

27. Korpimaki, T., et al., Engineering of a broad specificity antibody for simultaneous detection of 13 sulfonamides at the maximum residue level. *J Agric Food Chem*, 2004. **52**(1):40–47.
28. Korpimaki, T., et al., Further improvement of broad specificity hapten recognition with protein engineering. *Protein Eng*, 2003. **16**(1):37–46.
29. Bienenmann-Ploum, M., et al., Comparison of multi-sulfonamide biosensor immunoassays. *Anal Chim Acta*, 2005. **529**(1–2):115–122.
30. Altshuler, E.P., D.V. Serebryanaya, and A.G. Katrukha, Generation of recombinant antibodies and means for increasing their affinity. *Biochemistry (Mosc)*, 2010. **75**(13):1584–1605.
31. Sheedy, C., C.R. MacKenzie, and J.C. Hall, Isolation and affinity maturation of hapten-specific antibodies. *Biotechnol Adv*, 2007. **25**(4):333–352.
32. Maynard, J., and G. Georgiou, Antibody engineering. *Annu Rev Biomed Eng*, 2000. **2**:339–376.
33. Fitzgerald, J., et al., Light-chain shuffling from an antigen-biased phage pool allows 185-fold improvement of an anti-halofuginone single-chain variable fragment. *Anal Biochem*, 2011. **410**(1):27–33.
34. Kaul, Z., et al., Mortalin imaging in normal and cancer cells with quantum dot immuno-conjugates. *Cell Res*, 2003. **13**(6):503–507.
35. Myers, F.B., and L.P. Lee, Innovations in optical microfluidic technologies for point-of-care diagnostics. *Lab Chip*, 2008. **8**(12):2015–2031.
36. Sun, C.X., et al., Advances in the study of luminescence probes for proteins. *J Chromatogr B*, 2004. **803**(2):173–190.
37. Tang, D.P., et al., Ultrasensitive electrochemical immunoassay of staphylococcal enterotoxin B in food using enzyme-nanosilica-doped carbon nanotubes for signal amplification. *J Agric Food Chem*, 2010. **58**(20):10824–10830.
38. Goldman, E.R., I.L. Medintz, and H. Mattoussi, Luminescent quantum dots in immunoassays. *Anal Bioanal Chem*, 2006. **384**(3):560–563.
39. Li, Y., et al., Simultaneous electrochemical immunoassay of three liver cancer biomarkers using distinguishable redox probes as signal tags and gold nanoparticles coated carbon nanotubes as signal enhancers. *Chem Commun*, 2012. **48**(4):537–539.
40. Park, J.S., et al., A highly sensitive and selective diagnostic assay based on virus nanoparticles. *Nat Nanotechnol*, 2009. **4**(4):259–264.
41. Mayer, K.M., et al., A single molecule immunoassay by localized surface plasmon resonance. *Nanotechnology*, 2010. **21**(25).

42. Ng, A.H.C., U. Uddayasankar, and A.R. Wheeler, Immunoassays in microfluidic systems. *Anal Bioanal Chem*, 2010. **397**(3):991–1007.

43. Thaxton, C.S., et al., Nanoparticle-based bio-barcode assay redefines "undetectable" PSA and biochemical recurrence after radical prostatectomy. *Proc Natl Acad Sci U S A*, 2009. **106**(44):18437–18442.

44. Sano, T., C.L. Smith, and C.R. Cantor, Immuno-PCR: very sensitive antigen detection by means of specific antibody-DNA conjugates. *Science*, 1992. **258**(5079):120–122.

45. Niemeyer, C.M., M. Adler, and R. Wacker, Immuno-PCR: high sensitivity detection of proteins by nucleic acid amplification. *Trends Biotechnol*, 2005. **23**(4):208–216.

46. Barletta, J., Applications of real-time immuno-polymerase chain reaction (rt-IPCR) for the rapid diagnoses of viral antigens and pathologic proteins. *Mol Aspects Med*, 2006. **27**(2–3):224–253.

47. Malou, N., and D. Raoult, Immuno-PCR: a promising ultrasensitive diagnostic method to detect antigens and antibodies. *Trends Microbiol*, 2011. **19**(6):295–302.

48. Dirks, R.M., and N.A. Pierce, Triggered amplification by hybridization chain reaction. *Proc Natl Acad Sci U S A*, 2004. **101**(43):15275–15278.

49. Choi, J., et al., Immuno-hybridization chain reaction for enhancing detection of individual cytokine-secreting human peripheral mononuclear cells. *Anal Chem*, 2011. **83**(17):6890–6895.

50. Parida, M., et al., Loop mediated isothermal amplification (LAMP): a new generation of innovative gene amplification technique; perspectives in clinical diagnosis of infectious diseases. *Rev Med Virol*, 2008. **18**(6):407–421.

51. Lee, M.F., Y.H. Chen, and C.F. Peng, Evaluation of reverse transcription loop-mediated isothermal amplification in conjunction with ELISA-hybridization assay for molecular detection of *Mycobacterium tuberculosis*. *J Microbiol Methods*, 2009. **76**(2):174–180.

52. Mori, Y., and T. Notomi, Loop-mediated isothermal amplification (LAMP): a rapid, accurate, and cost-effective diagnostic method for infectious diseases. *J Infect Chemother*, 2009. **15**(2):62–69.

53. Ries, J., et al., Supercritical angle fluorescence correlation spectroscopy. *Biophys J*, 2008. **94**(1):221–9.

54. Kurzbuch, D., et al., A biochip reader using super critical angle fluorescence. *Sens Actuators, B*, 2009. **137**(1):1–6.

55. Ruckstuhl, T., and D. Verdes, Supercritical angle fluorescence (SAF) microscopy. *Opt Express*, 2004. **12**(18):4246–4254.
56. Rajan, J., Glorikian, H., Point-of-care diagnostics: market trends and growth drivers. *Blood*, 2009. **3**(1):1–4.
57. Beyette, F.R., et al., Point-of-care technologies for health care. *IEEE Trans Biomed Eng*, 2011. **58**(3):732–735.
58. Dell, N., et al. Towards a point-of-care diagnostic system: automated analysis of immunoassay test data on a cell phone. In *Proceedings of the 5th ACM workshop on Networked systems for developing regions*. 2011.
59. Point of care, in Available: http://www.bccresearch.com/report/point-of-care-diagnostics-market-hlc043c.html2012, BCC Research Market Forecasting.
60. Sia, S.K., and L.J. Kricka, Microfluidics and point-of-care testing. *Lab Chip*, 2008. **8**(12):1982–1983.
61. Weigl, B., et al., Towards non- and minimally instrumented, microfluidics-based diagnostic devices. *Lab Chip*, 2008. **8**(12):1999–2014.
62. Choi, S., et al., Microfluidic-based biosensors toward point-of-care detection of nucleic acids and proteins. *Microfluid Nanofluid*, 2011. **10**(2):231–247.
63. Lee, B.S., et al., Fully integrated lab-on-a-disc for simultaneous analysis of biochemistry and immunoassay from whole blood. *Lab Chip*, 2011. **11**(1):70–78.
64. Gubala, V., et al., Point of care diagnostics: status and future. *Anal Chem*, 2012. **84**(2):487–515.
65. Wong, A.P., et al., Egg beater as centrifuge: isolating human blood plasma from whole blood in resource-poor settings. *Lab Chip*, 2008. **8**(12):2032–2037.
66. St Ledger, K., et al., Analytical validation of a highly sensitive microparticle-based immunoassay for the quantitation of IL-13 in human serum using the Erenna (R) immunoassay system. *J Immunol Methods*, 2009. **350**(1–2):161–170.
67. Akerstedt, M., et al., Relationship between haptoglobin and serum amyloid A in milk and milk quality. *Int Dairy J*, 2008. **18**(6):669–674.
68. Bradbury, A.R.M., et al., Beyond natural antibodies: the power of in vitro display technologies. *Nat Biotechnol*, 2011. **29**(3):245–254.
69. Resch-Genger, U., et al., Quantum dots versus organic dyes as fluorescent labels. *Nat Methods*, 2008. **5**(9):763–775.

70. Waheed, S., J.M. Cabot, N.P. Macdonald, T. Lewis, R.M. Guijt, and M.C. Breadmore, 3D printed microfluidic devices: enablers and barriers. *Lab Chip*, 2016. **16**:1993–2013.

71. Mok, J., M.N. Mindrinos, R.W. Davis, and M. Javanmard, Digital microfluidic assay for protein detection. *Proc Natl Acad Sci*, 2014. **111**(6): 2110–2115.

72. Shim, J., R.T. Ranasinghe, C.A. Smith, S.M. Ibrahim, F. Hollfelder, W.T.S. Huck, D. Klenerman, and C. Abell, Ultrarapid generation of femtoliter microfluidic droplets for single-molecule-counting immunoassays. *ACS Nano*, 2013. **7**(7):5955–5964.

73. Vashist, S.K., P.B. Luppa, L.Y. Yeo, A. Ozcan, and J.H.T. Luong, Emerging technologies for next-generation point-of-care testing. *Trends Biotechnol*, 2015. **33**(11):1–14.

74. Mora, J., A. Given Chunyk, M. Dysinger, S. Purushothama, C. Ricks, K. Österlund, and V. Theobald, Next generation ligand binding assays—review of emerging technologies' capabilities to enhance throughput and multiplexing. *J Am Assoc Pharm Sci*, 2014. **16**(6):1175–1184.

75. Bylund, M. Automating and miniaturizing immunoassays: starting the switch to maximum productivity. *Genetic Engineering and Biotechnology News*, 2016.

Chapter 10

Recent Trends and the Future of Electrochemical Immunoassay Systems

Frank Davis and Seamus Higson
University of Chichester, College Lane, Chichester, West Sussex, PO19 6PE, UK
f.davis@chi.ac.uk, s.higson@chi.ac.uk

In this chapter we present an overview of the field of electrochemical immunosystems, concentrating on the most recent advances in this rapidly advancing field as well as attempting to extrapolate future trends within this area. We begin with a brief overview of immunoassay techniques and the advantages and disadvantages of the most widely used methods. This is followed by a description of the principles of electrochemical immunoassay systems and their advantages compared to other methods. Various methods used to improve sensitivity and specificity of electrochemical immunoassay systems are then discussed. These include the utilisation of nanostructured materials such as metal nanoparticles and carbon nanotubes. This is followed by a description of some methods used to construct immunosensor microelectrodes and arrays, the large enhancements in sensitivity that can be obtained using these techniques and the possibility of using them to quantify multiple analytes simultaneously. Various methods of imaging these arrays are discussed, including scanning electrochemical microscopy.

Immunoassays: Development, Applications and Future Trends
Edited by Richard O'Kennedy and Caroline Murphy

ISBN 978-981-4669-97-9 (Hardcover), 978-1-315-20654-7 (eBook)
www.panstanford.com

Finally, this chapter includes a summary of how electrochemical immunoassays are being used to address current problems such as the analysis of various environmental, clinical and food samples along with a discussion of the potential for these systems to become much more widely used in scientific and commercial applications.

10.1 Introduction to Electrochemical Immunoassays

Immunoassays are dependent on exploiting the complex interactions found in biological systems. Antibodies bind their antigens with a selectivity and specificity that is unrivalled by most other host-guest binding systems. The nature of these interactions has led to their incorporation in a number of assay systems. One of the earliest was the radioimmunoassay protocol developed by Yalow and Berson [1] in which known quantities of antibody and radioactivity-labelled antigen are combined and form a conjugate. Then a sample such as serum is added and any antigen present in the sample competes with, and displaces some of the bound radiolabeled antigen. The conjugates are then removed and the radioactivity of unbound labelled antigen in solution measured, which gives a quantification of the labelled antigen displaced and, therefore, how much unlabelled antigen was present in the sample.

A major drawback of this method is related to the safety and environmental drawbacks of radiolabelling which led to intensive research into alternative labels. One of the most widely used and commercially available formats is the enzyme-linked immunosorbent assay (ELISA). Enzymes are used as markers for binding events and are detected by their catalytic activity. ELISAs allow for the detection of binding events by using a variety of techniques. Enzymes are particularly suitable because they catalyse a variety of reactions with high activity and extreme selectivity. The presence of the enzyme label can be determined by exposing it to a substrate for which it catalyses its conversion to a product. The appearance of product or loss of substrate can be detected by a variety of methods including electrochemical, fluorescence-based or spectrophotometric approaches. Often the antibodies are chemically immobilised onto the wells of microtitre plates. A number of formats are commonly used such as displacement assays similar to the radioimmunoassay described above. These include competitive assays (antibody is exposed to samples spiked with labelled antigen which then competes with the native antigen for binding) or by the binding of antigen to the immobilised antibody and then exposing it to an enzyme-labelled secondary antibody, which in turn binds to a different epitope of the antigen (sandwich ELISA). ELISA assays offer a number of advantages related to ease-of-use; they are highly sensitive due to enzyme amplification, highly commercialised and are relatively inexpensive. They do require enzyme labelling and can be subject to interference effects from non-specific binding or matrix effects such as coloured solutions. Notwithstanding these potential drawbacks, however, ELISAs are presently the most used and successful technique for immunologically-based detection of a wide variety of antigens.

Another commonly used technique is via a lateral-flow assay, a simple method intended for detection of the presence (or absence) of a target analyte in a sample matrix. Lateral-flow assays tend to be utilised in a dipstick where the test sample is applied to an adsorbent pad and then is transmitted along a strip by capillary action. As the sample passes along the strip, it encounters a labelled reagent, to which it binds, then passes further along the strip where it encounters two lines, one containing immobilised specific antibody and a second line that contains immobilised control antibody. These then bind and immobilise the analyte and its markers produce a visual indication of the binding event. Unfortunately they are mainly qualitative in measurement and cannot accurately assess the level of analyte present leading to them being mainly used in applications where a simple yes/no answer is required, such as pregnancy testing.

It is obvious, therefore, that there is potential for a method where not only the presence but the level of an analyte in a matrix can be determined using a simple, inexpensive method. One solution to this is the development of immunosensors. Immunosensors exploit the exquisite selectivity of the immunosensing process by binding either an antibody or an antigen to a surface and monitoring the selective binding of its counterpart by a variety of approaches such as electrochemical, optical or mass change methods. One of the most common academic optical methods is via surface plasmon resonance (SPR) approaches. A detailed description of SPR is outside the remit of this chapter, however, the basic premise is to immobilise antibodies or antigens onto a gold surface such as a gold-coated microscope slide (see Chapter 11 of this book for further information). This is mounted on a prism and a laser beam directed through the prism onto the back of the gold film with the intensity of the reflected radiation being measured [2]. At a certain critical angle, surface plasmons are generated at the gold surface, with the energy required for this leading to a drop in intensity of the reflected laser light. Immobilisation of biological species and their interactions, such as binding of analytes, all affect this critical angle. This method is widely used to study immunological and other biological interactions since it is highly reliable and reproducible - and does not require any labelling. However, SPR is prone to interference from non-specific interactions, is relatively expensive and requires skilled operating personnel, all of which limit its use for point-of-care applications.

10.2 Electrochemical Immunoassays

The recorded use of electrochemical biosensors dates back to the 1960s. Early biosensors utilised enzymes, such as in the initial paper by Leyland Clark, where glucose oxidase was used to catalyse the reaction of glucose with oxygen, the consumption of which could then be measured by an oxygen electrode [3]. Electrochemical biosensors are the basis of much of the field of blood glucose sensing and the development of simple, home blood glucose testing devices now widely used in the management of diabetes [4]. Electrochemical biosensors have several major advantages in their favour; they are usually sensitive and easy-to-use, portable and less prone to interferences than ELISA (no problem with coloured samples). Also, the commercialisation of cheap screen printed technology and production of conductive ink formulations allows the mass production of electrochemical sensors with potential large cost savings and the possibility of formulating cheap, single-shot sensors, thereby solving any problems of cleaning and reuse or regeneration of sensor components such as chips or strips.

First generation enzymatic biosensors function by production or consumption of electroactive substrates such as oxygen or hydrogen peroxide, whereas the second-generation biosensors utilise electroactive mediators such as ferrocene compounds [4, 5]. Later work also involved direct 'wiring' of the enzyme to a substrate [4, 6] to give so-called third generation biosensors. However, all of these require electrochemical oxidation or reduction to occur at some stage. One major issue with immunosensors is that antibody–antigen interactions tend to be based on hydrogen bonding and other non-covalent interactions, meaning that there is no generation of electrochemically active species, which makes detection of such events more challenging. A variety of methods have been utilised to address this challenge, such as labelling of various components of the immunoassay or the use of 'label-free' electrochemical techniques such as AC impedance and these will be detailed within this chapter.

10.2.1 Principle of Electrochemical Immunoassay

A summary of the principle of electrochemical immunoassays and immunosensors is shown in Fig. 10.1. A recognition element (in this example an antibody) is bound onto an electrode. When exposed to a solution containing its antigen, a recognition event occurs where the antigen is bound. For detection of this binding, however, there must be a transduction event where this binding is converted into a signal. Transducers used can for example be optical (as in SPR), mass-based (as in quartz crystal microscopy) or electrochemical as shown in Fig. 10.1. They allow the transduction of the binding event into an electrical signal, which can then be quantified and used to assess the level of binding. The first description of an electrochemical immunosensor was published in 1991 and involves the co-deposition of a conductive polymer, polypyrrole, along with an antibody to human IgG [7]. Binding of the corresponding antigen (human IgG) led to the appearance of a new peak in the cyclic voltammagram of the polymer film. For a description of the

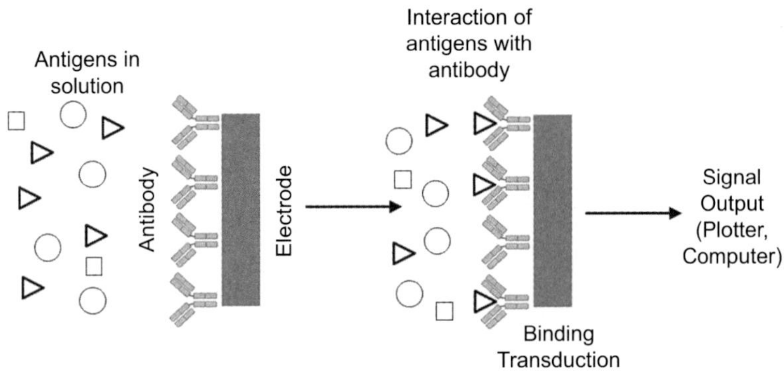

Figure 10.1 Schematic of an electrochemical immunosensor.

research up to 1997 the reader is referred to [8] while more recent information can be obtained in other reviews [9–12].

The advantages of electrochemical immunoassays and immunosensors are that they are relatively inexpensive compared to techniques such as SPR, rapid, quantitative (unlike lateral-flow assays) and do not suffer interference from coloured or turbid solutions. The base electrodes required for these tests can usually be mass-produced using inexpensive screen-printing technology. Also, often only very small amounts of what can be highly expensive biological reagents are required, minimising cost and potentially allowing the production of single use sensors, which do not have to be cleaned or regenerated. The regeneration process can lead to denaturation or degradation of the sensitive biological moieties used for many of these assays. These advantages potentially allow electrochemical techniques to be used for high throughput mass-screening projects.

10.2.2 Labelled Immunoassay Methods

For labelled immunoassays, one of the components of the assay is conjugated with a label of some kind. This can be a fluorescent molecule, a quantum dot, a redox active molecule or when using the same principle as an ELISA, an enzyme. They allow the detection of targets with a high sensitivity and low detection limits [10]. Electrochemical methods can be utilised in a variety of formats (direct, competitive, sandwich, etc.) and also in homogeneous and heterogeneous assays. Much of the work over the last number of years has combined flow cell technology with electrochemical detection to create a range of labelled immunoassays with a number of the earlier assays being summarised here [10].

The combination of electrochemical detection with the mature ELISA technology has allowed the development of high throughput methods to carry out a large number of assays in relatively short timeframes. For example, multiple immunological reactions can be carried out in a microtitre plate in a similar manner to classic ELISA except that instead of a coloured product, a redox active material is produced. This can then be detected electrochemically. Early work utilised horse radish peroxidase (HRP) as the enzyme label and a variety of substrates such as 1,4-diaminobenzene [13] or 1,2-diaminobenzene [14]. A miniature three-electrode system was used for detection purposes. This could be inserted sequentially into each plate well and used to determine the levels of an antigen. This system required about one minute to interrogate each sample, however, later work combined an eight-electrode arrangement (Fig. 10.2) with a multichannel potentiostat, along with an alkaline phosphatase label and 4-aminophenyl phosphate substrate to give an assay with a much more rapid throughput [15]. Other assays have also been developed, such as a competitive membrane-based immunoassay for the herbicide isoproturon utilising HRP as the enzyme label with a 1,2-diaminobenzene substrate [16] being used to determine isoproturon levels down to 0.84 ng mL^{-1}. This format also proved suitable for incorporation into a multi-flow cell allowing the measurement of four samples simultaneously. These systems, however, still require washing of electrodes between samples.

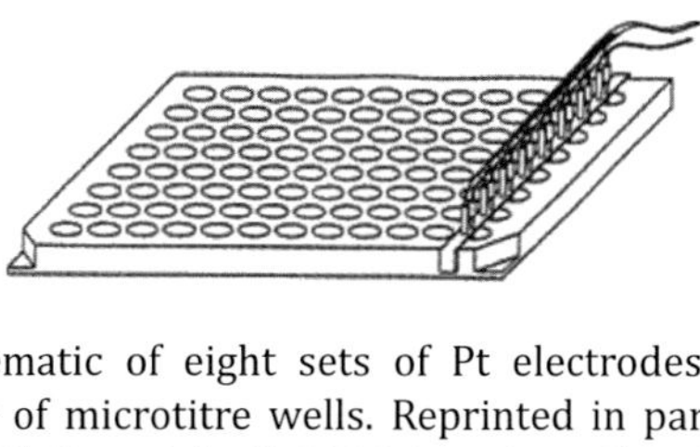

Figure 10.2 Schematic of eight sets of Pt electrodes being utilised to interrogate a row of microtitre wells. Reprinted in part with permission from Tang et al. [15]. Copyright © 2002 American Chemical Society.

In other work, screen-printed carbon electrodes coated with Nafion were situated within polystyrene microwells [17]. A sandwich immunoassay for human chorionic gonadotrophin could be carried out within these wells producing a cationic redox product that was adsorbed into the anionic polymer coating and could be detected by cyclic voltammetry. This allowed the detection of the target with a 10- to 40-fold enhancement of sensitivity over classical spectrometry-based techniques.

10.2.3 Label-Free Methods

One major disadvantage of labelled methods is the requirement for substitution of one of the components of the immunosensing reaction with a label such as an enzyme and it would be much simpler if the formation of an antibody/antigen reaction could be detected directly. The immunoreaction does not produce a directly measurable product such as a redox-active species, proton or electron - although methods do exist for the direct detection of the formation of an antibody-antigen complex on an electrode surface. Some of the earliest work in this field utilised a polypyrrole/anti-human serum albumin system combined with a pulsed amperometric technique [18] in which the current transients obtained during the electrical relaxation of the polypyrrole composite were measured after 520 ms. Later work using a repeating polarising waveform allowed the development of a label-less, reversible immunosensor for bovine serum albumin (BSA) and digoxin with a working concentration range of 0–50 mg L^{-1} [19].

Another interrogation method that was widely utilised as a protocol for the detection of antibody-antigen binding is AC impedance. This allows a continuous perturbation of the system by subjecting it to an AC waveform and monitoring the resultant current. The resulting behaviour can be plotted as a Nyquist plot which allows separate determination of the Faradaic or the resistive or real component (Z'), as well as the capacitive or imaginary (Z'') component. When combined with the use of a redox probe in solution, such as ferri/ferrocyanide, this also allows determination of some factors such as the probe to electrode electron transfer resistance. Much of the theory of AC impedance and its application to probing biomolecular interactions has been reviewed up to 2002 [20] as well as more recently [21].

We initially utilised this technique within our group [22] by using AC impedance on a polypyrrole/anti-BSA composite to develop immunosensors capable of detection of BSA within a range of between 0–75 μg mL^{-1}. In this initial work, the antibodies were simply entrapped within the polypyrrole; however, one problem with this technique is that it potentially leads to many of the antibodies being inaccessible to or in the wrong orientation for the binding of the antigen. In later work, the same group utilised polyaniline as the conducting polymer and chemically reacted the film to graft biotin moieties onto the surface [23]. This then allowed binding of neutravidin to the surface and further grafting of biotinylated antibodies. In these systems the antibodies are immobilised at the surface of the electrode rather than entrapped within a polymer matrix allowing them to be much more accessible to the antigen. Combined with an AC interrogation protocol, this allowed for the development of label-free immunosensors for BSA and digoxin [23], myelin basic protein [24] and internalin B, a surface protein of *Listeria monocytogenes* [25] with detection limits of the order of 1 ng mL^{-1}. Besides these large species, smaller molecules could also be detected; the antibiotic ciprofloxacin for example could be determined at ranges between 1–100 ng mL^{-1} in PBS [26] and also in a much more complex medium, milk [27].

AC impedance has also been used widely by other groups. Amongst the most recent investigations include the label-free detection of atrazine in a competitive assay, where an analogue of the pesticide is immobilised onto a gold electrode and then exposed to a solution of antibody and free antigen to give a sensor with a limit of detection of 40 ng mL^{-1} in water or 190 ng mL^{-1} in red wine [28]. A direct sensor assay for *Salmonella typhimurium* in milk could be constructed by casting anti-Salmonella antibodies onto gold electrodes with glutaraldehyde crosslinking, incubating with the sample and then measuring the AC characteristics in the presence of a redox couple [29], without any need for sample centrifugation or washing. Similarly, thiol-modified gold electrodes could be used as substrates to covalently immobilise antibodies to the antibiotic enrofloxacin with pg mL^{-1} limits of detection [30].

Gold SPEs could also be used as a platform for immobilisation via a cross-linker or directly using thiolated antibodies to give a label-free impedimetric sensor for *Escherichia coli* in river and tap water [31].

Other workers electrodeposited polyaniline/polystyrene sulphonates for use as a platform to immobilise aflatoxin B_1 antibodies and developed a label-free immunosensor with a detection limit of 0.1 μg mL^{-1} [32]. Polytyramine can also be electrodeposited onto gold and then glutaraldehyde used to couple anti-HSA to give a label-free capacitative sensor for HSA with a usable range of 1.84–368.6 ng mL^{-1} and a detection limit of 1.60 ng mL^{-1} [33]. One point of interest is that this array is stable upon acidic washing, allowing dispersal of the antibody–antigen complex and reuse of the sensor. Other groups used poly(1,2-diaminobenzene) to immobilise antibodies to generate an immunosensor for the detection of transferrin [34].

AC impedance has also been combined with labelling methods. For example, this approach was used in a study where transglutaminase was immobilised onto screen-printed gold electrodes coated with a polyelectrolyte layer of poly(styrenesulphonate) [35] and then used to determine anti-transglutaminase antibodies from human serum samples. The sensitivity was increased by using a sandwich type format, where a secondary antibody labelled with peroxidase was bound and then utilised to oxidise amino-9-ethylcarbazole to give an insoluble precipitate on the immunosensor surface, the presence of which could be detected by AC impedance.

MOSFETS (metal–oxide–semiconductor field-effect transistors) and ISFETs (ion-selective field-effect transistors) have also been used as the basis for labelled and label-free immunosensors. For example, peptide-based aptamers for cyclin-dependant kinase 2 were immobilised onto the gate of a MOSFET and the resultant immunosensor was shown to be capable of detecting the antigen at concentrations as low as 5 pg mL^{-1} which is a clinically significant concentration [36]. A variety of other **potentiometric** devices have also been developed. Polypyrrole, for example, can be electrodeposited onto a strip with up to fifty gold electrodes generated by spot casting. This polymer layer can then be used to immobilise antibodies which can then bind their targets. An enzyme-labelled secondary antibody which binds to a different epitope on the antigen is then utilised as a development step, allowing the detection of species such as hepatitis B surface antigen, troponin I, digoxin and tumour necrosis factor with detection limits as low as 50 fmol L^{-1} [37].

10.3 Use of Nanomaterials

One major focus in the entire field of biosensors research has been the incorporation of nanosized materials into various sensors and assays. Nanosized materials can be thought of as being a wide range of organic or inorganic structures where at least one dimension is <100 nm. Several advantages can be conferred onto sensors that incorporate these materials. Firstly, there is often a simple increase in roughness and/or porosity, leading to an increase in the effective surface area of the sensor. Many of the nanomaterials are conductive in nature and can enhance electron transport throughout an electrochemical sensor, as well as being capable of catalysing certain electrochemical reactions. Finally, since many of the materials are of a size comparable with the biological recognition elements used, there is an intimate mixing and in some cases the nanomaterial can effectively 'wire' the recognition species to the electrode. Two of the most popular examples of these types of materials are gold nanoparticles and carbon nanotubes.

10.3.1 Metal Nanoparticles

The field of metal nanoparticles as elements in immunosensors is dominated by gold nanoparticles. Gold has several qualities that makes it especially suitable. It is highly stable and does not react with oxygen or water, is easily synthesised in nanoparticular form with a wide range of sizes and shapes, is highly electrically conductive and can be easily immobilised by a series of methods one of which utilises the strong gold-thiol interaction. Since there are a wide range of papers on this subject, a full discussion of which would be beyond the scope of this chapter, only the most important and recent papers are summarised although there are other reviews which describe this field in more detail [38–40].

A sizable number of papers have recently been published which report that utilising nanogold within immunosensors leads to increases in sensitivity. Gold nanoparticles were incorporated into a layer-by-layer assembled film on a Nafion-modified gold electrode and then a layer of antibody for α-1-fetoprotein adsorbed on to this [41]. Levels of antigen in the range 1 to 250 ng mL^{-1} with a detection limit of 0.56 ng mL^{-1} could be quantified and the system could be regenerated up to eight times by washing with 4 M urea solution. In later work, capping the gold nanoparticles with the electroactive 1,1′-bis-(2-mercapto)-4,4′-bipyridinium dibromide [42] was shown to allow for the construction of a label-free **amperometric** α-1-fetoprotein immunosensor with a lower detection limit of 0.23 ng mL^{-1}. Gold nanoparticles could also be deposited onto sol-gel-coated electrodes by an electrochemical deposition procedure to give films onto which antibodies to transferrin could be adsorbed [43]. Both the resultant immunosensor and an analogue without gold nanoparticles were assessed, with the sensor containing the nanoparticles having both a lower detection limit of 0.05 ng mL^{-1} and a wider linear response range of 1–75 ng mL^{-1} compared to the analogue (detection limit 1 ng mL^{-1}). Colloidal gold solution and horseradish peroxidase-labelled anti-hCG antibody could be mixed and cast onto glassy carbon electrodes and coated with a titania sol-gel film by vapour deposition to give a labelled immunosensor with a detection range from 0.5 to 30 mIU mL^{-1} and a relatively low detection limit of 0.3 mIU mL^{-1} [44]. A simpler method for the production of immunosensors was to coat clean gold electrodes with mercaptoethyl amine, electrostatically adsorb citrate-modified gold nanoparticles onto the amine groups and then adsorb anti-IgG onto this surface [45] to give a **potentiometric** immunosensor with a detection limit of 12 ng mL^{-1} IgG.

Colloidal gold could be incorporated into carbon paste electrodes and then used to measure the electrochemistry of a HRP-labelled CA-19-9 antibody in solution [46], with the addition of the antigen causing formation of a complex and reduction of HRP activity. Human serum could be analysed for the antigen with greater accuracy than a classical immunometric assay. In a similar method

HRP-labelled antibody for interleukin-6 and colloidal gold were immobilised onto a screen-printed graphite electrode and inserted in a flow cell [47]. Inhibition of HRP activity by antigen binding led to an assay for interleukin-6 with a range of 5–100 pg mL^{-1} with a detection limit of 1.0 pg mL^{-1}.

The main advantage of the gold nanoparticle electrodes is their increased sensitivity. Limits of detection have been reduced to the pg mL^{-1} level. In this context gold nanoparticles, for example, could be included along with poly(terthiophene) and a polymeric dendrimer to give immunosensors for the lung cancer markers Annexin II and MUC5AC with pg mL^{-1} limits of detection [48]. A sandwich-type immunoassay was developed based on a gold nanoparticle/DNA-modified gold electrode which was then modified with hepatitis B antibody as well as a gold nanoparticle/HRP/secondary antibody conjugate to detect low levels of the antigen [49]. Utilisation of a gold nanoparticle-modified electrode to immobilise antibodies to biotin combined with a competitive assay using biotin-tagged liposomes with encapsulated ferricyanide ions allowed determination of biotin to levels as low as 9.1 pg [50]. A similar use of gold nanoparticle-tagged antibodies and modified electrodes was used to produce an immunoassay for hepatitis B with a detection limit of 2.3 pg mL^{-1} with good correlation with ELISA results when applied to serum samples but with 100-fold better sensitivity [51].

We have attempted here to give a brief overview on how the use of gold nanoparticles has allowed the development of highly sensitive immunosensors and a more detailed description of recent work is given in several reviews [38–40]. The relative ease of synthesis, stability and beneficial effects of gold nanoparticles will ensure their continuing use in many immunoassays.

10.3.2 Carbon Nanotubes

Carbon nanotubes (CNTs) have also been widely studied as they possess many properties which can be beneficial to biosensor performance. CNTs can be rendered electrically conducting, display a high aspect ratio of length to thickness, can catalyse several electrochemical reactions and are often of a similar 'size' to many biomolecules, which means they can potentially act as a direct contact between the electrode and one or a number of biomolecules. They can be synthesised as stable suspensions in a variety of solvents, including water. One advantage of CNTs is that they can be easily incorporated into screen-printed electrodes or many other types of electrodes, allowing the possibility for them to be used in inexpensive, mass produced sensors. In much of the early research they were simply cast onto planar electrodes, but other methods have been developed such as incorporation into conductive polymers or by growing them from suitable 'seeds' on an electrode surface to give forests of vertically orientated nanotubes. CNTs can also be relatively easily functionalised at their ends with carboxylic acid groups, allowing direct covalent attachment of biorecognition moieties to the ends of the nanotubes. Much of the work on CNTs in electrochemical biosensors and immunosensors has been reviewed [38–40, 52] and we will present just a brief overview of recent work in an attempt to demonstrate the versatility of these materials. From their facile incorporation into a variety of sensor formats it is likely that CNTs could well become a vital component of a wide range of immunosensors. Figure 10.3 shows the structure of both single and multi-walled carbon nanotubes. These could potentially be used to 'wire' immunosensors to an electrodes surface (Fig. 10.3c).

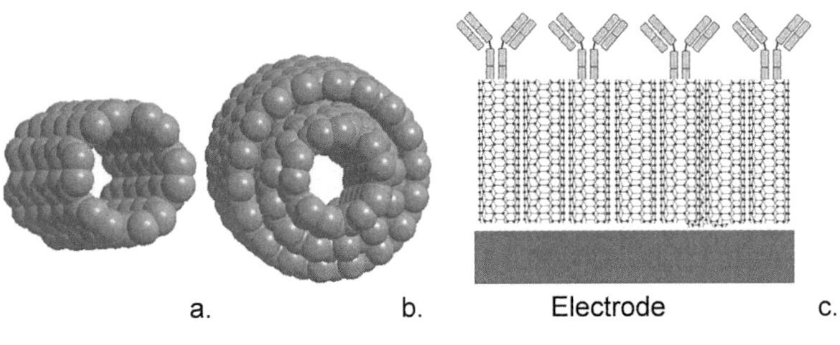

Figure 10.3 Structures of (a) single-walled and (b) multi-walled carbon nanotubes along with (c) a schematic of a potential CNT-based immunosensor.

In one example of CNT utilisation they were used as a substrate to immobilise antibodies against carcinoembryonic antigen as part of a field-effect transistor [53]. A number of other CNT-containing field-effect transistor–based immunosensors have been described [40]. Single-walled CNTs, polylysine and anti-biotin could be covalently linked to pyrolytic graphite electrodes and the resultant immunosensor shown to be capable of amperometrically detecting HRP-labelled biotin with a detection limit of 10 fmol mL^{-1} [54] and with an enhanced thermal stability compared to sensors which did not contain polylysine. Multi-walled CNTs could be cast onto glassy carbon electrodes and then conductive poly(3,4-ethylenedioxy thiophene) electropolymerised onto the surface along with cholera toxin antibody [55]. The resultant sensor was used in a competitive format with ganglioside-substituted liposomes containing encapsulated ferricyanide to give an immunoassay with a detection limit of 10^{-16} g of cholera toxin. Other workers have integrated CNTs into polysulphone screen-printed sensors containing rabbit IgG with the resultant sensor being utilised in competitive assays between free and labelled anti-rabbit IgG capable of antigen detection with limits of 1.66 μg mL^{-1}, a sensitivity five times that of a similar electrode containing graphite instead of CNTs and with lower levels of non-specific binding [56]. Multi-walled CNTs could also be cast, along with a polyethylene glycol/silane copolymer onto indium tin oxide electrodes and used to immobilise avidin [57]. The resultant composite could then be modified with biotinylated mouse antibody and used to bind mouse IgG followed by an enzyme-labelled secondary antibody. The enzyme (alkaline phosphatase) was used to generate p-aminophenol which was then electrocatalytically oxidised by the CNTs to give an immunoassay which could detect 10 pg mL^{-1} of mouse IgG as well as showing low levels of biofouling.

CNTs can be grown by chemical vapour deposition onto silicon wafers to give a vertically aligned array onto which hemagglutinins could be immobilised and used to detect their antibody with higher sensitivity than the corresponding ELISA method [58]. Likewise a vertically aligned single-walled CNT forest could be constructed on graphite discs and the CNTs then substituted with an antibody to prostate specific antigen (PSA). Exposure to PSA followed by further hybridisation with a HRP-labelled secondary antibody/multi-walled CNT conjugate allowed **amperometric** determination of PSA in the range 0.4—40 ng mL^{-1} [59], allowing detection throughout the clinical range of 4–10 ng mL^{-1}.

10.3.3 Other Nanomaterials

A wide variety of other nanoparticle systems have been utilised in biosensors [38–40] and so only a few specific examples will be given within this chapter. With the success of gold nanoparticles and carbon nanotubes in enhancing sensitivity of various biosensor systems, inevitably workers began to develop hybrid systems containing both types of nanostructure. Layer-by-layer assembly methods were used to construct films containing gold nanoparticles, multi-walled carbon nanotubes, thionine and chitosan on gold electrodes [60]. These films could be used as substrates to encapsulate anti-carcinoembryonic antigen/antibody and the resultant label-free immunosensor used to detect carcinoembryonic antigen (with a working range of 0.5–200 ng mL^{-1} and a lower limit of detection of 10 pg mL^{-1}) using a label-free cyclovoltammetric method. In other work, CNTs and gold nanoparticles were incorporated in a chitosan matrix to give a labelled immunosensor for human chorionic gonadotropin where the catalytic activity of the CNT towards hydrogen peroxide greatly amplified the electrochemical response of the sensor [61].

Inorganic oxides are also being widely investigated for their use in biosensors [62]. Individual indium oxide (In_2O_3) nanowires could be functionalised with anti-PSA antibody and then used for 'real-time', label-free detection of PSA (5 ng mL^{-1}); also within this work similar sensors were constructed using a mat of CNTs instead of the nanowires [63]. Magnetite nanoparticles functionalised with an antibody to human IgG have been utilised within a **potentiometric** immunosensor with the nanoparticles being held magnetically at a carbon paste electrode whilst glutaraldehyde crosslinking was used for covalent immobilisation. The sensor was capable of detecting human IgG with a linear range of 0.1–1.2 ng mL^{-1} [64]. Similar work utilised magnetite nanorods to generate an immunosensor for carcinoembryonic antigen with a range 1.5–80 ng mL^{-1}, and a detection limit of 0.9 ng mL^{-1} [65]. Comparable sensitivities were obtained for $CoFe_2O_4$ nanoparticle-containing immunosensors for α-fetoprotein, and were found to have good correlation with ELISA results from human serum samples [66].

Other nanoparticles that have been used include silver, for example, a label-free capacitive immunosensor for microcystin-LR, in which the nanoparticles were bound onto a thiourea-modified gold electrode and then used to immobilise anti-microcystin-LR antibody [67]. The resultant immunosensor was capable of detecting microcystin-LR toxin to provide a detection limit of 7.0 pg L^{-1} and a linear response between 10 pg L^{-1} and 1 μg L^{-1}.

10.4 Microarrays and Nanoarrays

Microelectrodes have several advantages over much larger planar electrodes. Whereas planar electrodes are often diffusion-limited, microelectrodes can experience hemi-spherical diffusion profiles (Fig. 10.4). This can lead to enhanced sensitivity and also responses that are independent of stirring or flow of the analyte. One challenge is that microelectrodes tend to generate smaller signals than larger electrodes, although this can be addressed by having an array of microelectrodes. The responses for these can be combined to give a much larger signal but, providing the microelectrodes are sufficiently spaced, their diffusion profiles do not overlap and they display the enhanced qualities of individual microelectrodes. A number of processes for the construction of microelectrode arrays exist such as, for example, by photolithography. These methods can however often become time consuming and expensive. Within our group we have pioneered a technique for forming microelectrode arrays using sonochemistry [68]. The process is shown schematically in Fig. 10.4. A suitable conductive electrode, such as gold or carbon, is used as a substrate for deposition of an insulating polymer such as poly(1,2-diaminobenzene). This material insulates the electrode so this process is self-limiting and an insulating layer of the order of 50 nm thickness is finally achieved. Sonochemical ablation is then used to pierce holes in the insulating polymer, with diameters in the range 0.1–3 μm, as clearly shown by scanning electron microscopy (Fig. 10.4d). These have been shown to act as a microelectrode array [68]. A further step is then to electrochemically grow conductive polyaniline 'mushrooms' (Fig. 10.4e) from these microelectrodes. Biological

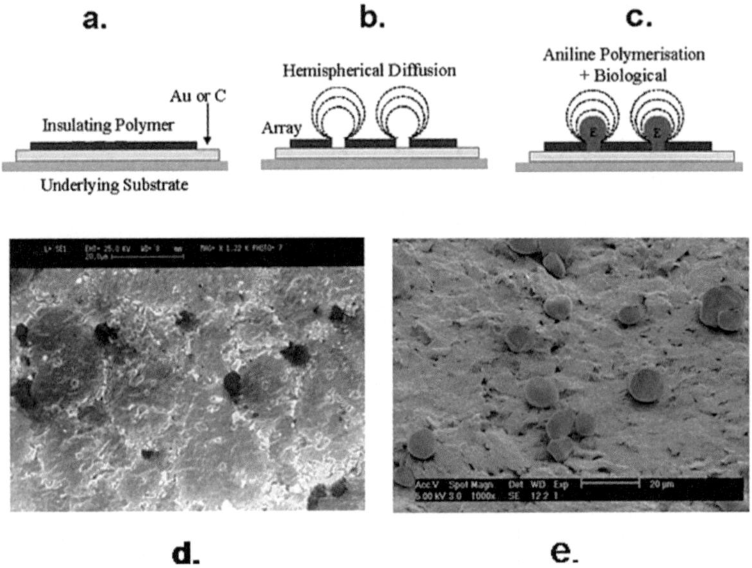

Figure 10.4 Generation of polyaniline microarrays consisting of (a) deposition of insulating layer, (b) sonochemical formation of pores, (c) electropolymerisation to form polyaniline electrodes. Scanning electron micrographs of sonochemically formed pores (d) and polyaniline mushrooms (e) are shown.

recognition moieties can be entrapped in these protrusions, for example glucose oxidase, thereby allowing construction of a glucose sensor [68].

Earlier in this chapter we described AC impedance-based techniques for studying conductive polymer films containing entrapped antibodies [22]. We attempted to demonstrate whether the use of these microarray electrodes would enhance sensitivity. Antibodies to BSA were entrapped in polyaniline mushrooms and compared to similar planar films. Enhancements from μg mL^{-1} to ng mL^{-1} limits of detection were observed with the use of the microelectrode arrays [23]. We had also observed [24–27] that planar electrodes containing antibodies that were selectively bound at the surface by an affinity protocol also displayed much higher sensitivities, with detection limits 2–3 orders of magnitude lower than analogues containing entrapped antibodies. We therefore combined these techniques, forming microarrays of conductive polyaniline mushrooms and then immobilising antibodies to various proteins on their surfaces. The two techniques were synergistic, allowing the construction of immunosensors for BSA, PSA, and the stroke marker proteins neuron specific enolase (NSE) and S100[β], with detection limits as low as 1 pg mL^{-1} [23, 69].

Other workers have fabricated microarrays using different techniques and have even incorporated nanoscale objects such as carbon nanotubes within their sensors to give nanoarray sensors. For example, photolithographic techniques were used to fabricate gold microelectrode arrays with a finger thickness of 5 μm, onto which thiols were adsorbed and used to covalently attach cortisol-specific monoclonal antibodies to give an immunosensor which could detect 1 pM–100 nM cortisol using a label-free electrochemical impedance technique [70]. Similarly, interdigitated gold electrodes with immobilised antibodies could be combined with AC impedance to determine levels of the avian influenza virus H5N1 [71]. Photolithographic methods were also used to fabricate five-by-five arrays of gold microelectrodes of dimensions 25 $\times$ 25 μm onto which diisocyanate-crosslinked antibodies could be deposited. A HRP-labelled competitive immunoassay could then be used for the detection of aflatoxin M_1 in milk with a detection limit of 8 pg mL^{-1} and a dynamic detection range of 10–100 pg mL^{-1} [72].

The ability to grow vertical 'forests' of carbon nanotubes led to their utilisation in nanoelectrode arrays. Carbon nanotubes up to 2 mm in length could be grown by chemical vapour deposition onto a silicon surface. They were grown in blocks 100 $\times$ 100 μm in size to give a microelectrode array of 'nanoforest' (Fig. 10.5). These could then be encapsulated in epoxy, the ends polished and then anti-mouse IgG covalently immobilised on the array [73]. The resultant immunosensor had a detection limit of 200 ng mL^{-1} and a dynamic range up to 100 μg mL^{-1}. Other groups grew vertical carbon nanotubes from a platinum substrate to give a nanoarray of CNTs onto which antibodies to PSA could be attached to give an immunosensor capable of detecting as little as 0.25 ng mL^{-1} of PSA using differential pulse voltammetry [74].

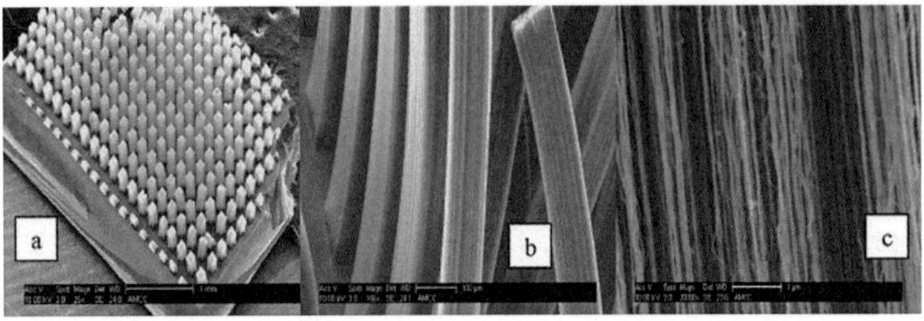

Figure 10.5 ESEM images of (a) aligned multi-wall carbon nanotube patterned arrays on Si substrate; (b) side view of the nanotube array; (c) high-resolution side view of nanotube array. Reproduced from Yun et al. [73] with permission from Elsevier.

10.5 Multiple Target Detection

Currently, most of the immunosensors described in the literature are specific for an individual antigen. This is sufficient if the user is specifically looking for a single target, but if the analysis is more complicated, for example, if looking at a blood sample to detect various disease markers (e.g. different cancers), the required test becomes much more complex. Rather than carrying out a sequence of single tests, it is much simpler and more convenient if a multiple array of sensors could be utilised, each capable of measuring an individual antigen. Examples of this include an immunosensor with separate electrodes that were modified with anti-human IgG, anti-rat IgG and anti-goat IgG, this being then incubated with a solution of one or a mixture of the three antigens and selective binding demonstrated [75]. Multiple detection was also demonstrated using a flow-injection device combined with four separate electrodes to potentially allow simultaneous analyses of four samples for one analyte, or by using four different electrodes, allowing determination of four analytes in one sample [16].

The deposition of multiple receptors onto a single substrate has been pioneered in the area of gene analysis. DNA-based chips and arrays have been constructed and are commercially available. They consist of a substrate, usually glass, which has a collection of microscopic single-stranded DNA spots (probe DNA) immobilised and can be used to simultaneously detect the presence of their counter-strands in complex mixtures by hybridisation. Fluorescence-based labelling in various formats is often utilised to signal a binding event. Tens of thousands of different DNA probes can be immobilised on a single chip. Typical applications include simultaneously genotyping multiple regions of a genotype or measuring expression of a large number of genes. Similar techniques have been used to construct protein microarrays. However, quantification can be difficult, with the detection of fluorescence tending to be qualitative rather than quantitative.

Electrochemical microarrays are being examined as a potential solution to this application. Microelectrode arrays have been developed by the Combimatrix Corporation which contain a large number of individually addressable microelectrodes. A variety of oligonucleotides can be assembled onto these microelectrodes and then used to immobilise antibodies tagged with the appropriate complementary strands, allowing simultaneous immobilisation of several antibodies. For example antibodies to human α-1-acid glycoprotein, ricin, M13 phage, *Bacillus globigii* spores, and fluorescein were all immobilised onto a commercial chip and shown to detect a wide range of antigen concentrations selectively in 50 μL mixed samples [76].

Other workers also constructed a microarray containing 36 platinum microelectrodes. Antibodies were selectively spotted onto the microelectrodes and then a labelled sandwich immunoassay protocol utilised to simultaneously determine levels of α-1-fetoprotein and β_2-microglobulin [77]. Another worker patterned dual indium oxide electrodes onto a glass substrate, immobilised antibodies onto these and could selectively detect any two antigens from goat IgG, mouse IgG, CEA, and AFP with detection limits of 1, 2, 1.2 and 1 ng mL^{-1}, respectively [78]. Screen-printed electrodes could also be constructed with antibodies to three different herbicides immobilised on them and a competitive 'ELISA-type' assay used to measure the presence of the herbicides individually and in mixtures [79].

Screen-printed carbon arrays have been successfully constructed and used to immobilise antibodies to carcinoembryonic antigen, α-fetoprotein, β-human choriogonadotropin and carcinoma antigen [80]. The resultant array was capable of analysing the four antigens with detection limits of 1.1 μg L^{-1}, 1.7 μg L^{-1}, 1.2 IU L^{-1} and 1.7 kIU L^{-1}, respectively. Other teams have also constructed gold electrode arrays on which they immobilised antigens to five hepatitis variants (hepatitis A to E); these proved capable of independently determining the concentrations of the viral antigens in mixed samples with limits of detection <1 ng mL^{-1} [81].

10.6 Imaging of Arrays and Scanning Electrochemical Microscopy (SECM)

The previous section described how multiple electrode arrays can be constructed, with a number of biological recognition elements being immobilised and utilised for simultaneous analysis for a variety of antigens. These systems are, however, much more difficult to construct than the simple coated glass slides used for many DNA microarray studies and this challenge increases with the number of antigens we wish to immobilise. A different approach would be simply to immobilise the recognition elements on a suitable surface using a dotting technique such as is used for DNA microarrays and then after incubation with the sample, scan across each dot using a technique that can detect the electrochemical changes that occur when the target species is bound. Such a technique is called scanning electrochemical microscopy (SECM).

SECM is a technique in which a probe is scanned above a surface in a similar approach to atomic force microscopy, except in this case both topographical information and high resolution electrochemical data are obtained [82]. Usually the probe will be a microelectrode, such as a thin platinum wire suitably encased in a non-conductive sheath, for example, glass or epoxy and this is then mounted on an XYZ stage. The surface is immersed into an electrolyte, often containing a redox probe such as ferrocene carboxylic acid with the microelectrode being scanned across the surface (Fig. 10.6). Most commonly the SECM is operated in feedback mode, where perhaps the redox probe is, for example, oxidised at the surface before diffusing through the solution to the probe where it can be reduced, or vice versa. SECM can be used to detect and image a

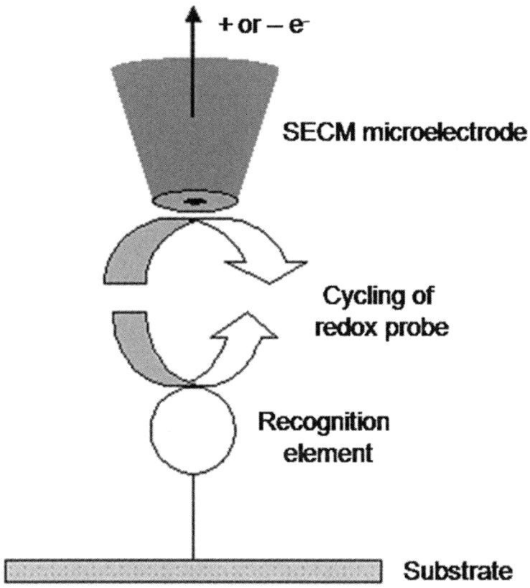

Figure 10.6 Schematic of the SECM operating in feedback mode.

wide range of biological moieties such as enzymes, antibodies, DNA or cells and has been reviewed extensively [82]. Labelled methods, where the species bound is labelled with an electrochemically active unit or an enzyme, such as HRP are known in addition to label-free techniques. SECM is especially effective if electroactive species are being generated at a surface, with the small size of the microelectrode allowing imaging of that process.

Since a detailed review of SECM is beyond of the scope of this chapter we shall just mention two pioneering studies that utilise this technique to image immunological activity. In early work, anti-digoxin antibody was immobilised as spots onto glass slides and exposed to solutions of the antigen conjugated to alkaline phosphatase [83]. The enzyme catalysed the reaction of 4-aminophenyl phosphate to 4-aminophenol which is redox active. Oxidation of this species occurred at the microelectrode tip and allowed imaging of the antibody spots.

Within our group we have also looked at SECM for both the formation and the 'label-free' imaging of antibody arrays [84]. The SECM was used first to form a 12-spot array by dotting solutions of anti-NSE (non-specific enolase [NSE] is a stroke marker protein) onto polyethyleneimine-modified screen-printed carbon electrodes. When the electrodes were placed in a 5 mM solution of ferrocene carboxylic acid and scanned, clear contrasts could be seen between dotted and non-dotted portions of the array, allowing for imaging of the antibody dots (Fig. 10.7). Comparison of images and line scans taken before and after exposure to the antibody showed clear changes (Fig. 10.7). This technique allowed determination of NSE concentrations with a linear range of 0.5 pg mL^{-1} to 200 pg mL^{-1} [84].

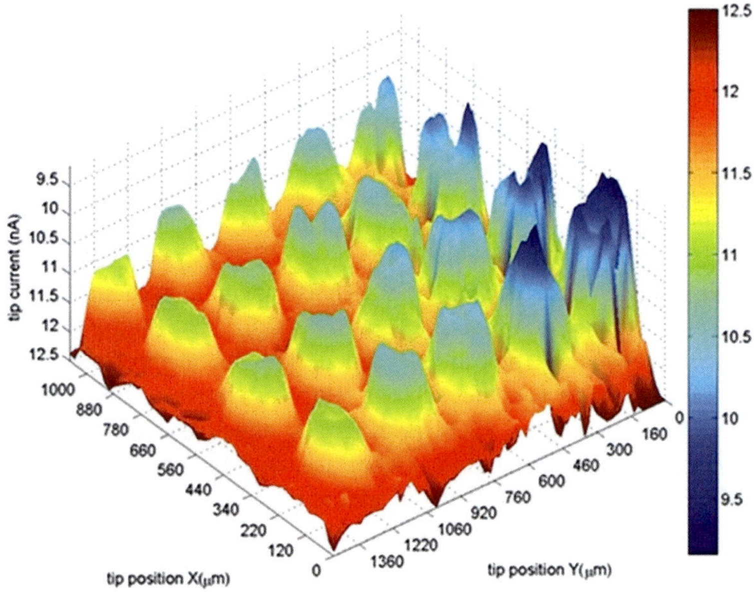

Figure 10.7 A typical scanning electrochemical microscope plot.

10.7 Conclusions and Future Prospects

We have, within this chapter attempted to discuss the most recent trends in electrochemical immunoassays and also what we feel will be the future trends in this field. Immunoassays really 'came of age' with the ELISA technique which allowed optical detection of a huge range of antigens without the need for such equipment intensive and expensive methods such as the various chromatographic and mass spectrometric methods that would otherwise be required. Other methods such as lateral-flow assay allowed simple home or point-of-care tests such as the pregnancy test to become feasible. However, these methods do have some associated challenges and electrochemical immunoassay systems have arisen which can address some of these. Many of the potential uses of electrochemical immunoassays have been reviewed elsewhere, such as for food screening [85].

One of the greatest needs is for point-of-care devices. The ideal device would be small, inexpensive, be capable of detecting a wide range of analytes and give rapid and quantitative results. It would be able to analyse a wide range of sample matrices (blood, sweat, etc.) and display high specificity, minimal biofouling and non-specific responses as well as being able to be used in turbulent systems. The electrochemical immunoassay goes some way towards addressing these challenges.

The unrivalled specificity of antibody-antigen interactions is the main driver for immunoassays of any type. These interactions allow the binding of antigens even when present in low concentrations, which combined with the high sensitivity of electrochemical techniques to changes at electrode surface allows detection of extremely low (pg mL^{-1}) levels of analyte. A major advantage of many of these electrochemical methods is that they are very rapid, with the actual measurement requiring minutes or seconds while many are label-free, which removes the need for costly and time consuming pre-treatment.

For many analytes, the immunoassay system is required to give an accurate result and be sensitive across a range of concentrations. We have shown that this range can be modified by the design of the immunoassay. The use of microelectrodes and microelectrode arrays will come to the fore in this due to the demonstrated increases in sensitivity attributed to these devices, along with their 'stir independence' and the ability to be used in 'high-resistance' media.

Although many immunoassays are just required for a single purpose (again the obvious one being the pregnancy test which is used more for confirmation rather than as a regular diagnostic check) immunoassays which can detect a range of analytes in a small sample volume, e.g. from a drop of blood, are likely to become more common, especially in the context of point-of-care devices. It would be highly advantageous to be able to scan a blood sample, for example, the ten most common markers for cancer as part of a general health check. Likewise, should a paramedic or other 'first-line' responder be called to the aid of an unconscious person, an assay which could simultaneously check, blood glucose, stroke markers and myocardial infarction markers would aid in rapid diagnosis and reduce the time required to apply appropriate remedial treatment. Apart from medical sensors, other applications would include analysing a river water sample for all common pesticides or milk for presence of antibiotics [27]. Other targets include mycotoxins [32, 55, 72], microcystins [67], bacterial contaminants [36, 71] and pathogens [49, 51, 81]. Electrochemical immunoassays have been applied to simultaneously detect a variety of analytes in a mixed sample and devices such as those produced by Combimatrix will become prominent.

We predict that in the future, the mature state of electronic technology will allow the miniaturisation of many of these devices. For this to be successful there will need to be integration with microfluidic technology to allow delivery of the sample to multiple assay electrodes for analysis of complex samples containing many antigens of interest. Label-free techniques will become more prevalent and will aid in reducing the cost and time of these assays, allowing them to be performed as point-of-care or even home tests. The low cost of screen-printed electrodes and the speed of many of these assays will allow high throughput screening of the large number of samples required for mass screening. Electrochemical immunoassay methods will join enzymatic glucose biosensors, ELISA and lateral-flow assays as major tools in the monitoring of human health and disease diagnosis, for quality control for our food and water supplies as well as for the protection of the environment.

In the academic field much research seems to be focussed on the incorporation of smart materials into immunoassay systems, with a number of recent books and reviews having been published on this [86–88]. We have already discussed the use of many of these materials such as metal nanoparticles and carbon nanotubes. Other materials that are being widely studied include inorganic nanoparticles because of their ability to catalyse reactions, this has made them of interest for such applications as the non-enzymatic determination of glucose and other targets without the need for expensive biological reagents [89, 90]. Another relatively new material graphene, is of great interest due to its high surface area to mass ratio, high conductivity and ability to catalyse electrochemical reactions. A number of biochemical assays and immunoassays have been reported as reviewed here [91–93]. Although a relatively new material, there is now much research being carried out on graphene and other carbon nanomaterials. Although both are made up mainly of sp^2 hybridised carbon, their difference in shape makes carbon nanotubes and graphene very different indeed [94]. For example, graphene has lower cost, higher purity, lower electrical noise and can be more processable. However, the high aspect ratio of carbon nanotubes allows them to be used as electrical wires, formulated into nanotube "forests" or used as individual nanoelectrodes. Hydrogels are also being studied because of their ability to change their properties in response to many stimuli and also their high biocompatibility and ability to stabilise complex biological molecules without denaturation [95].

On the commercial side, the future market for electrochemical immunoassays looks set to increase, for example a recent report [96] predicts a 6% annual increase in the clinical immunoassay analyser market. The US is the largest medical device market, predicted to reach $155 billion in 2017, approximately 43% of the world market. The top market vendors include companies such as Abbott Diagnostics, Beckman Coulter, bioMerieux, Roche Diagnostics and Siemens Healthcare with the fastest growing market predicted to be in the oncology and endocrinology field. They also estimate that instruments will be 75% of the market share by 2020. Other technologies allowing the wireless communication of data, driven by the computing and mobile phone industries, will also be applied to these devices allowing remote use. Paper-based immunoassays are being widely studied in an attempt to reduce the costs of assays. Should the combination of reduced sizes, reduced costs and increased ease-of-operation prove attainable, it looks likely that hand-held instruments for determining clinical, veterinary and environmental targets will become common, in the same way that glucose testing for diabetes has gone from being a hospital-based laboratory procedure to the simple hand-held devices allowing home monitoring.

References

1. Yalow, R.S., and S.A. Berson, Immunoassay of endogenous plasma insulin in man. *J Clin Invest*, 1960. **39**:1157–1175.
2. Frazier, R.A., Tudos, A.J., ed. *Handbook of Surface Plasmon Resonance*. 2008, Royal Society of Chemistry.
3. Clark, L.C., Jr., and C. Lyons, Electrode systems for continuous monitoring in cardiovascular surgery. *Ann N Y Acad Sci*, 1962. **102**:29–45.
4. Wang, J., Glucose biosensors: 40 years of advances and challenges. *Electroanalysis*, 2001. **13**(12):983–988.
5. Cass, A.E., et al., Ferrocene-mediated enzyme electrode for amperometric determination of glucose. *Anal Chem*, 1984. **56**(4):667–671.
6. Degani, Y., and Heller, A., Direct electrical communication between chemically modified enzymes and metal electrodes. I. Electron transfer from glucose oxidase to metal electrodes via electron relays, bound covalently to the enzyme. *J Phys Chem*, 1987. **91**:1285–1289.
7. John, R., et al., Development of a polypyrrole-based human serum-albumin sensor. *Anal Chim Acta*, 1991. **249**(2):381–385.
8. Hock, B., Antibodies for immunosensors - a review. *Anal Chim Acta*, 1997. **347**(1–2):177–186.
9. Cosnier, S., Affinity biosensors based on electropolymerized films. *Electroanalysis*, 2005. **17**(19):1701–1715.
10. Diaz-Gonzalez, M., M.B. Gonzalez-Garcia, and A. Costa-Garcia, Recent advances in electrochemical enzyme immunoassays. *Electroanalysis*, 2005. **17**(21):1901–1918.
11. Rodriguez-Mozaz, S., M.J.L. de Alda, and D. Barcelo, Biosensors as useful tools for environmental analysis and monitoring. *Anal Bioanal Chem*, 2006. **386**(4):1025–1041.
12. Centi, S., S. Laschi, and M. Mascini, Strategies for electrochemical detection in immunochemistry. *Bioanalysis*, 2009. **1**(7):1271–1291.

13. Jiao, K., et al., Application of p-phenylenediamine as an electrochemical substrate in peroxidase-mediated voltammetric enzyme immunoassay. *Anal Chim Acta*, 2000. **413**(1–2):71–78.
14. Sun, W., K. Jiao, and S.S. Zhang, Electrochemical ELISA for the detection of cucumber mosaic virus using o-pheneylenediamine as substrate. *Talanta*, 2001. **55**(6):1211–1218.
15. Tang, T.C., A.P. Deng, and H.J. Huang, Immunoassay with a microtiter plate incorporated multichannel electrochemical detection system. *Anal Chem*, 2002. **74**(11):2617–2621.
16. Baskeyfield, D.E.H., et al., A membrane-based immunosensor for the analysis of the herbicide isoproturon. *Anal Chim Acta*, 2011. **699**(2):223–231.
17. Bagel, O., et al., Enzyme affinity assays involving a single-use electrochemical sensor. Applications to the enzyme immunoassay of human chorionic gonadotropin hormone and nucleic acid hybridization of human cytomegalovirus DNA. *Electroanalysis*, 2000. **12**(18):1447–1452.
18. Sadik, O.A., and G.G. Wallace, Pulsed amperometric detection of proteins using antibody-containing conducting polymers. *Anal Chim Acta*, 1993. **279**(2):209–212.
19. Grant, S., et al., Labeless and reversible immunosensor assay based upon an electrochemical current-transient protocol. *Anal Chim Acta*, 2003. **495**(1–2):21–32.
20. Katz, E., and I. Willner, Probing biomolecular interactions at conductive and semiconductive surfaces by impedance spectroscopy: routes to impedimetric immunosensors, DNA-sensors, and enzyme biosensors. *Electroanalysis*, 2003. **15**(11):913–947.
21. Prodromidis, M.I., Impedimetric immunosensors - a review. *Electrochim Acta*, 2010. **55**(14):4227–4233.
22. Grant, S., et al., Label-free and reversible immunosensor based upon an AC impedance interrogation protocol. *Anal Chim Acta*, 2005. **537**(1–2):163–168.
23. Barton, A.C., et al., Labeless AC impedimetric antibody-based sensors with pg/ml sensitivities for point-of-care biomedical applications. *Biosens Bioelectron*, 2009. **24**(5):1090–1095.
24. Tsekenis, G., et al., Label-less immunosensor assay for myelin basic protein based upon an AC impedance protocol. *Anal Chem*, 2008. **80**(6):2058–2062.

25. Tully, E., S.P. Higson, and R. O'Kennedy, The development of a 'labeless' immunosensor for the detection of *Listeria monocytogenes* cell surface protein, Internalin B. *Biosens Bioelectron*, 2008. **23**(6):906–912.
26. Garifallou, G.Z., et al., Labeless immunosensor assay for fluoroquinolone antibiotics based upon an AC impedance protocol. *Anal Lett*, 2007. **40**(7):1412–1422.
27. Tsekenis, G., et al., Detection of fluoroquinolone antibiotics in milk via a labeless immunoassay based upon an alternating current impedance protocol. *Anal Chem*, 2008. **80**(23):9233–9239.
28. Ramon-Azcon, J., et al., An impedimetric immunosensor based on interdigitated microelectrodes (ID mu E) for the determination of atrazine residues in food samples. *Biosens Bioelectron*, 2008. **23**(9):1367–1373.
29. Pournaras, A.V., T. Koraki, and M.I. Prodromidis, Development of an impedimetric immunosensor based on electropolymerized polytyramine films for the direct detection of *Salmonella typhimurium* in pure cultures of type strains and inoculated real samples. *Anal Chim Acta*, 2008. **624**(2):301–307.
30. Wu, C.C., C.H. Lin, and W.S. Wang, Development of an enrofloxacin immunosensor based on label-free electrochemical impedance spectroscopy. *Talanta*, 2009. **79**(1):62–67.
31. Escamilla-Gomez, V., et al., Gold screen-printed-based impedimetric immunobiosensors for direct and sensitive *Escherichia coli* quantisation. *Biosens Bioelectron*, 2009. **24**(11):3365–3371.
32. Owino, J.H.O., et al., Modelling of the impedimetric responses of an aflatoxin B-1 immunosensor prepared on an electrosynthetic polyaniline platform. *Anal Bioanal Chem*, 2007. **388**(5–6):1069–1074.
33. Wu, Z.S., et al., A sensitive immunoassay based on electropolymerized films by capacitance measurements for direct detection of immunospecies. *Anal Biochem*, 2005. **337**(2):308–315.
34. Liu, Z., et al., A novel capacitive immunosensor using electropolymerized insulating poly (o-phenylenediamine) film on a glass carbon electrode for probing transferrin. *Anal Lett*, 2004. **37**(11):2283–2301.
35. Balkenhohl, T., and F. Lisdat, Screen-printed electrodes as impedimetric immunosensors for the detection of anti-transglutaminase antibodies in human sera. *Anal Chim Acta*, 2007. **597**(1):50–57.
36. Estrela, P., et al., Label-free sub-picomolar protein detection with field-effect transistors. *Anal Chem*, 2010. **82**(9):3531–3536.
37. Purvis, D., et al., An ultrasensitive and stable potentiometric immunosensor. *Biosens Bioelectron*, 2003. **18**(11):1385–1390.

38. Pandey, P., M. Datta, and B.D. Malhotra, Prospects of nanomaterials in biosensors. *Anal Lett*, 2008. **41**(2):159–209.

39. Merkoci, A., Nanoparticles-based strategies for DNA, protein and cell sensors. *Biosens Bioelectron*, 2010. **26**(4):1164–1177.

40. Siangproh, W., et al., Nanoparticle-based electrochemical detection in conventional and miniaturized systems and their bioanalytical applications - a review. *Anal Chim Acta*, 2011. **690**(1):10–25.

41. Zhuo, Y., et al., Amperometric enzyme immunosensors based on layer-by-layer assembly of gold nanoparticles and thionine on Nafion-modified electrode surface for alpha-1-fetoprotein determinations. *Sens Actuators B*, 2006. **114**(2):631–639.

42. Liang, W.B., et al., A novel, label-free immunosensor for the detection of alpha-fetoprotein using functionalised gold nanoparticles. *Clin Biochem*, 2009. **42**(15):1524–1530.

43. Yin, T.J., et al., A novel capacitive immunosensor for transferrin detection based on ultrathin alumina sol-gel-derived films and gold nanoparticles. *Sens Actuators B*, 2006. **117**(1):286–294.

44. Chen, J., et al., A gold nanoparticles/sol-gel composite architecture for encapsulation of immunoconjugate for reagentless electrochemical immunoassay. *Biomaterials*, 2006. **27**(10):2313–2321.

45. Fu, Y.Z., et al., Study on the immobilization of anti-IgG on Au-colloid modified gold electrode via potentiometric immunosensor, cyclic voltammetry, and electrochemical impedance techniques. *Colloids Surf B*, 2005. **40**(1):61–66.

46. Du, D., et al., Reagentless amperometric carbohydrate antigen 19-9 immunosensor based on direct electrochemistry of immobilized horseradish peroxidase. *Talanta*, 2007. **71**(3):1257–1262.

47. Liang, K.Z., and W.J. Mu, Flow-injection immuno-bioassay for interleukin-6 in humans based on gold nanoparticles modified screen-printed graphite electrodes. *Anal Chim Acta*, 2006. **580**(2):128–135.

48. Kim, D.M., et al., Immunosensors for detection of Annexin II and MUC5AC for early diagnosis of lung cancer. *Biosens Bioelectron*, 2009. **25**(2):456–462.

49. Wu, S., et al., Gold nanoparticle-labeled detection antibodies for use in an enhanced electrochemical immunoassay of hepatitis B surface antigen in human serum. *Microchim Acta*, 2009. **166**(3–4):269–275.

50. Ho, J.A.A., et al., Gold-nanostructured immunosensor for the electrochemical sensing of biotin based on liposomal competitive assay. *J Nanosci Nanotechnol*, 2009. **9**(4):2324–2329.

51. Ding, C.F., et al., Electrochemical immunoassay of hepatitis B surface antigen by the amplification of gold nanoparticles based on the nanoporous gold electrode. *Talanta*, 2010. **80**(3):1385–1391.
52. Ahammad, A.J.S., J.J. Lee, and M.A. Rahman, Electrochemical sensors based on carbon nanotubes. *Sensors*, 2009. **9**(4):2289–2319.
53. Park, D.W., et al., Detection of tumor markers using single-walled carbon nanotube field effect transistors. *J Nanosci Nanotechnol*, 2006. **6**(11):3499–3502.
54. Cataldo, V., A. Vaze, and J.F. Rusling, Improved detection limit and stability of amperometric carbon nanotube-based immunosensors by crosslinking antibodies with polylysine. *Electroanalysis*, 2008. **20**(2):115–122.
55. Viswanathan, S., et al., Electrochemical immunosensor for cholera toxin using liposomes and poly(3,4-ethylenedioxythiophene)-coated carbon nanotubes. *Anal Chem*, 2006. **78**(4):1115–1121.
56. Sanchez, S., M. Pumera, and E. Fabregas, Carbon nanotube/polysulfone screen-printed electrochemical immunosensor. *Biosens Bioelectron*, 2007. **23**(3):332–340.
57. Aziz, M.A., et al., Amperometric immunosensing using an indium tin oxide electrode modified with multi-walled carbon nanotube and poly(ethylene glycol)-silane copolymer. *Chem Commun*, 2007(25): 2610–2612.
58. Takeda, S., et al., Application of carbon nanotubes for detecting anti-hemagglutinins based on antigen-antibody interaction. *Biosens Bioelectron*, 2005. **21**(1):201–205.
59. Yu, X., et al., Carbon nanotube amplification strategies for highly sensitive immunodetection of cancer biomarkers. *J Am Chem Soc*, 2006. **128**(34):11199–11205.
60. Ou, C.F., et al., A novel amperometric immunosensor based on layer-by-layer assembly of gold nanoparticles-multi-walled carbon nanotubes-thionine multilayer films on polyelectrolyte surface. *Anal Chim Acta*, 2007. **603**(2):205–213.
61. Li, N., et al., Sensitive immunoassay of human chorionic gonadotrophin based on multi-walled carbon nanotube-chitosan matrix. *Bioprocess Biosyst Eng*, 2008. **31**(6):551–558.
62. Liu, A.H., Towards development of chemosensors and biosensors with metal-oxide-based nanowires or nanotubes. *Biosens Bioelectron*, 2008. **24**(2):167–177.

63. Li, C., et al., Complementary detection of prostate-specific antigen using $In_{(2)}O_{(3)}$ nanowires and carbon nanotubes. *J Am Chem Soc*, 2005. **127**(36):12484–12485.

64. Li, J.P., and H.D. Gao, A renewable potentiometric immunosensor based on Fe_3O_4 nanoparticles immobilized anti-IgG. *Electroanalysis*, 2008. **20**(8):881–887.

65. Fu, X.H., et al., Label-free electrochemical immunoassay of carcinoembryonic antigen in human serum using magnetic nanorods as sensing probes. *Microchim Acta*, 2009. **165**(3–4):437–442.

66. Wang, L., and X.X. Gan, Antibody-functionalized magnetic nanoparticles for electrochemical immunoassay of alpha-1-fetoprotein in human serum. *Microchim Acta*, 2009. **164**(1–2):231–237.

67. Loyprasert, S., et al., Label-free capacitive immunosensor for microcystin-LR using self-assembled thiourea monolayer incorporated with Ag nanoparticles on gold electrode. *Biosens Bioelectron*, 2008. **24**(1):78–86.

68. Barton, A.C., et al., Sonochemically fabricated microelectrode arrays for biosensors offering widespread applicability: Part I. *Biosens Bioelectron*, 2004. **20**(2):328–337.

69. Collyer, S.D., F. Davis, and S.P.J. Higson, Sonochemically fabricated microelectrode arrays for use as sensing platforms. *Sensors*, 2010. **10**(5):5090–5132.

70. Arya, S.K., et al., Dithiobis(succinimidyl propionate)-modified gold microarray electrode-based electrochemical immunosensor for ultrasensitive detection of cortisol. *Biosens Bioelectron*, 2010. **25**(10):2296–2301.

71. Wang, R.H., et al., Interdigitated array microelectrode-based impedance immunosensor for detection of avian influenza virus H5N1. *Talanta*, 2009. **79**(2):159–164.

72. Parker, C.O., et al., Electrochemical immunochip sensor for aflatoxin M(1) detection. *Anal Chem*, 2009. **81**(13):5291–5298.

73. Yun, Y., et al., A nanotube array immunosensor for direct electrochemical detection of antigen-antibody binding. *Sens Actuators B*, 2007. **123**(1):177–182.

74. Okuno, J., et al., Label-free immunosensor for prostate-specific antigen based on single-walled carbon nanotube array-modified microelectrodes. *Biosens Bioelectron*, 2007. **22**(9–10):2377–2381.

75. Yu, X.B., et al., An impedance biosensor array for label-free detection of multiple antigen-antibody reactions. *Front Biosci*, 2006. **11**:983–990.

76. Dill, K., et al., Immunoassays based on electrochemical detection using microelectrode arrays. *Biosens Bioelectron*, 2004. **20**(4):736–742.
77. Kojima, K., et al., Electrochemical protein chip with arrayed immunosensors with antibodies immobilized in a plasma-polymerized film. *Anal Chem*, 2003. **75**(5):1116–1122.
78. Wilson, M.S., Electrochemical immunosensors for the simultaneous detection of two tumor markers. *Anal Chem*, 2005. **77**(5):1496–1502.
79. Kasna, A., and P. Skladal, A four-channel electrochemical immunosensor for detection of herbicides based on phenoxyalkanoic acids. *Int J Environ Anal Chem*, 2003. **83**(2):101–109.
80. Wu, J., et al., A disposable multianalyte electrochemical immunosensor array for automated simultaneous determination of tumor markers. *Clin Chem*, 2007. **53**(8):1495–1502.
81. Tang, D.P., et al., Simultaneous determination of five-type hepatitis virus antigens in 5 min using an integrated automatic electrochemical immunosensor array. *Biosens Bioelectron*, 2010. **25**(7):1658–1662.
82. Roberts, W.S., et al., Advances in the application of scanning electrochemical microscopy to bioanalytical systems. *Biosens Bioelectron*, 2007. **23**(3):301–318.
83. Wittstock, G., et al., Imaging of immobilized antibody layers with scanning electrochemical microscopy. *Anal Chem*, 1995. **67**(19):3578–3582.
84. Holmes, J.L., et al., A new application of scanning electrochemical microscopy for the label-free interrogation of antibody-antigen interactions. *Anal Chim Acta*, 2011. **689**(2):206–211.
85. Ricci, F., et al., A review on novel developments and applications of immunosensors in food analysis. *Anal Chim Acta*, 2007. **605**(2):111–129.
86. Honeychurch, K.J., ed. *Nanosensors for Chemical and Biological Applications: Sensing with Nanotubes, Nanowires and Nanoparticles*. 2014, Woodhead.
87. Li, S., Ge, Y., and Li, H., *Smart Nanomaterials for Sensor Application*, 2012, Bentham.
88. Choi, S., Tripathi, A., and Singh, D.J., Smart nanomaterials for biomedics. *Biomed Nanotech*, 2014. **10**:3162–3188.
89. Malhotra, B.D., Das, M., and Solanki, P.R., Opportunities in nanostructured metal oxides based biosensors. *J Phys Conf Ser*, 2012. **358**:012007-1/8.

90. Solanki, P.R., Kaushik, A., Agrawal, V.V., and Malhotra, B.D., Nanostructured metal oxide-based biosensors. *NPG Asia Mater*, 2011. **3**:17–24.
91. Fang, Y., and Wang, E., Electrochemical biosensors on platforms of graphene. *Chem Commun*, 2013. **49**:9526–9539.
92. Wu, S., et al., Graphene-based electrochemical sensors. *Small*, 2013. **9**:1160–1172.
93. Wisitsoraat, A., and Tuantranont, A., Graphene-based chemical and biosensors. In *Applications of Nanomaterials in Sensors and Diagnostics*. 2013, Springer-Heidelberg, New York.
94. Yang, W.K., et al., Carbon nanomaterials in biosensors: should you use nanotubes or graphene? *Angew Chem Int Ed*, 2010. **49**:2114–2138.
95. Xiong, X., et al., Responsive DNA-based hydrogels and their applications. *Macromol Rapid Commun*, 2013. **34**:1271–1283.
96. Clinical Immunoassay Analyzer Market in the US 2016–2020. Published by Technavio 2016. http://www.technavio.com/report/usa-life-science-research-tools-clinical-immunoassay-analyzer-market. Accessed on: Jan 2017.

Chapter 11

Optical Signal Transduction with an Emphasis on the Application of Surface Plasmon Resonance (SPR) in Antibody Characterisation

Caroline Murphy, Aoife Crawley, Hannah Byrne, Kara Moran, Jenny Fitzgerald, and Richard O'Kennedy
School of Biotechnology and Biomedical Diagnostics Institute, Dublin City University, Collins Avenue, Dublin 9, Ireland
caroline.s.murphy@dcu.ie

Optical immunosensors utilise properties of light, such as **refraction**, production of **evanescent waves** and **reflection**. They measure changes in these properties during biomolecular interactions. This chapter looks at the different facets of optical signalling technology and its use in immunoassays. The use of a variety of approaches utilising optical labels and associated detection approaches was previously described in Chapter 1. Finally, one of the most commonly used methods of optical signal transduction, surface plasmon resonance (SPR), is described and its key role in antibody characterisation is discussed.

Immunoassays: Development, Applications and Future Trends
Edited by Richard O'Kennedy and Caroline Murphy

ISBN 978-981-4669-97-9 (Hardcover), 978-1-315-20654-7 (eBook)
www.panstanford.com

11.1 The Fundamentals of Optical Signal Transduction

Optical sensing can be carried out using 'labelled' or 'label-free' systems. Labelled systems make use of luminescent elements, while label-free do not. The uses of label-free optical monitoring systems have increased in popularity due to an associated 'ease-of-construction', low cost, and superior performance in complex matrices while maintaining high sensitivities. Label-free optical detection can facilitate 'real-time' monitoring of bio-molecular interactions; however, they are pre-disposed to problems such as non-specific binding and reduced sensitivities to low molecular weight analytes [1]. Optical sensors can be easily combined with microfluidic systems, to provide a convenient method for sample delivery and measurement.

The refractive index (RI) of light is a measure of how light bends (refracts) when it moves through a medium. Materials such as glass, quartz, diamond, polymer films and polymer fibres exhibit high refractive indices and hence make useful waveguides [1, 2]. Waveguides function to guide electronic waves such as light along a medium. The RI of light comes into play when utilising sensors that take advantage of total internal reflection (TIR). Incident light is shone between two media of different optical densities (light travels from the more optically dense [high RI, e.g. glass] medium towards the less optically dense [low RI, e.g. water]). Depending on the angle at which incident light hits the interface of the two media, some light is refracted and some light is internally reflected back into the medium of higher optical density. Finally, at a certain angle of incidence there is no further refraction and all of the light is totally internally reflected. This phenomenon results in the penetration of an evanescent wave into the medium of lower optical density (lower RI), where the biomolecular sensing occurs [1, 2].

The process of **total internal reflection fluorescence (TIRF)** is a useful analytical technology that uses both TIR and fluorescence. The evanescent wave propagates into the biological layer influencing (and/or exciting) the adsorbed biological molecules [1]. The fluorescently tagged molecules (antibodies or analyte) are excited and emit fluorescence that is recorded using a fluorimeter. This tool has proved very useful for visualising live cellular events, and allowing measurement of these events specifically at the plasma membrane, such as exocytosis, single-molecular interactions and ionic changes during signal transduction [3]. Boulanger and colleagues devised a method to view cellular processes at the plasma membrane of live adherent cells in three dimensions. They computationally reconstructed three-dimensional images using multi-wavelength azimuthal averaging and incidence angle scanning. This approach allows investigation of several dynamic processes in the cell at a depth of up to 800 nm from the plasma membrane [4].

Optical waveguide lightmode spectroscopy (OWLS) is an alternative optical sensor platform that utilises waveguide technology. Linearly polarised light (using a He-Ne laser) is incoupled at a specific angle into a waveguide. Light is guided along the waveguide layer by TIR to the ends of the sensor chip. The association or dissociation of biomolecules at the surface of the waveguide impact on the RI of the medium. Changes at the sensor surface result in changes in the incoupling resonance, which is measured by a photodiode [5, 6]. OWLS-based immunosensors are routinely employed in food quality monitoring for the detection of toxins [5, 6] enzymes [7] antibiotics [8] and bacteria [9].

Ellipsometry is an additional optical detection technique that recognises changes in the thickness of ultrathin films. It achieves this by measuring changes in light reflection intensity when biomolecules bind to the surface [10]. Wang et al. used this technique to analyse the interaction of tropomyosin allergens with specific antibodies and compared the technique to ELISA [10]. The ellipsometric method was found to perform a fast, label-free analysis. Ellipsometry is routinely used for characterisation of materials employed in technological applications such as protective and functional coatings, sensors, microelectronics, surface modification, membrane separations and even batteries [11, 12]. The main advantages of this technique include the very high precision and accuracy achievable, combined with the fact that it is non-intrusive and can be used with both transparent and non-transparent substrates [13]. Wang found that the technique was amenable to multiplexing and performing 'on-site' analysis. An alternative evanescent wave-based device was described by Gupta and colleagues [14], whereby a **resonant mirror** was used to detect 'real-time' 'protein-protein' interactions using anti-IgG and IgG as a model system. A resonant mirror is an optical sensing system that probes the sensing surface to which an evanescent wave has been applied. A simple system was described that used a silica sol–gel spacer layer on a standard microscope glass slide. Using an evanescent polystyrene waveguide system and a dielectric resonant structure, the bio-molecular interactions at the sensing layer were investigated and measured by ellipsometry [14, 15].

Fibre-optic technology can be used in simple and 'easy-to-develop' biosensors. Fibre-optic immunosensors have been reported for numerous analytes [16–20]. Antibody or analyte immobilised on the end (proximal and distal ends have been described) of an optical fibre are excited by TIR that propagates the length of the fibre from a light source.

Finally, surface plasmon resonance (SPR) is an optical signal transduction system that is commonly used to determine the binding of antibody/antigen partners. It has become an integral part of antibody characterisation and is the cornerstone of label-free biosensing applications. SPR is described in more detail in the following section.

Within these systems, further signal enhancement is also possible through the use of functionalised nanomaterials. Optical nanoparticle probes such as fluorescence energy transfer nanobeads and quantum dots (QDs) provide significant advantages in comparison to organic dyes or fluorescent particles in terms of signal brightness, photostability, and multicolour-light emission [21].

11.2 Description and Evaluation of the Use of Surface Plasmon Resonance in Immunoassays

Surface plasmon resonance (SPR) is a phenomenon that occurs at the interface between a metal surface and a liquid when a light beam strikes at a particular angle. SPR is sensitive to changes in mass that occur at the sensor surface when an antibody binds to its antigen (Fig. 11.1) [22]. This technique is valuable in the determination of affinity parameters for biomolecular interactions [23]. SPR-based methods are favourable as the binding events can be monitored in real-time and without the requirement of ancillary labels. These key attributes facilitate accurate kinetic measurements, rapid analysis times, reduced additional costs, and avoids possible heterogeneities or other complications that may arise when using labelled interactants [24].

The fundamental mechanics of SPR start when polarised light is shone through a prism onto a metal surface at a certain angle and light is reflected (Fig. 11.1). At a certain angle at which the light passes through the prism, total internal reflection (TIR) occurs. Photons of light that are totally internally reflected create an **evanescent wave** at the interface between the gold film and the reaction medium. The evanescent wave moves exponentially and excites what are known as **plasmons** (electron charged density waves) at the gold surface. This excitation causes a decrease in the intensity of the reflected light. The angle at which this occurs is called the resonance angle or SPR angle. This angle is intrinsically affected by changes in the RI, which occur between the gold surface and the liquid medium. Upon accumulation of biomolecules at the gold/liquid interface, the RI changes, thus causing a shift in the SPR angle, which can be seen in Fig. 11.1A (shifting from a red to a blue line). This shift is measured, recorded, and is displayed in real-time on a sensorgram. When a biomolecular interaction occurs at the sensor surface, a change in mass occurs. These changes at the interface are directly proportional to concentrations in the picomolar to nanomolar range [25, 26]. SPR capabilities go beyond the quantitative and qualitative measurement of intermolecular reactions, and, as the shift in resonance angle can be measured over time, kinetic data can be obtained. This can be utilised to generate information relating to the affinity and specificity of the measured biomolecular interaction [25].

A number of SPR-based systems exist on the market today (e.g. Horiba Scientific, Reichert Technologies, Affinity Sensors, Biosensing Instruments, Texas Instruments and Corning [27]). The most prominent is the Biacore^{TM} system from GE Healthcare and will

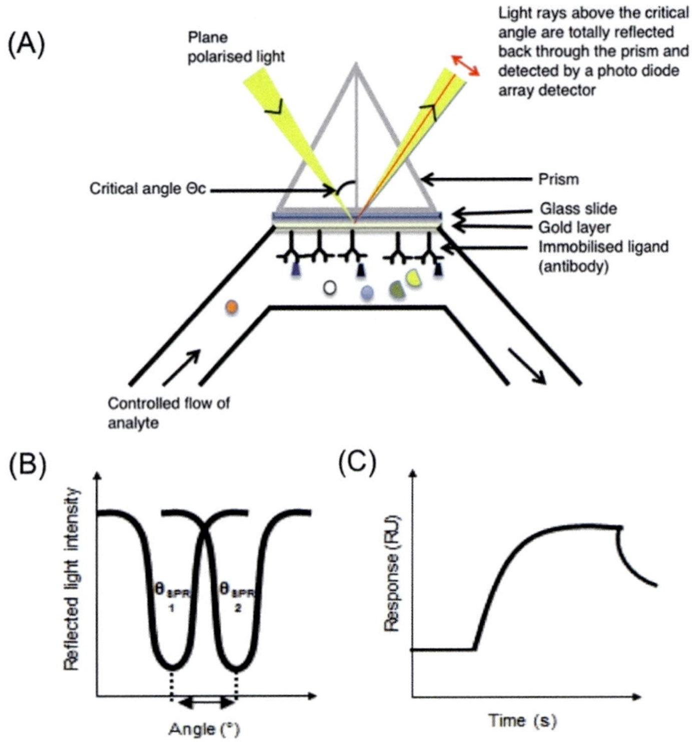

Figure 11.1 (A) Schematic representation of the 'flow-through' mechanism of a SPR-based system. SPR occurs on a thin layer of gold, which is sandwiched between a glass slide and the sample solution flowing through a specially designed microfluidic cartridge. Plane polarised light is directed onto the back of the sensor chip at a specific angle, which allows TIR to occur. When the light hits the gold at the critical angle (θ_c), not only does it internally reflect, but it also leaks an evanescent wave which moves exponentially across the gold interface exciting plasmons (electron charge density waves). This is seen as a drop in the intensity in the reflected light measured by the photo diode array detector. When analyte binds to the sensor surface a mass change occurs near the surface of the sensor chip. The refractive index near the sensor chip surface changes and this in turn changes the angle at which the SPR occurs. The photo diode array detects the change in SPR angle and displays the change in 'real-time' on a sensorgram. (B) When molecules bind to the sensor surface, plasmons form with a different angle of incidence and a SPR curve shift is observed from θ_{SPR1} to θ_{SPR2}. (C) Association and dissociation are measured in arbitrary units and are displayed in a graph called a sensorgram. The example shown consists of association, steady state and dissociation phases of an exponential molecular interaction.

be the focus of this chapter [25]. Biacore™ developed one of the first instruments that utilises SPR for real-time analysis of biomolecular interactions in a label-free environment. SPR technology offers the potential of obtaining a comprehensive understanding of the antibody/antigen binding interactions. The following section of this chapter outlines some of the fundamental aspects of SPR technology.

The use of SPR-based biosensors has seen tremendous growth over the last two decades, and this trend is predicted to continue as the technology becomes more accessible and its applications more diverse. SPR has emerged as one of the most prominently favoured and intrinsically valuable technologies for monitoring molecular interactions. Table 11.1 gives an overview of SPR-based biosensors for the analysis of a plethora of analytes.

11.2.1 Optical Platforms Used in SPR

SPR-based sensors employ several different methods for optical excitation of surface plasmons. The coupling of the light emitted to the surface plasmon wave requires, for electromagnetic reasons, a high-index prism or a periodic grating surface [44]. Prism couplers represent the most frequently used method for optical excitation of surface plasmons. Prism coupling can be achieved with simple optical elements and can also be combined with any type of modulation, making it highly convenient [28]. The use of diffraction grating-based systems for SPR sensing was investigated as an alternative to prism-based systems. The grating replaces the need for a glass prism traditionally used in SPR. Compatibility with mass production makes a grating coupler an attractive approach for fabrication of low-cost SPR sensing platforms [28].

As the prism coupling method is not amenable to miniaturisation and integration, other alternative methods such as optical fibres and waveguide structures are increasingly becoming prevalent.

Song and colleagues [45] reported a novel waveguide-coupled SPR. This system had simply designed waveguide-coupled SPR chips and, when compared to conventional SPR chips, proved to have higher sensitivity as well as better resolution. They also reported that the waveguide layer can be adjusted in its thickness and RI,

Table 11.1 Overview of SPR-based biosensors (adapted from Homola [28])

Analyte	Sensor system	Limit of detection	Ref.
Cancer biomarkers			
Prostate specific antigen (PSA)	Custom-built LSPR lab-on-a-chip	1 ng mL^{-1}	[29]
PSA	Biacore 2000	1 ng mL^{-1}	[30]
PSA-ACT complex	Biacore 2000	18.1 ng L^{-1}	[31]
Total PSA (tPSA)	Custom-built point-of-care SPR immunosensor	0.29 ng mL^{-1}	[32]
Vascular endothelial growth factor (VEGF)	Custom-built SPRI	1 pM	[33]
Carcinoembryonic antigen (CEA)	Autolab Springle	0.5 ng mL^{-1}	[34]
Interleukin-8 (IL-8)	Biacore X	2.5 pM	[35]
Carbohydrate antigen (CA 19-9)	Spreeta	66.7 U mL^{-1}	[36]
Cardiac markers			
B-type natriuretic peptide (BNP)	Custom-built nanoparticle-enhanced SPR biosensor	1 aM	[37]
Cardiac troponin (cTnI)	Custom fibre-optic	68 ng L^{-1}	[38]
Troponin T	SPR Navi 200	100 μg mL^{-1}	[39]
Drug and drug induced antibodies			
Warfarin	Biacore 3000	4 ng mL^{-1}	[40]
Insulin	SPR-670	1 ng mL^{-1}	[41]
Anti-insulin	Biacore 2000	0.6 μg mL^{-1}	[42]
Anti-V-adnectin	Biacore T100	0.93 nM	[43]

SPRI, surface plasmon resonance imaging; LSPR, localised surface plasmon resonance.

and polymers or inorganic matrix can be applied during production, deeming it more flexible in design and easier in fabrication than other kinds of SPR structures. Ahn applied a waveguide-coupled SPR mode to a fibre-optic sensor [46]. This novel approach made it possible to precisely tune the resonance wavelength in a broad range from the visible to infrared region and to generate multiple modes, which may be selectively used for suitable applications.

In an SPR-based fibre-optic sensor, the prism can be replaced by the core of an optical fibre. In this fibre-optic format, all the guided rays are launched and hence, instead of angular interrogation, spectral interrogation is used. The light from a polychromatic source is launched into one of the ends of the optical fibre. The evanescent field produced by the guided rays excites the surface plasmons at the metal-dielectric sensing layer interface. The coupling of an evanescent field with surface plasmons strongly depends on wavelength, fibre parameters, probe geometry, and the metal layer properties [47].

A major limitation previously noted in fibre-optic SPR systems is in the successful adhesion of the gold layer to the fibre-optic core. Aghir et al. reported a more robust method of adhesion by introducing a silane compound prior to adhesion. This silanised fibre-optic sensor showed enhanced stability under chemical, mechanical and thermal stress, which may pave the way for more robust and reusable fibre-optic sensors in the future [48].

11.3 Fundamental Steps in SPR-Based Analysis

In SPR, the term *ligand* refers to the molecule that is attached to the surface and the term *analyte* refers to the molecule that is found in the sample and binds to the ligand (Fig. 11.1). The ligand is bound to the sensor surface using a number of different immobilisation techniques (see Chapter 3 of this book for immobilisation strategies). The sample analyte is injected into the system and is passed over the sensor surface. The analyte moves across the sensor surface in a continuous flow (1–100 μL min^{-1}). The analyte encounters and binds the ligand. This causes an increase in the refractive index (RI), which is measured in real-time. Importantly, a control reference surface containing no ligand or an irrelevant ligand is also included, and the analyte also flows over this and any binding is recorded. The binding response is monitored, measured and the output is displayed as a sensorgram (Fig. 11.1C). The readout is plotted as response units (RU) versus time. A response of 1000 RU is approximately equivalent to a change of 0.1° in the SPR angle, which correlates to about 1 ng/mm^2 in surface protein concentration [49]. When equilibrium is reached, the flow is switched to buffer devoid of interacting molecule. The change in mass is measured in RU and is directly proportional to the concentration of molecules bound on the surface. The change in RI from the control/reference cell is also measured. The values are subtracted from the analytical sample to give an accurate reading that takes into account non-specific binding. Following binding measurement, the bound analyte is removed during a process called **regeneration**. Regeneration must occur without damaging the immobilised ligand and prepares the surface for a new round of analyte measurement. See Section 11.7 of this book for further reading.

11.4 Surfaces Used in SPR Immunoassay Development

The SPR-based Biacore™ instruments employ a sensor chip with integrated microfluidics, an auto-sampler and an optical detection unit with control software. The sensor chip is comprised of a glass surface covered with a thin uniform layer of gold onto which a number of different materials can be applied. The following section highlights the intricacies of gold surface layer modification. A layer of gold (~50 nm) is used because of its inert properties in the presence of physiological buffers, and its suitability for providing the requisite physical conditions necessary for SPR [25]. It is also amenable to covalent bonding of surface matrix layers. The gold surface layer is functionalised to aid in biomolecular binding and to reduce non-specific binding. This is carried out by covalently binding a layer of alkanethiol molecules to the gold surface. The alkanethiol surface is strongly hydrophobic, and in some cases (Biacore™ sensor chip HPA) can be used when working with lipid monolayers. The hydrophobic monolayer of alkanethiol molecules are then coated with a hydrogel layer of flexible carboxymethylated dextran. This provides the three-dimensional surface to facilitate ligand attachment [50]. Commercial SPR biosensors are generally capable of detecting 1 pg/mm^2 of absorbed analytes. This sensitivity is strongly dependent on many parameters, but it is particularly dependent on surface functionalisation [49].

11.4.1 Dextran-Coated Sensor Chips: The Carboxymethylated Series

A sensor chip that incorporates a carboxymethylated (CM) dextran layer (25–200 nm depending on the type of sensor chip) covalently attached to the alkanethiol monolayer effectively acts as a three-dimensional surface for the molecules (ligands) to attach [25]. The favourable properties of the dextran matrix provides (i) a hydrophobic environment to which most proteins will attach, (ii) a well-defined environment which facilitates covalent attachment, (iii) negatively charged carboxymethyl groups which allow electrostatic concentration of positively charged molecules and (iv) flexibility of the polymer chains, which allows the 'surface-attached' molecules to move in relative freedom in the dextran layer, thereby facilitating greater access of the analyte to the ligand.

Sensor chips that are coated in this unbranched carboxymethylated dextran surface include CM5 [51, 52], CM4 and CM3 [53]. More information regarding the use of these chips can be found in Table 11.2. Sensor chip L1 is composed of a carboxymethyl (CM) dextran layer, to which lipophilic residues have been covalently attached [25]. L1 is coated with alkane chains, which act as lipophilic anchors which insert into the cellular lipid bilayers, thus allowing the capture of intact cells and associated membrane or transmembrane proteins. This may help to reduce the likelihood of structural change occurring in membrane-associated proteins and helps to maintain the functionality of these proteins. The chip can also directly capture lipid vesicles or liposomes by inserting the lipophilic residues associated with the chip into the membrane. Hodnik and Anderluh describe in detail a protocol for capturing liposomes on L1 sensor chips [54].

11.4.2 Sensor Chip with Pre-immobilised Surfaces: Capture Applications

Sensor chips with pre-immobilised surfaces can be readily used for capture applications. Sensor chip SA is pre-immobilised with streptavidin and readily binds to biotinylated molecules (proteins, peptides, nucleic acids, etc.) [54, 57]. Poly-histidine tagged

Table 11.2 Range of Biacore™ chips and surfaces available (this information was sourced from the *Biacore Surface Handbook*, GE Healthcare [25])

	Sensor chip	Surface type	Uses	Ref.
Carboxymethylated Series	CM5	CM-dextran	General purpose; very versatile for binding haptens, proteins, DNA and carbohydrates	[25, 53, 55]
	CM4	CM-dextran, 30% lower concentration of dextran than CM5, less negative charge on surface	Binding of large molecules; exhibits reduced immobilisation capacity and reduced non-specific binding	[25, 56]
	CM3	CM-dextran, shorter dextran matrix than CM5, but has same degree of carboxylation	Facilitates binding of large molecules and particles (cells, viruses and multicomponent complexes); exhibits low immobilisation levels	[25]
	L1	CM-dextran (similar to CM5) covalently attached to lipophilic residues	Used for capture of lipid vesicles and liposomes and helps retain the lipid bilayer structure.	[25]
Capture Applications	SA	CM-dextran pre-immobilised with streptavidin	Used for the capture of biotinylated molecules such as proteins, peptides, nucleic acids, carbohydrates and lipids.	[25, 54, 57]
	NTA	CM-dextran pre-immobilised with nitriloacetic acid (NTA)	Aids in the capture of poly-histidine tagged recombinant molecules via metal chelation; controls the orientation of the molecule for optimal exposure of the binding site	[25, 58]

Special Applications	C1	No dextran matrix; flat carboxylated surface	Facilitates the binding of large particles, whole cells and viruses; the lack of dextran means particles are not free to move within surface layer	[25]
	HPA	Flat hydrophobic surface, alkanethiol molecules directly attached to gold film	Captures lipid monolayers and membrane associated proteins	[25, 59, 60]
	Au	Unmodified gold surface mounted on chip support	Facilitates custom design chemistry	[25, 61]
	SIA kit Au	Unmodified gold surface not mounted on chip support	Surface modifications outside Biacore™ systems	[25]

CM, carboxymethylated; L1, lipophilic; NTA, nitriloacetic acid; SA, streptavidin; C, carboxylated; HPA, long-chain hydrophobic alkane thiols; Au, gold; SIA, surface interaction analysis.

recombinant proteins can also be captured on the surface of Sensor Chip NTA [58]. The NTA sensor chip is pre-immobilised with $NiCl_2$-activated nitriloacetic acid (NTA) groups. Capture molecules can be easily removed with the addition of ethylenediaminetetraacetic acid (EDTA) [62, 63].

11.4.3 Sensor Chips for Specialised Applications

The C1 sensor chip is solely composed of a carboxylated surface without a dextran matrix. It is commonly called a 'matrix-free' chip and it can be used to develop new sensor-chip functionalisation methods. The sensor chip has similar properties to carboxymethyl-coated chips in that it can be derivatised using the same methods. However, the lack of the CM dextran layer means that it has lost its dimensionality and has a significantly reduced surface area. It is used primarily to bind large structures such as whole cells or viruses [25, 64, 65]. Roussille and colleagues outlined the used of a C1 sensor chip to demonstrate the development of new technologies. They developed a novel functionalisation technique that could be applied to both SPR and their newly developed optical microscopy technology based on surface-enhanced ellipsometric contrast (SEEC). The chip was functionalised with a dense layer of carboxyl (–COOH) groups followed by the addition of a self-assembled monolayer (SAM) of 16-mercaptohexadecanoic acid (MHDA) [65]. The binding capacity of the chip was compared to a CM5 chip (chip containing a gold film covered in carboxymethylated dextran hydrogel), and antibody-antigen and biotin-labelled anti-body to streptavidin binding was also assessed. The C1 SAM-MHDA chip displayed a better signal-to-noise ratio and lower non-specific binding when compared to the CM5 chip [65].

The HPA sensor chip is coated in a monolayer of covalently bound alkanethiol molecules. It is a flat hydrophobic surface, which is amenable to the formation of lipid monolayers (whereas chip L1 is more suitable for bilayer formation) [59, 60]. The HPA Biacore^{TM} chip was used successfully by Stokes et al. [60] to monitor the binding of the outer membrane-bound transferrin binding proteins, TbpA, TbpB and human transferrin. TbpA and TbpB were reconstituted into liposomes and fused onto HPA chips, where they formed stable monolayers. Kinetic data was obtained for the interaction between the Tbps and human transferrin [60]. HPA chips have also been used in a screening method to identify anti-lipopolysaccharide (LPS) recombinant antibodies [59]. The HPA chip was coated with LPS and recombinant antibodies were passed over the surface. The association and dissociation rates of the antibodies were obtained. Three antibodies with low dissociation rates were chosen for further immunoassay development [59].

Au and SIA sensor chips consist of bare gold surfaces. They are customisable surfaces which can be used in projects seeking to optimise different surface chemistries [61].

11.4.4 Functionalisation of SPR Surfaces

There are two major ways of functionalising SPR chips: (1) carboxylated dextran (CM-dextran) layers and (2) self-assembled monolayers (SAMs) on gold surfaces using a range of different thiolated organic chemicals. Several reports of novel SPR surfaces with increased detection limits have been described in the literature. A novel and sensitive molecularly imprinted SPR sensor for detection of oxytocin in milk samples was prepared by fabricating a self-assembling monolayer of allyl-mercaptane on a gold chip surface. Subsequently, an oxytocin-imprinted poly (2-hydroxyethyl methacrylate–methacryloylamidoglutamic acid) nanofilm was applied onto the allyl-mercaptane-modified chip. The imprinted SPR sensor was found to be sensitive and selective. The detection limit of this novel sensor was calculated to be as low as 0.003 ng mL^{-1} [66]. Huang and colleagues reported a novel SPR sensor for sensitive detection of concanavalin A (ConA). In this sensing platform, dextran-capped gold nanoparticles (Dex-Au NPs) were initially synthesised and utilised as an amplification reagent. After deposition of graphene oxide (GO) on the SPR gold film, phenoxy-derivatised dextran (DexP) was assembled onto the GO-modified gold chip surface through π–π interactions. The resultant GO/DexP sensing interface could specifically capture ConA which could further react with Dex-Au NPs through the specific interaction between ConA and Dex, forming a sandwich configuration. The newly developed sandwich-based SPR sensor successfully achieved the sensitive detection of ConA in the range of 1.0–20.0 μg mL^{-1} with a detection limit of 0.39 μg mL^{-1}. Compared to the direct assay format, the prepared sandwich SPR sensor led to an improvement of 28.7-fold in the sensitivity [67]. To overcome high surface backgrounds previously observed for DNA/protein interactions in SPR, Pillet and colleagues built a pseudo-three-dimensional surface on the gold surface by functionalising the biosensor with synthesised phosphorous dendrimers. These 'branch-like' polymer structures significantly improved selectivity of the detection of protein–DNA interactions. They showed that amino–gold surface functionalisation with phosphorus dendrimers allowed complete coverage of the gold surface and an increase in surface roughness. Using this dendrimer-functionalised surface, the specificity of the SPR response was significantly improved allowing discrimination between protein and DNA interactions of different strengths [68].

Aldehyde groups were used to functionalise gold nanorod-Fe_3O_4 nanohybrids and used in a wavelength modulation SPR biosensor for mouse IgG detection. The functionalised nanorods were shown to possess unique magnetic properties, exceptional optical properties and good biocompatibility, which can be used as an immobilisation matrix for biomolecules. These gold nanorods-Fe_3O_4 nanohybrids could be easily immobilised on the sensor surface by a magnetic pillar and were demonstrated to be an ideal support for the sensitive detection of biomolecules [69].

Graphene oxide sheet (GOS)-based SPR chips generated a highly sensitive immunoassay sensor. The sensing film, which is formed by chemically modifying a GOS surface, has covalent bonds that strongly interact with bovine serum albumin (BSA), creating a higher sensitivity. This GOS film-based SPR chip has a BSA concentration detection limit that is 100 times higher than that of the conventional Au-film-based sensor. The affinity constants on the GOS film-based SPR chip were shown to be 5.2 times higher than the conventional SPR chip. Their results demonstrate that the GOS film is a promising tool for use in high sensitivity clinical diagnostic applications [70].

A highly efficient SPR-based immunosensor is described by Singh using a functionalised single graphene layer on a thin gold film. The aim of this approach was to amplify the SPR signal by growing graphene through chemical vapour deposition and to control the immobilisation of biotinylated cholera toxin antigen on copper coordinated nitrilotriacetic acid (NTA) using graphene as an ultrathin layer [71].

New sensing SPR platforms which consist of Cu(II) complexes of a pentetic acid thiol ligand (DPTA-Cu(II)) and of a thiol derivative of dipyrromethene DPM-Cu(II) were created on the surface of gold SPR discs. These complexes form a self-assembled monolayer using a gold-sulphur linkage. The surfaces were applied to orientated immobilisation of His-tagged Janus kinase 2 (GST-His$_6$-JAK2). This method is based on the covalent bond formation between histidine from a His-tag chain of a protein and Cu(II) centres from the complexes. Kinetic and thermodynamic analysis proved stable immobilisation of His-tagged kinase JAK2 on these new sensing platforms. Binding capacity for these new SPR sensing platforms were comparable to NTA-modified dextran layers [72].

11.4.5 The Use of Reference/Control Surfaces in SPR Immunoassays

The use of reference surfaces in assays is incorporated to account for matrix effects caused by bulk refractive index changes [25, 28]. Reference surfaces used in SPR studies must be as similar as possible to the ligand surface used in the assay [26, 73]. Having such a reference surface records the background response and the level allows one to determine the degree of non-specific binding [26].

Reference surfaces to be included in SPR-based assays may include:

- an unmodified surface, used to identify non-specific binding to the dextran matrix
- an activated surface in the absence of ligand (the flow cell surface is treated with the same coupling chemistry as the working flow cell in the absence of ligand)
- a surface containing an antibody of identical species, for example, of the same class and subtype but with different specificity

The highest concentration of analyte to be used should be injected over the reference chip and any binding recorded. This can be subsequently subtracted from the analyte response and this yields the true specific binding values of the ligand for the analyte.

11.5 Determination of Kinetic Parameters between Binding Partners Using SPR

All life depends on biomolecular interactions, and for scientists to better understand these interactions it is important to know more about their behaviour. Critical to this, is the rate at which molecules (e.g. analyte/ligand) associate and dissociate. When carrying out kinetic measurements using SPR, the lowest concentration of ligand that will achieve a measurable response should be used. The most typical analyte–ligand interaction is a reversible reaction between a surface-bound ligand (A) and an analyte (B) in solution (Fig. 11.2 and Eq. 11.1), and can be described as follows:

$$[A]^{k_a}_{k_d} + [B] \rightleftharpoons [AB] \quad (11.1)$$

$[A]$ and $[B]$ represent concentrations of A (ligand) and B (analyte),
$[AB]$ the concentration of the newly formed complex,
k_a the association rate, and
k_d the dissociation rate.

The association kinetics of an interaction provides information on how fast an interaction occurs, i.e. how fast molecules A and B bind together. This is known as the association rate (k_a). The dissociation rate (k_d) gives information on how fast the molecules

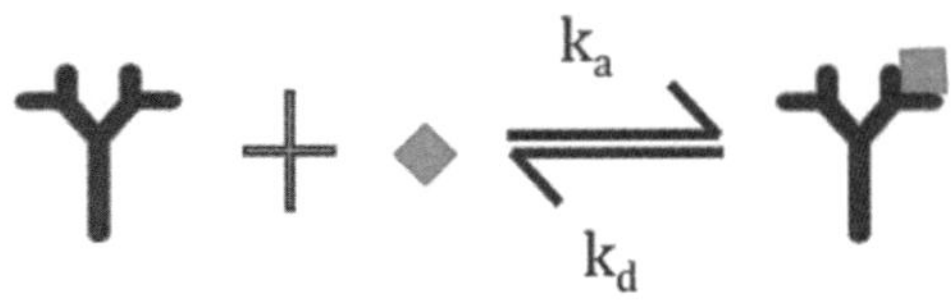

Figure 11.2 Diagrammatic representation of the antibody–antigen interaction. The forward reaction rate is known as k_a (association rate), while the reverse reaction is known as k_d (dissociation rate).

come apart and on how strong an interaction is. The association and dissociation rates are time-dependent and are written as follows:

Association constant:

$$K_A = \frac{k_a}{k_d} = \frac{[AB]}{[A]\,[B]} \tag{11.2}$$

The equilibrium association constant is $K_A = M^{-1}$.
M represents molarity.

Dissociation constant:

$$K_D = \frac{k_d}{k_a} = \frac{[A][B]}{[AB]} \tag{11.3}$$

The equilibrium dissociation constant is $K_D = M$.

In order to define association and dissociation kinetics ('on' and 'off' rates) of a molecular interaction, the analyte must be of as high purity as possible and the concentration of the analyte must be known with great accuracy [26]. During a rate determination assay, the sample is passed over the sensor surface and the bound molecules cause an increased response, as shown on the sensorgram (see Fig. 11.1C). This is followed by the injection of buffer devoid of sample over the surface. The bound molecules start to dissociate and the dissociation is visualised on the sensorgram.

Using a SPR-based instrument, kinetic values can be obtained using three methods:

- *Multi-cycle.* Injection of a series of known analyte concentrations over the sensor surface. The surface is regenerated after each concentration of analyte to be ready for the next cycle.
- *Single-cycle.* Injection of analyte with increasing concentrations in a single cycle but with no surface regeneration. The single-cycle kinetic parameter identification has many advantages in that it reduces time spent determining regeneration conditions (as regeneration conditions are redundant). It allows the identification of molecular interactions that were previously unobtainable due to difficulties associated with finding suitable regeneration conditions.

- *'2-over-2' kinetics.* Developed to optimise antibody screening and characterisation using Biacore™ A100 (now known as Biacore™ 4000). Two different concentrations of antibodies are captured on one half of an entire flow cell, and two different concentrations of antigen are injected over the antibody (Fig. 11.3). The data obtained provides a number of curves per clone for the software to fit, thus providing improved reliability of the values obtained. 2-over-2 kinetics is preferentially used to obtain kinetic data for antibody clones in the screening process as the run time is substantially reduced (up to 50%). Little sample preparation is required as crude sample analyte can be used.

The concentration of an analyte can be determined using SPR, by monitoring its interaction with its cognate binding ligand on a prepared sensor surface in the presence of excess (known concentration) analyte in solution [24, 25]. Concentrations for either purified or crude samples can be determined in the nanomolar range. Concentrations are determined by interpolation of the binding responses on a calibration curve or using the 'calibration-free' concentration analysis (CFCA) method, developed by Biacore™.

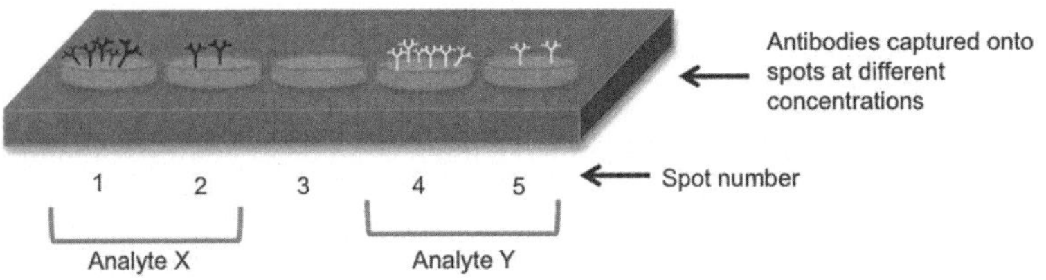

Figure 11.3 Diagrammatic representation of 2-over-2 kinetics. Two concentrations of antibodies are captured on two different spots, a higher concentration is captured on to spots 1 and 4, and a lower concentration is captured onto spots 2 and 5. Two different concentrations of analyte (X and Y) are injected over different flow channels of the sensor surface. Spot number 3 is used as a reference.

11.6 Immobilisation of Ligands onto Sensor Surfaces

The ligand must be immobilised onto the sensor surface without compromising its integrity. The ligand can be immobilised either by direct covalent coupling or indirect covalent coupling onto the sensor surface. A number of different immobilisation strategies can be used and are indicated as follows:

- Streptavidin – Biotin – SA chips
- Nickel (Ni^{2+})/NTA – Polyhistidine tag – NTA chips
- Anti-biotin
- Anti-GST
- Species specific antibody
- Anti-HA

Covalent immobilisation takes advantage of the presence of CM groups on the sensor chip surface. A relatively small amount of protein is required for immobilisation (~5–10 μg). The protein must be relatively pure and have a high level of activity as all the protein present in the preparation will be coupled to the sensor chip surface. It is important to note that all types of immobilisations can be carried out directly using Biacore™ technology. For Biacore, immobilisation is usually carried out at low flow rates (5–10 μL min^{-1}), while the concentration of ligand usually used is in the range of 1–100 μg mL^{-1}.

The following points may help to determine which immobilisation strategy is suitable for ligand capture:

- If the ligand is impure, a capture immobilisation strategy would be advisable.
- If the ligand is unstable, a capture immobilisation strategy would be advisable as the docking of the ligand onto a binding partner may help to prevent its degradation or may slow down the degradation process.
- If covalently coupling your ligand to the matrix results in the loss of ligand activity, reconsider changing the

immobilisation strategy, possibly changing from amine- to thiol-coupling.

For further information on the covalent immobilisation of molecules to sensor surfaces, please see Section 12.5.8 (Immobilisation Strategies for Biomolecules onto Solid Surfaces) of this book.

11.6.1 Electrostatic Pre-concentration of the Protein onto the Sensor Chip

The function of the pre-concentration step is to concentrate the protein to high levels (>100 mg mL^{-1}) at the dextran matrix, thereby facilitating the coupling reaction thus reducing or minimising the amount of protein required for coupling reactions [26]. Pre-concentration is an important step in SPR assay development as it controls the immobilisation level of ligand for experimental optimisation and efficiency. The principle behind electrostatic pre-concentration exploits the tendency of the electropositive proteins to be attracted to the electro-negatively charged carboxylated dextran matrix. See associated protocol in Chapter 12 of this book for pre-concentration of ligands onto surfaces.

11.7 Regeneration of Surfaces

Regeneration refers to the process whereby analyte is removed from the ligand on the sensor-chip surface in preparation for the next round of analysis. This must occur without damaging the bound ligand or decreasing its activity [25, 71]. The choice of regeneration solution must also be compatible with the running buffer used during the analysis (e.g. $MgCl_2$ causes precipitation in phosphate buffers and sodium dodecyl sulphate (SDS) may precipitate in a running buffer with a high potassium content) [25]. It is important to spend time developing a successful regeneration strategy, as efficient regeneration will greatly increase the performance of the subsequent assay.

Solutions used can be subdivided into four categories:

- High ionic strength solution (NaCl [1 M] or $MgCl_2$ [2–4 M])

- Low pH (glycine–HCl [10 mM, pH 1.5–3], phosphoric acid [10–100 mM])
- High pH (NaOH [1–100 mM])
- Detergents (up to 0.5% [w/v] SDS)

(For further information on regeneration solutions please see the SPR Handbook from GE Healthcare [25].)

Each regeneration step must be tailored for every immunoassay. In order to limit the damage to the bound ligand during the search for a suitable regeneration solution, it is advisable to start with the mildest and move to harsher conditions. Upon finding suitable regeneration conditions, the effect of the regeneration buffers on the ligand's activity and binding capacity over time must be determined. The ligand is exposed to repeated cycles of regeneration [25, 71]. When suitable regeneration conditions have been determined, a surface performance test is carried out. The binding/regeneration cycle is repeated for 30 to 40 cycles and the ligand stability and baseline over time is monitored. Combinations of solutions have also been shown to be very effective for regeneration. For example, combining low pH with high ionic strength (e.g. 10 mM glycine, pH 2.0 and 1 M sodium chloride), basic with chaotropic solutions (e.g. 10 mM sodium hydroxide and 500 mM sodium thiocyanate), low pH solutions combined with detergents (e.g. 10 mM glycine, pH 2.0 and 0.05% [v/v] polysorbate 20) have been found to be highly successful [25]. If the baseline appears to increase over time, then more stringent regeneration conditions are required. If the ligand activity is being reduced (capacity to bind analyte is being lost) then milder regeneration conditions are required. If the analyte binding response is consistent following repeated injections and the read-out is within 10% of the level of the first injection then acceptable regeneration conditions have been attained.

11.8 Advances in SPR Immunoassays

Developments in SPR sensors have expanded the scope for SPR applications; these range from biomarker screening to drug delivery [74]. These advances are a consequence of the need for faster and more flexible, label-free immunoassays, with the ability to rapidly detect analytes in complex matrices [75].

A particular aspect of SPR technology that has received much attention is the improvement of surface functionalisation to aid in the specific orientation of ligands. Different functionalisation methods such as the use of graphene and alkanethiol monolayers have been successful [76]. Graphene is a carbon-based monolayer that is easily functionalised to aid in targeted immobilisation and it displays excellent light transmittance properties (transmits 97.7% of light) [77]. A study to detect β-agonists used an immunosensor surface composed of a self-assembled alkanethiol monolayer. The immunosensor exhibited exquisite sensitivities and a robust surface for repeated regeneration cycles (100 cycles) was achieved [78].

SPR sensors are also being constructed using silver sensing layers (as opposed to gold). Gold requires a layer of titanium (Ti) or chromium (Cr) between it and the glass, so the thicker sensing layer causes a broadening of the SPR signal. Silver attaches easily to glass substrates and hence the SPR signal produced has a very sharp curve and therefore displays better sensitivities. Unfortunately, when using silver, harmful sulphidisation and oxidation may affect the ligand if the silver is not properly protected using 11-mercaptoundecanoic acid (11-MUA) [78]. The prism configuration of SPR imaging is limited by physical constraints and can result in poor spatial resolution. A solution that has shown promise, proposes an 'objective-type surface plasmon resonance imaging (SPRI)' approach that utilises a high numerical aperture oil immersion objective and an inverted microscope [79].

An interesting study generated a SPR-based competitive immunoassay to detect amikacin [80]. Previous detection methods included HPLC and other time consuming technologies. The SPR immunoassay was portable, label-free, capable of real-time measurement and is widely applicable to all kinds of drugs [80]. A four-channel miniature SPR biosensor was developed for the direct analysis of methotrexate in patients who are undergoing chemotherapy treatments. It is apparent that SPR biosensors may be a more suitable detection method for therapeutic drug monitoring (TDM) than the standard technologies [81]. The refractive index of any liquid is temperature dependant. Therefore, it is essential that the detection unit in these smaller devices is temperature controlled to ensure the temperature of the sample will not affect the data reading. Within SPR assays, reagents must be sensitive, reliable and of a high affinity. Peng and colleagues exploited antibody mixtures to make low affinity antibodies into viable capture reagents. The approach used a sensor surface termed 'bi-epitope', where different pairs of antibodies against the target (in this case ephrin type A receptor (EphA2)) were immobilised using amine coupling. The bi-epitope was then compared to the single-epitope approach by binding affinity and detection sensitivity. The bi-epitope surface showed significant increase in binding affinity ($\sim$10–100-fold), an improved dissociation rate and an enhanced limit of detection [82].

In a bid to enhance SPR sensitivities, the use of gold nanoparticles was employed. A study on the detection of cardiac troponin T for acute myocardial infarction (AMI) utilised gold nanoparticles (AuNPs) to amplify the signal by sandwich assay format with consequent success [83]. The conjugation of antibodies to AuNPs for enhanced SPR response has been frequently and positively reported in SPR assays for a variety of other diseases such as, acute coronary syndrome (ACS) [84].

A novel SPR-based assay was developed for the assessment of bispecific antibodies (bsAb) [85]. In this assay, the bsAbs bind to both specific targets thus providing parallel analysis in a single assay. The assay has two vital elements; firstly, a sensor chip, which is coated in one of the antigens for which the bsAb is specific, captures the bsAb, and secondly, the remaining specific antigen is added and will bind to the captured bsAb. The concentration of the binding molecules will be reflected by the bridging signal, which is translated into dose-response curves [85]. This advance is of particular importance due to the increased use of bsAb as therapeutic agents.

A notable disadvantage of traditional immunoassays is their time-consuming nature. SPR biosensors have been developed to become far more time efficient in recent years. In a study, nine different SPR assays for protein quantification, using the Biacore™ systems, were developed and compared to traditional ELISAs. The SPR assays were found to be robust, allowing the immobilised antibody surface to retain performance for up to a week, and could determine protein concentrations in a very short time-frame. During cell culture experiments, SPR was used for quick analysis (in 10 minutes) to determine optimum conditions, proving that SPR advances can greatly improve time usage within laboratories [86]. As such, it is imperative that improvements in SPR-based immunoassays are continual so that SPR may, in the future, outperform the analytical abilities of current conventional methods.

A highly innovative SPR-based sensing platform for the detection of clinically relevant analytes is SPINIT®, developed by Biosurfit [87]. It utilises a customised recombinant antibody (developed by Dublin City University) incorporated into a compact-disc microfluidic-based platform, which is capable of detecting C-reactive protein (CRP), an indicator of inflammation, in less than 5 minutes. In this assay, a drop of blood is manually added to the disc, which is then sealed and inserted into the analyser. The combination of centrifugal forces, optimised microfluidics for reagent/sample handling, linked to SPR detection demonstrates the capacity for such systems to be used for point-of-care analyses.

SPR-based instruments such as Biacore (3000, 4000 and T100) provide excellent systems for high-throughput antibody selection and characterisation. The Biacore 4000 has additional capacity for throughput and sophisticated kinetic analysis, which is very useful for selection of high-performance antibodies and has been used to rank multiple specific epitopes on troponin I [88]. The design and implementation of the selection approach is of key importance to maximise the discovery and selection of the most appropriate antibodies for the applications envisaged.

Indeed in the use of Biacore™ and other instruments in the design and implementation of appropriate assay formats is of great importance. Frequently, the reported use of such systems for monitoring ligand interactions (including derivation of kinetic properties of antibodies) has demonstrated inherent errors [89]. Optimisation of chip immobilisation for specific ligands, choice of appropriate concentrations (e.g. of immobilised ligand and antibody), choice of buffer, use of correct reference surfaces, use of regeneration solutions, choice of correct models for interpreting ligand binding, regular servicing of instruments, knowledge of the effects of environmental factors (e.g. temperature, salt, pH) and the need for critical evaluation of results by experienced users are all key features that must be addressed carefully to ensure optimal SPR experimentation.

11.9 Conclusions

Advances and developments of SPR-based immunosensors have shown vast improvements over the past few years. Their limitations are being addressed and SPR confers comparable analytical capabilities to the conventional methods used in clinical analysis. Its label-free, high-throughput, cost-effectiveness, and speed render it a powerful analytical tool. Emphasis on instrument miniaturisation, further reduction of cost and increased ease-of-use could translate current bulky SPR immunosensors into convenient portable instruments for in-field analysis, point-of-care diagnostics and daily routine clinical analyses.

References

1. Luppa, P.B., L.J. Sokoll, and D.W. Chan, Immunosensors - principles and applications to clinical chemistry. *Int J Clin Chem*, 2001. **314**(1–2): 1–26.
2. Conroy, P.J., et al., Antibody production, design and use for biosensor-based applications. *Semin Cell Dev Biol*, 2009. **20**(1):10–26.
3. Loder, M.K., T. Tsuboi, and G.A. Rutter, Live-cell imaging of vesicle trafficking and divalent metal ions by total internal reflection fluorescence (TIRF) microscopy. *Methods Mol Biol*, 2013. **950**:13–26.
4. Boulanger, J., et al., Fast high-resolution 3D total internal reflection fluorescence microscopy by incidence angle scanning and azimuthal averaging. *Proc Natl Acad Sci*, 2014. **111**(48):17164–17169.
5. Adanyi, N., et al., Development of immunosensor based on OWLS technique for determining Aflatoxin B1 and Ochratoxin A. *Biosens Bioelectron*, 2007. **22**(6):797–802.
6. Adanyi, N., et al., Optical waveguide lightmode spectroscopy immunosensor for detection of carp vitellogenin. *Sens Actuators B*, 2013. **176**:932–939.

7. Kim, N., and W.Y. Kim, Measurement of polyphenol oxidase activity using optical waveguide lightmode spectroscopy-based immunosensor. *Food Chem*, 2015. **169**:211–217.
8. Kim, N., D.-K. Kim, and W.-Y. Kim, Sulfamethazine detection with direct-binding optical waveguide lightmode spectroscopy-based immunosensor. *Food Chem*, 2008. **108**(2):768–773.
9. Cooper, I.R., et al., The rapid and specific 'real-time' detection of *Legionella pneumophila* in water samples using optical waveguide lightmode spectroscopy. *J Microbiol Methods*, 2009. **78**(1):40–44.
10. Wang, W., et al., Analysis of the interaction between tropomyosin allergens and antibodies using a biosensor based on imaging ellipsometry. *Anal Chem*, 2013. **85**(9):4446–4452.
11. Ogieglo, W., et al., In situ ellipsometry studies on swelling of thin polymer films: a review. *Prog Polym Sci*, 2015. **42**:42–78.
12. McArthur, M.A., S. Trussler, and J.R. Dahn, In situ investigations of SEI layer growth on electrode materials for lithium-ion batteries using spectroscopic ellipsometry. *J Electrochem Soc*, 2012. **159**(3):A198–A207.
13. Vörös, J., et al., Optical grating coupler biosensors. *Biomaterials*, 2002. **23**(17):3699–3710.
14. Gupta, R., and N.J. Goddard, A polymeric waveguide resonant mirror (RM) device for detection in microfluidic flow cells. *Analyst*, 2013. **138**(11):3209–3215.
15. Zourob, M., et al., Label-free detection with the resonant mirror biosensor, in *Biosensors and Biodetection*, A. Rasooly and K. Herold, eds. 2009, Humana Press, pp. 89–138.
16. Herrmann, S., et al., Chemiluminescent optical fiber immunosensor for the detection of anti-West Nile virus IgG. *Talanta*, 2005. **66**(1):6–14.
17. Long, F., et al., Portable optical immunosensor for highly sensitive detection of microcystin-LR in water samples. *Biosens Bioelectron*, 2009. **24**(8):2346–2351.
18. Mendonca, M., et al., Highly specific fiber optic immunosensor coupled with immunomagnetic separation for detection of low levels of *Listeria monocytogenes* and *L. ivanovii*. *BMC Microbiol*, 2012. **12**:275.
19. Xing, W.L., et al., Portable fiber-optic immunosensor for detection of methsulfuron methyl. *Talanta*, 2000. **52**(5):879–883.
20. McCormack, T., et al., Optical immunosensing of lactate dehydrogenase (LDH). *Sens Actuators B*, 1997. **41**(1–3):89–96.

21. Lei, J., and H. Ju, Signal amplification using functional nanomaterials for biosensing. *Chem Soc Rev*, 2012. **41**(6):2122–2134.

22. Englebienne, P., A. Van Hoonacker, and M. Verhas, Surface plasmon resonance: principles, methods and applications in biomedical sciences. *Spectroscopy*, 2003. **17**(2–3):255–273.

23. Phizicky, E.M., and S. Fields, Protein-protein interactions - methods for detection and analysis. *Microbiol Rev*, 1995. **59**(1):94–123.

24. Leonard, P., S. Hearty, M. Hui, and R. O'Kennedy, Measuring protein-protein interactions using Biacore. *Methods Mol Biol*, 2017. **1485**:339–354.

25. Biacore Sensor Surface Handbook (web) G. Healthcare, ed., GE Healthcare, pp. 1–100.

26. Van Der Merwe, P.A., ed. Surface plasmon resonance, in *Protein-Ligand Interactions: Hydrodynamics and Calorimetry*. Practical Approach Series, 2001, eds. S.E. Harding and B.Z. Chowdhry: Oxford University Press, pp. 137–170.

27. Rich, R.L., and D.G. Myszka, Survey of the year 2005 commercial optical biosensor literature. *J Mol Recognit*, 2006. **19**(6):478–534.

28. Homola, J., Surface plasmon resonance sensors for detection of chemical and biological species. *Chem Rev*, 2008. **108**(2):462–493.

29. Aćimović, S.S., et al., LSPR chip for parallel, rapid, and sensitive detection of cancer markers in serum. *Nano Lett*, 2014. **14**(5):2636–2641.

30. Wu, L.P., et al., Visual detection of Sudan dyes based on the plasmon resonance light scattering signals of silver nanoparticles. *Anal Chem*, 2006. **78**(15):5570–5577.

31. Cao, C., et al., A strategy for sensitivity and specificity enhancements in prostate specific antigen-alpha1-antichymotrypsin detection based on surface plasmon resonance. *Biosens Bioelectron*, 2006. **21**(11):2106–2113.

32. Uludag, Y., and I.E. Tothill, Cancer biomarker detection in serum samples using surface plasmon resonance and quartz crystal microbalance sensors with nanoparticle signal amplification. *Anal Chem*, 2012. **84**(14):5898–5904.

33. Li, Y., H.J. Lee, and R.M. Corn, Detection of protein biomarkers using RNA aptamer microarrays and enzymatically amplified SPR imaging. *Anal Chem*, 2007. **79**(3):1082–1088.

34. Tang, D.P., R. Yuan, and Y.Q. Chai, Novel immunoassay for carcinoembryonic antigen based on protein A-conjugated immunosensor chip by

surface plasmon resonance and cyclic voltammetry. *Bioprocess Biosyst Eng*, 2006. **28**(5):315–321.

35. Yang, C.Y., et al., Detection of picomolar levels of interleukin-8 in human saliva by SPR. *Lab Chip*, 2005. **5**(10):1017–1023.
36. Chung, J.W., et al., Additive assay for the repeated measurements of immunosensor without regeneration step. *Sens Actuators B*, 2006. **114**(2):1007–1012.
37. Jang, H.R., et al., Ultrasensitive and ultrawide range detection of a cardiac biomarker on a surface plasmon resonance platform. *Anal Chem*, 2014. **86**(1):814–819.
38. Kwon, Y.C., et al., Development of a surface plasmon resonance-based immunosensor for the rapid detection of cardiac troponin I. *Biotechnol Lett*, 2011. **33**(5):921–927.
39. Liu, J.T., et al., Surface plasmon resonance biosensor with high anti-fouling ability for the detection of cardiac marker troponin T. *Anal Chim Acta*, 2011. **703**(1):80–86.
40. Fitzpatrick, B., and R. O'Kennedy, The development and application of a surface plasmon resonance-based inhibition immunoassay for the determination of warfarin in plasma ultrafiltrate. *J Immunol Methods*, 2004. **291**(1–2):11–25.
41. Gobi, K.V., H. Iwasaka, and N. Miura, Self-assembled PEG monolayer based SPR immunosensor for label-free detection of insulin. *Biosens Bioelectron*, 2007. **22**(7):1382–1389.
42. Kure, M., et al., A trial to assess the amount of insulin antibodies in diabetic patients by surface plasmon resonance. *Intern Med*, 2005. **44**(2):100–106.
43. Barbosa, M.D., et al., Altering drug tolerance of surface plasmon resonance assays for the detection of anti-drug antibodies. *Anal Biochem*, 2013. **441**(2):174–179.
44. Raether, H., Surface plasmons on smooth and rough surfaces and on gratings. *Springer Tracts in Modern Physics*. Springer-Verlag, 1988. **111**.
45. Song, L., et al., Waveguide coupled surface plasmon resonance imaging measurement and high-throughput analysis of bio-interaction. *Sens Actuators B*, 2013. **181**:652–660.
46. Ahn, J.H., et al., Fiber-optic waveguide coupled surface plasmon resonance sensor. *Opt Express*, 2012. **20**(19):21729–21738.
47. Gupta, B.D., and R.K. Verma, Surface plasmon resonance-based fiber optic sensors: principle, probe designs, and some applications. *J Sens*, 2009. **2009**:1–12.

48. Arghir, I., et al., Improved surface plasmon resonance biosensing using silanized optical fibers. *Sens Actuators B*, 2015. **216**:518–526.

49. Stenberg, E., et al., Quantitative determination of surface concentration of protein with surface plasmon resonance using radiolabeled proteins. *J Colloid Interface Sci*, 1991. **143**(2):513–526.

50. Schasfoort R., B., M., and Tudos A., J., ed. *Handbook of Surface Plasmon Resonance*. 2008, RCS Publishing.

51. Baxter, G.A., et al., Detection of streptomycin residues in whole milk using an optical immunobiosensor. *J Agric Food Chem*, 2001. **49**(7):3204–3207.

52. Quinn, J.G., and R. O'Kennedy, Biosensor-based estimation of kinetic and equilibrium constants. *Anal Biochem*, 2001. **290**(1):36–46.

53. Drake, A.W., et al., Biacore surface matrix effects on the binding kinetics and affinity of an antigen/antibody complex. *Anal Biochem*, 2012. **429**(1):58–69.

54. Hodnik, V., and G., Anderluh, Capture of intact liposomes on Biacore sensor chips for protein-membrane interaction studies. *Methods Mol Biol*, 2010. **627**:201–211.

55. Avramis, V.I., et al., Immunogenicity of native or pegylated *E. coli* and Erwinia asparaginases assessed by ELISA and surface plasmon resonance (SPR-biacore) assays of IgG antibodies (Ab) in sera from patients with acute lymphoblastic leukemia (ALL). *Anticancer Res*, 2009. **29**(1):299–302.

56. Abdiche, Y.N., et al., Expanding the ProteOn XPR36 biosensor into a 36-ligand array expedites protein interaction analysis. *Anal Biochem*, 2011. **411**(1):139–151.

57. Piletska, E.V., and S.A. Piletsky, Size matters: influence of the size of nanoparticles on their interactions with ligands immobilized on the solid surface. *Langmuir*, 2010. **26**(6):3783–3785.

58. Chen, J., et al., G protein beta(1)gamma (2) subunits purification and their interaction with adenylyl cyclase. *Sci China, Ser C Life Sci*, 2003. **46**(2):212–223.

59. Yuan, Q., et al., Screening of high-affinity scFv from a ribosome displayed library using BIAcore biosensor. *Appl Biochem Biotechnol*, 2009. **152**(2):224–234.

60. Stokes, R.H., et al., Meningococcal transferrin-binding proteins A and B show cooperation in their binding kinetics for human transferrin. *Infect Immun*, 2005. **73**(2):944–952.

61. Wikstrom, A., and J. Deinum, Probing the interaction of coagulation factors with phospholipid vesicle surfaces by surface plasma resonance. *Anal Biochem*, 2007. **362**(1):98–107.
62. Jason-Moller, L., M. Murphy, and J. Bruno, Overview of Biacore systems and their applications, in *Current Protocols in Protein Science*, 2006. John Wiley & Sons, Inc.
63. Nieba, L., et al., Biacore analysis of histidine-tagged proteins using a chelating NTA sensor chip. *Anal Biochem*, 1997. **252**(2):217–228.
64. Khan, S.H., et al., A versatile method to measure the binding to basic proteins by surface plasmon resonance. *Anal Biochem*, 2012. **421**(2):385–390.
65. Roussille, L., et al., Surface characterization and efficiency of a matrix-free and flat carboxylated gold sensor chip for surface plasmon resonance (SPR). *Anal Bioanal Chem*, 2011. **401**(5):1601–1617.
66. Yola, M.L., N. Atar, and A. Erdem, Oxytocin imprinted polymer based surface plasmon resonance sensor and its application to milk sample. *Sens Actuators B*, 2015. **221**:842–848.
67. Huang, C.-F., et al., Graphene oxide and dextran capped gold nanoparticles based surface plasmon resonance sensor for sensitive detection of concanavalin A. *Biosens Bioelectron*, 2013. **50**:305–310.
68. Pillet, F., et al., Dendrimer functionalization of gold surface improves the measurement of protein-DNA interactions by surface plasmon resonance imaging. *Biosens Bioelectron*, 2013. **43**:148–154.
69. Zhang, H., et al., Studies of gold nanorod-iron oxide nanohybrids for immunoassay based on SPR biosensor. *Talanta*, 2014. **125**:29–35.
70. Chiu, N.-F., et al., Graphene oxide-based SPR biosensor chip for immunoassay applications. *Nanoscale Res Lett*, 2014. **9**(1):445.
71. Andersson, K., M. Hamalainen, and M. Malmqvist, Identification and optimization of regeneration conditions for affinity-based biosensor assays. A multivariate cocktail approach. *Anal Chem*, 1999. **71**(13):2475–2481.
72. Kurzątkowska, K., et al., Immobilization of His-tagged kinase JAK2 onto the surface of a plasmon resonance gold disc modified with different copper (II) complexes. *Talanta*, 2014. **130**:336–341.
73. Ober, R.J., and E.S. Ward, The choice of reference cell in the analysis of kinetic data using BIAcore. *Anal Biochem*, 1999. **271**(1):70–80.
74. Wong, C., and M. Olivo, Surface plasmon resonance imaging sensors: a review. *Plasmonics*, 2014. **9**(4):809–824.

75. Riedel, T., et al., Surface plasmon resonance: advances of label-free approaches in the analysis of biological samples. *Bioanalysis*, 2014. **6**(24):3325–3336.

76. Suherman, K. Morita, and T. Kawaguchi, Highly selective and sensitive detection of β-agonists using a surface plasmon resonance sensor based on an alkanethiol monolayer functionalized on a Au surface. *Biosens Bioelectron*, 2015. **67**(0):356–363.

77. Singh, M., et al., Noncovalently functionalized monolayer graphene for sensitivity enhancement of surface plasmon resonance immunosensors. *J Am Chem Soc*, 2015. **137**(8):2800–2803.

78. Karabchevsky, A., et al., Study of immobilization procedure on silver nanolayers and detection of estrone with diverged beam surface plasmon resonance (SPR) imaging. *Biosensors*, 2013. **3**(1):157–170.

79. Nguyen, H.H., et al., Surface plasmon resonance: a versatile technique for biosensor applications. *Sensors (Basel)*, 2015. **15**(5):10481–10510.

80. Losoya-Leal, A., et al., Design of a surface plasmon resonance immunoassay for therapeutic drug monitoring of amikacin. *Talanta*, 2015. **141**:253–258.

81. Zhao, S.S., et al., Miniature multi-channel SPR instrument for methotrexate monitoring in clinical samples. *Biosens Bioelectron*, 2015. **64**:664–670.

82. Peng, L., et al., Bi-epitope SPR surfaces: a solution to develop robust immunoassays. *PLoS One*, 2014. **9**(11):e112070.

83. Pawula, M., Z. Altintas, and I.E. Tothill, SPR detection of cardiac troponin T for acute myocardial infarction. *Talanta*, 2016. **146**:823–830.

84. Li, G., et al., A gold nanoparticles enhanced surface plasmon resonance immunosensor for highly sensitive detection of ischemia-modified albumin. *Sensors (Basel)*, 2013. **13**(10):12794–12803.

85. Gassner, C., et al., Development and validation of a novel SPR-based assay principle for bispecific molecules. *J Pharm Biomed Anal*, 2015. **102**:144–149.

86. Frostell, A., et al., Nine surface plasmon resonance assays for specific protein quantitation during cell culture and process development. *Anal Biochem*, 2015. **477**:1–9.

87. SPINIT. Biosurfit. 2010–2016, Available from: http://www.biosurfit.com.

88. Conroy, P.J., R.J. O'Kennedy, and S. Hearty, Cardiac troponin I: a case study in rational antibody design for human diagnostics. *Protein Eng Des Sel,* 2012. **25**(6):295–305.

89. Hearty, S., P. Leonard, and R. O'Kennedy, Measuring antibody-antigen binding kinetics using surface plasmon resonance. *Methods Mol Biol,* 2012. **907**:411–442.

Chapter 12

Protocols for Key Steps in the Development of an Immunoassay

Caroline Murphy and Richard O'Kennedy

School of Biotechnology and Biomedical Diagnostics Institute, Dublin City University, Collins Avenue, Dublin 9, Ireland

caroline.s.murphy@dcu.ie, richard.okennedy@dcu.ie

Immunoassays can be immunometric or competitive systems. They can be further sub-divided into direct, indirect, competitive or sandwich immunoassay formats. The selection of a suitable antibody or antibody fragment to detect the analyte of choice with high sensitivity and selectivity is a key element of assay development. Practical protocols for some of the most commonly used immunoassay techniques described in this book are outlined in this chapter along with information on preliminary tasks to be undertaken before commencing immunoassay development.

12.1 Introduction: Immunoassay Protocols

The protocols described in this chapter relate, firstly, to pre-assay preparation and, secondly, to the assay steps involved. Antibody selection involves choosing either polyclonal, monoclonal or recombinant antibodies. Figure 12.1 outlines the key steps in

Immunoassays: Development, Applications and Future Trends
Edited by Richard O'Kennedy and Caroline Murphy

ISBN 978-981-4669-97-9 (Hardcover), 978-1-315-20654-7 (eBook)
www.panstanford.com

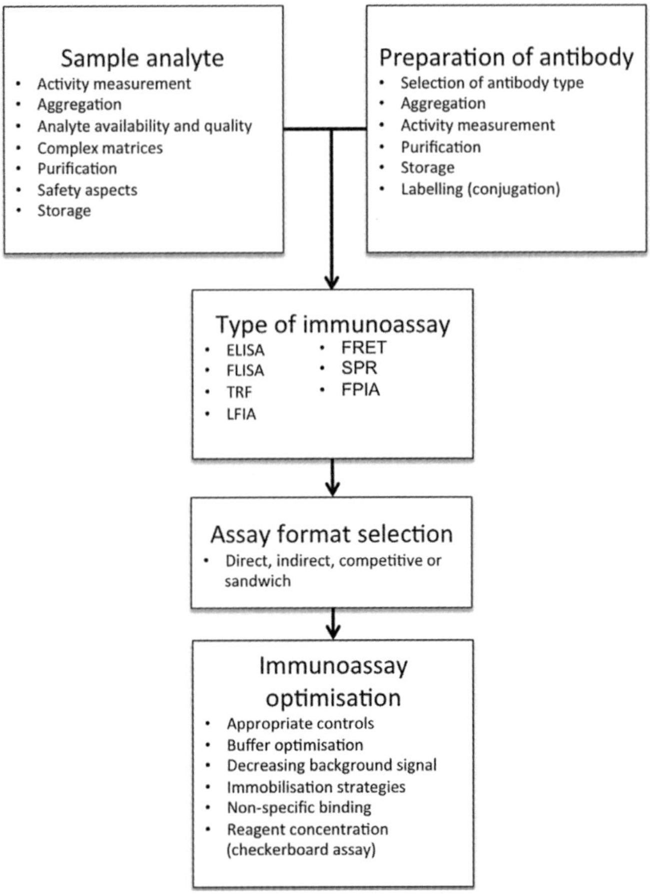

Figure 12.1 Key steps in the development of immunoassays. ELISA, enzyme-linked immunosorbent assay; FLISA, fluorescence-linked immunosorbent assay; TRF, time-resolved fluorescence; LFIA, lateral flow immunoassay; FRET, fluorescence resonance energy transfer; SPR, surface plasmon resonance; FPIA, fluorescent polarisation immunoassay.

the development of an immunoassay and forms the backbone of this chapter, as it outlines important points to be addressed before carrying out an immunoassay or optimisation of assay protocols. Finally, a section on trouble-shooting during immunoassay development is included.

12.2 Preparation of Sample Analyte from Complex Matrices

The analyte of interest is usually in a complex biological matrix. Biological matrices (foodstuffs, seawater, serum, milk, blood, egg yolk, sputum, saliva, urine, ascites fluid, cell culture supernatant or plant-derived extracts, etc. [1]) comprise many components such as lipids, crystals, unwanted cells (mammalian, fungal or bacterial), minerals and proteins, all of which may impact on the sensitivity and reproducibility of the immunoassay [2]. In some cases, the availability of analyte is also an issue. For example, fungal mycotoxins metabolised by plants may become undetectable using conventional assays, such as enzyme-linked immunosorbent assay (ELISA) (due to modifications to the toxin's epitope by metabolic changes or conjugation to glucuronides or by binding to proteins) or high-performance liquid chromatography (HPLC)-based methods (due to changes in polarity that will impact on the solvents used during extraction) [3].

A clever way to avoid assay interference is to separate the analyte from its source matrix. Separating the analyte physically using either affinity or size exclusion chromatography will have a marked impact due to removal of the effects of many interferants [4].

Rapid, simple and effective matrix management solutions and sample preparation methods include:

- Dilution of the sample: This is suitable for reducing matrix interference where detection of the required analyte still remains feasible. Dilution is particularly useful in cases of drug detection in urine, due to the usually high concentration of drug often present [2].
- Protein precipitation (PPT): This is achieved using ammonium sulphate (Protocol 12.1), octonic acid or polyethylene glycol [5]. It is particularly valuable for removing large protein contaminants (by selective use of concentrations/pHs, e.g. in antibody purification). However, limitations of PPT methods include an inability to fully remove all salts and the continued

presence of endogenous molecules such as lipids, phospholipids and fatty acids [2, 6].

- Centrifugation to remove particulates and protein aggregates.

If the aforementioned techniques are not sufficient, it is possible to use:

- Size exclusion chromatography (Protocol 12.2), affinity chromatography (Protocol 12.3) or ion-exchange chromatography.

12.3 Purification of Antibodies

Descriptions of the use of a precipitation (PPT) method (Protocol 12.1) to crudely concentrate antibodies and size exclusion chromatography (Protocol 12.2) and affinity chromatography methods (Protocol 12.3) to clean up the preparations follow.

Protocol 12.1
Purification and concentration of antibodies by precipitation

Note 1: *Reducing the number of hydrogen bonds that occur between a protein (e.g. immunoglobulin) and the solvent in which it is dissolved will cause the protein to precipitate out of solution. Increasing the concentration of ammonium sulphate in a sample causes any antibodies present to become less soluble and precipitation is initiated. The protocol presented here is a more specific form of the process known as 'salting out'. Antibodies precipitate at lower concentrations of ammonium sulphate compared to most other proteins in serum, thus allowing the other proteins to be removed. Ammonium sulphate precipitation allows the reversible precipitation of the antibody. This protocol is frequently used to concentrate polyclonal and monoclonal antibodies from ascites fluid, serum or cell culture supernatants.*

Note 2: *Ammonium sulphate crystals must not be poured directly into the supernatant at once, as this may result in the 'salting out' of all the proteins present in solution. Instead, ammonium sulphate should be added as a solution, thus allowing an incremental increase in the concentration of ammonium sulphate in the supernatant.*

Note 3: *All precipitation techniques are influenced by environmental parameters such as temperature and pH and by the concentration of the sample. To obtain reproducible results these parameters must be controlled* [7].

Note 4: *It is important not to allow the mixture to foam when mixing, as this may lead to protein denaturation. Foaming is prevented by adding the ammonium sulphate slowly and mixing the solution gently.*

Reagents required:

- Media containing antibody to be purified.
- Ammonium sulphate (a 100% (w/v) saturated solution of ammonium sulphate is approximately 4.32 M but this varies with temperature. The required amount of ammonium sulphate is added to 100 mL water and gently heated while stirring until dissolved [8]). Care is needed in the prepartion and use of these solutions to ensure the correct concentrations are used.
- Tris-base buffer (0.3 g Tris-base, 0.4 g NaCl), pH 8.
- Neutral buffer (20 mM Tris-HCl, pH 7.5, 20 mM NaCl, 10 mM $MgCl_2$).
- PBS (150 mM NaCl, 2.5 mM KCl, 10 mM Na_2HPO_4, 18 mM KH_2PO_4), pH 7.5.

Experimental

(1) Centrifuge serum/ascites fluid/cell culture media containing crude antibody at 10,000 g for 30 minutes to remove any large aggregates, pool all supernatants and place in a beaker. Carry out steps at 4°C.

(2) Make up a solution of ammonium sulphate, and filter sterilise through a 0.45 μm membrane.

(3) Slowly add the ammonium sulphate solution to the supernatant while continuously stirring the mixture.

(4) The addition of the slightly acidic ammonium sulphate solution to the supernatant will reduce the pH, and therefore monitoring

of the pH and buffering with tris-base buffer may be required throughout the procedure.

(5) At between 40% and 50% ammonium sulphate saturation, immunoglobulins should start to precipitate out. Stir the solution gently for 4 hours at room temperature or 16 hours at 4°C.
(6) The precipitated immunoglobulins are then removed by centrifugation at 10,000 g for 30 minutes at room temperature.
(7) Remove the supernatant and gently resuspend the pellet in a suitable volume of neutral buffer (20 mM tris-HCl, pH 7.5, with 20 mM NaCl and 10 mM $MgCl_2$).
(8) At this point, the immunoglobulin can be stored for extended periods at −80°C in a minimal volume of buffer (this can be achieved as the ammonium sulphate acts to stabilise the IgG structure with minimal degradation or effect on binding). Alternatively, dialyse the immunoglobulin using several changes of 1 L of buffer (e.g. PBS) at 4°C for 16 hours to remove salts and store aliquots at −80°C.

Ammonium sulphate precipitation yields antibody of purity that is suitable for most applications; however, if further purification is required, consider using size-exclusion, affinity or ion-exchange chromatography.

12.3.1 Purification of Antibodies by Chromatography

High-resolution purification using chromatographic methods can be used as a final polishing step following initial purification procedures. Size exclusion chromatography (SEC) or gel filtration uses a cross-linked beaded form of agarose (or other material) as a separation media for molecules based on their size. There are many types of chromatographic media and GE Healthcare provides a range of these to facilitate antibody purification. SEC can be used for 'group separation' and 'fractionation'. Group separation is used to remove high or low molecular weight contaminants (e.g. desalting), while fractionation is used to purify biomolecules according to their size. To perform SEC, a column is packed with porous spherical particles (e.g. agarose or sepharose). A suitable equilibration buffer is added to the column, which fills the spheres and the space between. A heterogeneous sample (containing antibody) is added to the column, the molecules move through the column at varying speeds according to their size. The smaller molecules move into the porous spheres, slowing their progress through the column, while the larger molecules move into and out of the beads to a lesser degree, therefore passing through the column at greater speed. A protocol using SEC for the purification of antibody follows (Protocol 12.2).

Affinity chromatography is a separation technique that facilitates purification of antibody by means of the reversible binding of the antibody to the cognate antigen immobilised on a solid phase. Other commonly used methods of affinity chromatography for antibody purification are based on specific-ligand or bacterial-receptor interactions. Some examples of specific ligands used for affinity chromatography of antibodies include antibody-binding proteins, lectins or anti-antibodies. Bacterial-receptor-based affinity chromatography has been widely exploited due to the high affinities attributed to certain immunoglobulins for the bacterial-receptors [1, 9]. The most commonly used bacterial-receptors are known as Staphylococcal protein (A) (or protein A), Streptococcal protein G (or protein G) and protein L derived from *Peptostreptococcus magnus*. Protein A and G display high affinities for the Fc region of IgG, and protein L binds to the kappa (κ) light chain of the antibody variable region. Protein A is more commonly used in affinity chromatography procedures due to protein G's tendency to cross-react with other protein such as albumin and kinogen [1, 10]. However, the emergence of genetic engineering and the production of protein A and G recombinantly means this issue is largely overcome. Affinity chromatography using protein A is a commonly employed procedure for the purification of IgG and is presented in Protocol 12.3. Please refer to a detailed review by Ayyar and colleagues [1] which describes in greater detail the use of affinity chromatography for the purification of antibodies.

Monoclonal IgM and the avian immunoglobulin IgY can be purified by thiophilic adsorption media using 2-mercaptopyridine coupled to sepharose high-performance beads as the ligand [1].

Protocol 12.2
Purification of antibodies using size exclusion chromatography (SEC) by fast protein liquid chromatography (FPLC)

This protocol outlines the use of Superdex® resin from GE Healthcare for the purification of antibodies by fast protein liquid chromatography (FPLC). A number of different purification resins are available from GE Healthcare; and each one is tailored for a particular application:

- Sephacryl or Sepharose—wide ranges of fractionation procedures
- Superdex for high-resolution purification
- Sephadex LH for separation of small molecules in organic solvents

Superdex prepacked columns from GE Healthcare are commonly used for additional purification of recombinant, polyclonal and monoclonal antibodies. The following columns are available from GE Healthcare for fast protein liquid chromatography (FPLC) using ÄKTA design systems [11].

- Superdex 30 is ideal for use with proteins $M_r < 10{,}000$ Da (columns can be purchased from GE Healthcare in pack sizes of 150 mL, 1 L or 5 L (no further information available on bed volume, sample volume or flow rate).
- Superdex 75 is most commonly used for the purification of proteins with molecular weights of between 3000 to 70,000 Da, such as recombinant antibodies (columns can be purchased from GE Healthcare in bed dimensions of 10 × 300 mm and 5 × 150 mm)
    - 10 × 300 mm column: 24 mL bed volume; 25–500 μL sample volume; 0.5–1 mL min^{-1} flow rate
    - 5 × 150 mm column: 3 mL bed volume; 4–50 all sample volume; 0.15–0.6 ml min^{-1} flow rate
- Superdex 200 is ideal for the purification or separation of larger molecular proteins (such as monoclonal antibodies) with M_r 10,000 to 600,000 Da (columns can be purchased from

GE Healthcare in bed dimensions of 10 × 300 mm and 5 × 150 mm).

- 10 × 300 mm column: 24 mL bed volume; 25–500 μL sample volume; 0.25–0.75 mL min^{-1} flow rate
- 5 × 150 mm column: 3 mL bed volume; 4–50 μL sample volume; 0.15–0.6 mL min^{-1} flow rate

Reagents required:

- PBS, filtered through 0.2 μm and degassed (150 mM, pH 7.4) (Table 12.2)
- Antibody sample to be purified; filtered through 0.2 μm filter membrane
- Superdex column (75 or 200) depending on type of antibody or antibody fragment to be purified
- 20% (v/v) ethanol; degassed.

Experimental

(1) Degas 1 L of PBS (150 mM, pH 7.4) (or buffer suitable to your particular antibody) for 30 minutes.
(2) Centrifuge antibody sample at 4°C for 10 minutes at 10,000g to remove any aggregates. Filter the sample through a 0.2 μm syringe filter.
(3) Equilibrate the column (e.g. Superdex 75 or 200) with 50 mL PBS at a flow rate of 0.5 mL min^{-1} at room temperature.
(4) Inject the sample (2 mL) into the FPLC system and run the sample through at a flow rate of 0.5 mL min^{-1}.
(5) Monitor the absorbance of sample fractions that are eluted from the column spectrophotometrically at 280 nm.
(6) Observe the chromatograph for protein peaks and collect the corresponding (0.5–5 mL) fractions.
(7) Wash the column with 50 mL PBS followed by 100 mL 20% (v/v) degassed ethanol. The column can be stored in 20% (v/v) degassed ethanol.

Antibodies can be further or alternatively purified using ion-exchange chromatography (IEC) or affinity chromatography (Protocol 12.3).

Protocol 12.3
Purification of IgG using protein A affinity chromatography

Note 1: *Affinity chromatographic methods are based on the ability of ligand bound to resin (usually agarose) to reversibly bind to specific antibodies in a complex mixture, thus, separating them from other proteins that may be present in a sample. Essentially, antibody diluted in a 'mobile phase' is added to a column pre-packed with 'stationary phase' (ligand-bound agarose). As the binding reaction is reversible, this allows the release of antibodies following elution (either by altering the pH or salt content in the column)* [9]. *The antibodies are usually eluted into neutralisation buffer to preserve their structural and functional integrity. Protein A is a surface protein derived from Staphylococcus aureus. It has a molecular weight of approximately 46.7 kDa and has five immunoglobulin binding sites. It is used for the purification of IgG (e.g. human IgG1, 2 and 4) through its Fc region. Binding varies depending on class and species of antibody.*

Note 2: *This protocol has been adapted from Peptide antibodies: Methods and Protocols by Ma and O'Kennedy* [12], *Essential Techniques: Antibody Production by P.J. Delves* [13] *and Immunology Methods Manual by I. Lefkovits* [14].

Note 3: *When carrying out affinity chromatography it is important not to let the column dry out as this will negatively impact the performance of the purification.*

Reagents required:

- Protein A agarose
- Serum containing the antibody of interest
- Sterile filtered (through a 0.2 μm membrane filter) PBS: 150 mM NaCl, 2.5 mM KCl, 10 mM Na_2HPO_4, 18 mM KH_2PO_4, pH 7.4
- Binding/washing buffer: PBS (as above)
- Elution buffer: 100 mM glycine-HCl, pH 2.5–3.0
- Neutralisation buffer: 1M tris-HCl, pH 8.0–9.0

Experimental

(1) Before commencing purification, remove any debris present in the supernatant by centrifugation at 3220 g for 10 minutes at 4°C and filtering through a 0.2 μm filter.

(2) To a 20 mL column, add 2 mL of protein A agarose and equilibrate with 10 mL. Allow the PBS to flow-through the column.
(3) Add 5 mL of the serum supernatant (from point 1), to the equilibrated protein A column. Cap the top and bottom of the column. Mix gently on a roller mixer overnight at 4°C.
(4) Place the column over a 50 mL tube and collect the 'flow-through'. Add the 'flow-through' back into the column and repeat this step 3 times to ensure that as much IgG as possible has bound to the column.
(5) Wash the column five times with 10 mL PBS to remove non-specifically bound proteins.
(6) Add 10 mL elution buffer to the column and collect the 'flow-through' into a clean 50 mL tube containing 1 mL neutralisation buffer.
(7) Buffer exchange the neutralised IgG three times using 5 mL volumes of PBS and a 10,000 MWCO spin column by centrifugation at 3,220 g at 4°C.
(8) Confirm the concentration of the purified IgG and dispense in 100–500 μL volumes into clean 1.5 mL microtubes, and store at 4°C for short-term storage or −20 or −80°C for longer term storage.

12.3.2 Antibody Storage Considerations

Antibodies, like most proteins need to be stored over long periods of time without losing significant functionality or being structurally compromised. Please refer to Fig. 12.2 for a guide to recommendations for antibody storage.

Antibodies can be stored at 4°C for up to a week without losing significant functionality, provided the storage buffer was filter-sterilised and a suitable antimicrobial agent had been included. For longer-term storage, antibodies can be stored at –20°C or –80°C. It is recommended to aliquot the antibodies into small volumes (100 μL to 1 mL) suitable for subsequent assay procedures. Dispensing antibodies into smaller volumes avoids freezing and thawing, thereby reducing the risk of degradation. Additionally, antibodies must not be stored in buffers at very low or very high pH as this may cause denaturation. Additional steps can be taken to avoid proteolytic degradation. It is recommended to store the antibodies in concentrations above 0.5 mg mL^{-1} and to store them in glass or low-protein binding microfuge tubes. The antibodies can be stored in stabiliser—e.g. bovine serum albumin (BSA) (or there are several commercially available materials)—which increases the concentration of protein in the aliquot and reduces the probability of the antibody binding to the surface of the storage vial and thereby undergoing degradation [15].

Cryoprotectants such as glycerol and ethylene glycol can be added to the storage buffer. Cryoprotectants act to reduce the freezing temperature of the storage buffer; in this case, glycerol and ethylene glycol can be added (25–50% v/v) to prevent the formation of ice crystals upon storage at –20°C. Antimicrobials such as sodium azide (0.02–0.05% w/v) or thimerosal (0.01% w/v) can be included to prevent microbial growth. However, these agents need to be carefully handled, as there are potential health-associated issues.

Protease inhibitors can be added to prevent protein degradation [16]. Serine protease inhibitors, for example, target proteases that break down peptide bonds in proteins where serine serves as the active site. Some examples of protease inhibitors (and their working concentrations) include:

- Serine proteases inhibitors
    - Phenylmethylsulphonyl fluoride (PMSF) 0.1–1 mM
    - Benzamidine 1 mM
    - Aprotinin 5 μg mL^{-1}
- Acid protease inhibitor
    - Pepstatin A 1 μg mL^{-1}
- Thiol protease inhibitor
    - Leupeptin 1 μg mL^{-1}

12.3.3 Antibody Conjugation

Antibodies are frequently conjugated to labels that enable detection of antibody-antigen binding. Additional amplification of the signal can be achieved by using a secondary antibody that binds to the

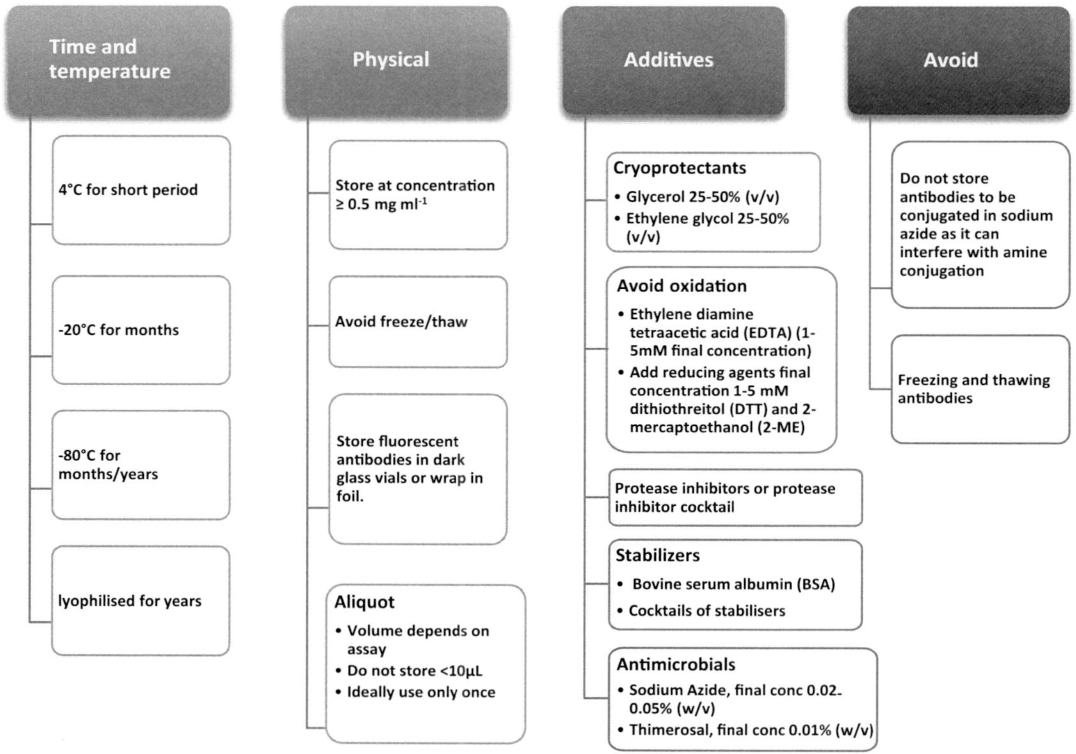

Figure 12.2 Overview guide to antibody storage and handling.

primary antibody recognising the antigen. Signalling molecules, such as enzymes (horse radish peroxidase (HRP) or alkaline phosphatase (AP)) fluorescent markers or quantum dots (QDs) can be attached. The following protocols outline the coupling of antibodies to an enzyme label (alkaline phosphatase) (Protocol 12.4), fluorescent label (protocol 12.5) or quantum dots (QDs) (protocols 12.6 and 12.7).

Protocol 12.4
Conjugation of alkaline phosphatase to antibody molecules

Note 1: *This protocol was adapted from a 'Procedure for the conjugation of alkaline phosphatase to antibody and other proteins' provided by Sigma-Aldrich* [17, 18].

Reagents required:

- 10 mg of purified antibody to be conjugated
- 5 mg alkaline phosphatase (Sigma-Aldrich)
- 0.1 M sodium phosphate, pH 6.8
- 1 % (v/v) glutaraldehyde
- 1 M ethanolamine, pH 7.0
- PBS (150 mM NaCl, 2.5 mM KCl, 10 mM Na_2HPO_4, 18 mM KH_2PO_4), pH 7.4
- Storage solution: 50% (v/v) glycerol, 1 mM $ZnCl_2$, 1 mM $MgCl_2$ and 0.02% (w/v) sodium azide

Experimental

(1) Add 10 mg of purified antibody to 5 mg high-activity alkaline phosphatase to a total volume of 1 mL.
(2) Dialyse the antibody/alkaline phosphatase mix in 0.1 M sodium phosphate buffer, pH 6.8 to remove any amine-containing compounds (overnight at 4°C).
(3) Gently stir the antibody/alkaline phosphatase mix in a fume hood and add 0.05 mL 1% (v/v) glutaraldehyde. Stir for 5 minutes.
(4) Stop stirring and incubate for 3 hours at room temperature.

(5) Add 0.1 mL 1 M ethanolamine, pH 7.0.
(6) Incubate for 2 hours at room temperature.
(7) Dialyse overnight at 4°C against three volumes of PBS.
(8) Place in a clean 1.5 mL centrifuge tube and centrifuge at 40,000 g for 20 minutes to remove precipitate.
(9) Keep in storage solution (see Fig. 12.2 for additives that may be included) at 4°C.

Protocol 12.5
Conjugation of fluorophore (e.g. fluorescein isothiocyanate (FITC)) to antibody molecules

Note 1: *This protocol was adapted from Immunocytochemical Methods and Protocols* [19].

Note 2: *In general, when conjugating an antibody to a label, the antibody preparation should be as pure as possible. Otherwise, the conjugation reagent will also bind to any contaminating proteins. Therefore, use antibody purified either by gel filtration or affinity chromatographic methods.*

Note 3: *Avoid the use of buffers that contain contaminating amines, such as Tris, sodium azide, glycine or ammonia as they will compete with the ligand for binding. If any of these substances are present in the sample, it is advisable to dialyse your sample into a more suitable buffer such as PBS or sodium carbonate buffer.*

Reagents required:

- IgG (3 mg mL^{-1}) in sodium carbonate buffer
- Sodium carbonate buffer: 1.0 M $NaHCO_3$-Na_2CO_3, pH 9.5
- Fluorescein isothiocyanate (FITC) (5 mg mL^{-1}) in ethanol
- Absolute ethanol
- 0.02% (w/v) sodium azide

Experimental

(1) Prepare the antibody to be functionalised; the concentration should be at least 3 mg mL^{-1} in 1 M sodium carbonate buffer at room temperature.

(2) Prepare a fresh solution of 5 mg mL^{-1} fluorescein isothiocyanate (FITC) in ethanol and protect from light to avoid photobleaching.
(3) The FITC should be added at 10-fold molar excess compared to antibody at room temperature.
(4) Mix the FITC with the antibody solution, and incubate in the dark at room temperature for 30 minutes with gentle shaking.
(5) Add the reaction mixture to a gel filtration column to separate the 'free' FITC from the FITC-labelled antibody.
(6) The antibody-conjugate can be stored in 0.02% (w/v) sodium azide in PBS at 4°C away from light, or can be snap frozen and stored at −20°C.
(7) It is important not to refreeze the antibody-conjugate once it has been thawed as this could compromise its binding capacity.
(8) The degree of fluorescein conjugation that occurs per molecule can subsequently be determined.

$$\text{Fluorescein conjugated IgG concentration}$$
$$= (A_{280\text{nm}} - 0.35 \times A_{493\text{nm}}) \div 1.4$$

The molar ratio FITC/Protein ratio (F/P) can be determined, based on a molar extinction coefficient of M_r 73,000 for the fluorescein group.

$$F/P = (A_{280}/73,000) \times (15,000/Fl\ \text{IgG Concentration})$$

12.3.3.1 Conjugation of quantum dots to antibodies

Antibody-conjugated quantum dots (QDs) can be used as detection molecules in sandwich and indirect immunoassays. Three QD conjugation strategies are most commonly used i.e. (1) direct covalent coupling, (2) electrostatic and (3) indirect capture [20, 21].

Direct covalent coupling of the carboxyl (–COOH) groups on the QD surface can be achieved using *N*-ethyl-*N*′-(3-(dimethylamino)propyl)carbodiimide hydrochloride (EDC), with subsequent attachment to protein via amine groups. Direct covalent coupling between carboxyl groups and sulfhydryl groups (catalysed by maleimide) or between aldehyde and hydrazine [22] can also be used. Amine-carboxyl linkages are commonly used for QD conjugation due to the availability of primary amines and carboxyl groups on most proteins (Protocol 12.6). Low reproducibility and aggregation sometimes occur during the chemical modification of the QDs, as the QD-COOH groups may cross react, with multiple amines on biomolecules [23].

Alternatively, antibodies can also be covalently linked to QDs by oxidising the carbohydrate groups on the Fc portion of the antibody. Following oxidation, the carbohydrate forms a reactive aldehyde group, which is then covalently linked to QDs. This approach may facilitate site-specific orientation of the antibody onto the QD (Protocol 12.7).

Protocol 12.6
Direct covalent coupling of antibodies to QDs: carboxyl–amine coupling

Note 1: *This protocol has been adapted from* Nature Protocols *and* Analytical and Bioanalytical Chemistry [22, 23].

Reagents required:

- Quantum dots (QDs) (8 μM)
- *N*-ethyl-*N′*-(3-(dimethylamino)propyl)carbodiimide hydrochloride (EDC) (2.2 mM in methanol)
- *N*-hydroxysuccinimide (NHS) (4 mM in methanol)
- Antibody (1 mg mL^{-1}) in PBS (150 mM NaCl, 2.5 mM KCl, 10 mM Na_2HPO_4, 18 mM KH_2PO_4, pH 7.4)

Experimental (A)
Activation of QD with EDC/NHS in methanol

(1) Add 3 μL EDC and 3 μL NHS to 15 μL QDs.
(2) Add 9 μL methanol.
(3) Incubate at room temperature for 30 minutes to generate activated QDs.

Experimental (B)
Direct conjugation of activated QD to antibodies by amine–carboxylic acid coupling

(1) Mix activated QDs (from protocol 12.6(A)) with antibody (1 mg mL^{-1}) and incubate for 4 hours at room temperature.
(2) The amount of methanol must be kept below 4–5% of total reaction volume.
(3) QD:antibody molar ratio should be 1:30. However, a variety of ratios have been used and trials to determine the optimal ratio to use may be required.
(4) Separate QD-antibody conjugates from unconjugated antibodies using gel filtration (Superdex 200 column).
(5) Measure the eluted fractions by UV-visible absorption and fluorescence microscopy. Wavelengths chosen depend on the QDs.

Protocol 12.7
Conjugation of QDs through oxidised Fc-carbohydrate groups on antibodies

Note 1: *This protocol has been edited from* Nature Protocols [22].

Reagents required:

- QDs (8 μM)
- EDC (N-(3-dimethylaminopropyl)-N′-ethylcarbodiimide hydrochloride) (5 mM)
- Adipic acid dihydrazide (ADH) solution
- Sodium phosphate (0.01 M) in water
- NaCl (0.15 M) in water, pH 7.2
- Sodium periodate in water (final concentration of 0.1 M); protect from light (wrap tube in aluminium foil)
- PBS (150 mM NaCl, 2.5 mM KCl, 10 mM Na_2HPO_4, 18 mM KH_2PO_4, pH 7.2)
- Dialysis tubing (MWCO: 50 kDa)

Experimental

(1) Add required volume of carboxylated QD stock (to achieve a final concentration of 100 mM) to 4 μL of 5 mM EDC stock

(final concentration 20 μM) and 5.1 μL ADH solution (3.2 μg μL^{-1} (w/v) dissolved in PBS).

(2) Mix the solution well and incubate for 4 hours at room temperature.

(3) Dialyse in 2 L PBS overnight to remove excess EDC and ADH (size exclusion chromatography can be carried out if preferable).

(4) Antibody is dissolved in 0.01 M sodium phosphate, 0.15 M NaCl, pH 7.2 (final concentration 10 mg mL^{-1}).

(5) The sodium periodate is dissolved in water (final concentration 0.1 M) and protected from light.

(6) Quickly add 100 μL sodium periodate to 10 mL antibody solution (1.5 mg mL^{-1}).

(7) Mix to dissolve and protect from light.

(8) Incubate in the dark for 30 minutes at room temperature.

(9) Dialyse overnight in 2 L PBS.

(10) Mix QD-hydrazide and periodate-oxidised antibodies at QD:antibody molar ratio of 1:30 and incubate the reaction for 2 hours at room temperature.

(11) Concentrate the reaction solution to 20 μL or less, using spin filters, before continuing to the next step.

(12) Separate QD-Ab conjugates from free antibodies by gel filtration using Superdex 200 columns (5 × 150 mm column; bed volume 3 mL; sample volume 4–50 μL).

(13) Collect the first ten drops of coloured eluted material which should contain the QD-Ab conjugates.

(14) Apply a few microlitres onto a microscope slide and examine by fluorescence microscopy to determine the quality of the QD-Ab conjugates.

12.3.4 Preparation of Biotinylated Antibodies

The use of biotin as an antibody conjugate is ubiquitous as the reaction between biotin and its binding partner avidin is the strongest currently known non-covalent interaction between a protein and ligand ($K_a = 10^{15}\ M^{-1}$) [24]. Biotin is a small (244 Da) B vitamin found in the body and reacts with avidin, streptavidin and NeutrAvidin. Due to its small size, it rarely negatively impacts on the conjugated protein's functionality or causes steric hindrance.

The biotin/avidin interaction is used in a wide variety of applications from affinity chromatography to signal detection. Thermo Scientific have a wide range of biotinylation reagents to suit different applications, with varying lengths to reduce steric hindrance effects. The most commonly used reactive biotinylation products are *N*-hydroxy-succinimide (NHS)-biotin and sulfo-NHS-biotin. Both are ester molecules which interact with N-terminal amines or amines found in lysines. Thermo Scientific's sulfo-NHS-long-chain (LC)-biotin molecule is most commonly used for antibody conjugation as it is the most simplest and is usually most effective. Alternative methods of antibody-biotinylation include the use of NHS-PEG_4-biotin which is also amine reactive and increases solubility of the biotinylated molecule. Finally, biotin-PEG_4-hydrazine from Thermo Scientific reacts with carbohydrate and is commonly used for the conjugation of biotin molecules to polyclonal antibodies. Protocols 12.8 and 12.9 outline the biotinylation of antibodies and their subsequent capture onto streptavidin-coated QDs.

Protocol 12.8
Preparation of biotinylated antibodies

Note 1: *This protocol has been adapted from Tully and colleagues* [25]. *Biotinylation labelling kits are available from Thermo Scientific* [16].

Reagents required:

- Antibody (1 mL IgG at 10 mg mL^{-1} in 0.1 M sodium phosphate buffer pH 7.2) to be biotinylated at suitable purity
- Dimethylsulphoxide (DMSO)
- Sulpho-NHS-LC-Biotin (Ideal for use with monoclonal and polyclonal antibodies. A long spacer arm is used to reduce steric hindrance between the biotin and avidin molecules.) (Sulpho-NHS-LC-LC-biotin molecules with extra-long spacer arms are also available to further reduce steric hindrance) [24].

Experimental

(1) Dialyse antibodies overnight to remove any traces of sodium azide as it can interfere with the amine reaction.

(2) Prepare stock solution of long-chain biotin by dissolving 1 mg of biotin in 1 mL DMSO.
(3) Add a volume of biotin to the prepared antibody solution at the appropriate concentration to give a molar ratio of 20:1 biotin to antibody. The amount of biotin to be added is calculated each time with respect to the amount of antibody and the size of the antibody to be used.
(4) Rotate the solution overnight at 4°C.
(5) Pass the biotin-conjugate through a PD-10 Sephadex G25 column (GE Healthcare) to remove any unbound biotin. This also stops the biotinylation reaction.

Protocol 12.9
Indirect capture of biotinylated antibodies onto streptavidin-coated QDs

Note 1: *This protocol has been edited from* Nature Protocols [22].

Reagents required:

- Biotin-long chain (LC)-hydrazide
- Oxidised antibody (biotin/antibody molar ratio is 4:1)
- PBS (150 mM NaCl, 2.5 mM KCl, 10 mM Na_2HPO_4, 18 mM KH_2PO_4, pH 7.4)
- 50 kDa MWCO spin columns
- QD-streptavidin nanocrystals (Invitrogen)

Experimental

(1) Mix biotin-LC-hydrazide with oxidised antibody, with a final biotin-hydrazide concentration of 5 mM.
(2) Incubate the reaction for 2 hours at room temperature.
(3) Purify the solution three times using spin filters (MWCO: 50 kDa or dialyse in 2 L PBS over night at 4°C), centrifuge at 5,000 rpm and dilute 1:10 with PBS.
(4) Mix biotinylated antibody with streptavidin coated QDs (volume ratio 1:1), and incubate for 1 hour at room temperature.
(5) Separate QD-antibody conjugates from free antibody using a gel filtration Superdex 200 column.
(6) The eluted QD-antibody conjugates are now ready for use.

12.4 Protein Aggregation

Protein aggregates result from the clumping together of mis-folded proteins or protein degradation products. They are caused by different stresses being applied to the protein such as temperature, agitation, differing ionic strengths, exposure to different interfaces (air, solid), and high protein concentrations [26]. It should be assessed whether aggregation readily occurs and under what conditions. If aggregation does occur there are a number of actions that can be taken to minimise it, for instance, adding co-solvents or changing buffers.

Many different forms of protein aggregates can be found in sample analytes. Aggregates can be found in both soluble and insoluble forms, and can be caused by the presence of covalent and non-covalent bonding. They can be reversible or irreversible or can be caused by the denaturation of the analyte concerned [27, 28].

Noteworthy point:

Insoluble aggregates visible to the naked eye can be removed using a 0.2 μm filter. Larger aggregates can be removed by centrifugation.

Covalent bonding can occur as a result of the formation of disulphide bonds between thiols, but can be avoided by introducing dithiothreitol (DTT) or β-mercaptoethanol [26]. Non-covalent bonding can occur in a solution of protein in equilibrium. However, if the pH, temperature or concentration of protein are altered, the balance can be shifted, causing the formation of dimer or trimer aggregates [27, 28]. The exposure of internal residues to surfaces and to solvents during the denaturation of proteins can also lead to aggregation [27, 28]. Physical and mechanical activities such as freezing and exposing the protein to metal surfaces or oxygen can lead to aggregation, and should be avoided [29].

12.4.1 Prevention of Protein Aggregation

Table 12.1 highlights a number of buffer additives that can be used to prevent protein aggregation. The presence of partially folded protein intermediates can cause further protein aggregation. By diluting the

Table 12.1 Additives that can be used to prevent protein aggregation

Effects	Additives	Effects	Refs.
Kosmotropes	$MgSO_4$ (0–0.4 M), $(NH_4)_2SO_4$ (0–0.3 M), Na_2SO_4 (0–0.2 M), NaCl (0–1 M), KCl (0.1 M)	Stabilise native state of proteins; tighten inter- and intramolecular structure making interactions in aqueous solutions	[26, 33]
Chaotropes	$CaCl_2$ (0–0.2 M), $MgCl_2$ (0–0.2 M), Urea (0–1.5 M)	Destabilise protein structure; loosen inter- and intramolecular interactions	[34]
Amino acids	Glycine (0.5–2% w/v) L-Arginine (0–5 M)	Glycine and proline are small polar molecules that enhance protein stability. Arginine increases the solubility of aggregation-prone molecules; most effective suppressor of heat-induced aggregation. It reduces the aggregation of folding intermediates	[31, 35, 36]
Osmolytes	Polyols, glycine, betaine, proline and ectoines	Protectant role	[37, 38]
Detergents	Tween-80 (0–0.2%, v/v) Tween-20 (0–120 μM) Nonidet P-40 (0–1%, v/v)	Decrease hydrophobic interactions	[29, 39, 40]
	Sodium dodecyl sulphate	Denatures protein by adhering to hydrophobic regions of peptides	[31]
Reducing agents	DTT, $\beta-$mercaptoethanol	Break up non-native disulphide bonds	[26]
Polyhydric alcohols and sugars	Sucrose, glucose, lactose, glycerol	Increase protein solubility	[41]

concentration of protein intermediates, protein aggregation should be reduced [26, 30].

The addition of low concentrations of salts can help to stabilise proteins [31]. **Kosmotropic** agents (their name derives from the word 'kosmotrope' (order-making)) function to stabilise proteins and hydrophobic aggregates in solution. They form strong hydrogen bonds and act to exclude hydrophobic residues (usually forming the internal structure of the protein) from the solvent, thereby maintaining the structural integrity of the protein. Too high a concentration of kosmotropic reagents will cause the protein to 'salt out'. Therefore, a balance must be achieved. **Chaotropic** agents get their name from the word 'chaotrope' (disorder-making) and function to destabilise proteins. They break up hydrogen bonds and increase the solubility of proteins in aqueous solutions. This encourages the protein to denature. **Amino acids:** During the production of recombinant proteins, arginine can be used to enhance the amount of appropriately refolded proteins. Arginine, used at high concentrations (2M) has the capacity to suppress aggregation of partially folded intermediates [32].

12.5 Immunoassay Optimisation

To quantify biological molecules with great accuracy, sensitivity and specificity, optimisation of different facets of the immunoassay must be carried out.

12.5.1 Immunoassay Buffers

The antibody/antigen interaction is designed to work most efficiently under physiological conditions. Therefore, it makes sense to use a physiological pH and ionic strength. The most commonly used buffers in immunoassays are phosphate buffered saline (PBS) and tris-buffered saline (TBS) (Table 12.2). To minimise non-specific binding, as discussed previously in this chapter, chaotropic salts or surfactants can be added to remove weakly bound interactants.

12.5.2 Decreasing Background Signal

In order to determine the concentration of a target analyte, the signal generated in the assay must be clearly determinable above blank values. In addition, issues such as non-specific binding and matrix effects can cause interference or 'background noise'. The use of washing and blocking steps can help to eliminate background

Table 12.2 Buffers suitable for immunoassay development

Application	Buffer*	pH	Ref.
Coating	150 mM phosphate buffered saline (PBS): (10 mM) 1.4 g of Na_2HPO_4, (18 mM) 0.2 g KH_2PO_4, (150mM) 8 g NaCl, (2.5 mM) 0.2 g KCl, 800 mL deionised H_2O, adjust to pH 7.4 with HCl and add H_2O to 1 L	7.4	[42–44]
	50–100 mM carbonate/bicarbonate: sodium carbonate 0.7 g, sodium bicarbonate 1.5 g, bring to 1 L with deionised H_2O	9.6	[43]
	10 mM Tris-HCl: 1.21 g Tris in 900 mL diH_2O, pH to 8.5 with HCl, add diH_2O to 1000L	8.5	[43]
Washing buffer	PBS (as above), 0.05% (v/v) 0.5 mL Tween-20	7.4	[42, 43]
Blocking buffer	PBS (as above) containing 1–5% (w/v) bovine serum albumin, milk marvel, casein, gelatin or other proteins	7.4	[42, 43]
Reagent diluent	PBS (as above) containing 1% (w/v) blocking reagent	7.4	[45]
Tris buffer	Tris base buffer: Tris base 3 g, NaCl 4 g, pH to 10.3 with NaOH, bring to 1 L with diH_2O	10.3	[8]

*Buffer reagents are supplied by Sigma-Aldrich or Fluka. All buffers must be prepared in double-distilled water. di: deionised.

noise. The choice of coating buffer, frequency of wash steps and composition of the washing buffer can be altered and, finally, the extent to which blocking of non-specific reaction sites is required must be considered. The following sections address some of these ideas.

12.5.3 Coating Buffer

Coating buffers used must facilitate the homogenous deposition of antibodies, for example, onto slightly hydrophobic polystyrene 96-well plates. Buffers that have a pH value above the pI of the antibody are ideal. Commonly used buffers are listed in Table 12.2.

12.5.4 Inclusion of Wash Steps

The main objective of incorporating washing steps into immunoassays is to separate unwanted and non-specific proteins from specifically bound protein, thus helping to reduce background noise.

Antibodies bind to their respective analyte with the highest affinity, however, antibodies may also bind to other proteins with lower affinities. These non-specific antibody interactions can be removed or significantly reduced by a number of different approaches:

- Introduction of **chaotropic salts** such as NaCl, Na_2SO_4, $MgCl_2$, $MgSO_4$ and $CaCl_2$ [34]
- The introduction of surfactants such as Tween-20 or Triton-X100 [1] will decrease hydrophobic interactions
- Organic solvents such as methanol and ethylene glycol will decrease hydrophobic interactions

Buffers most commonly used for washing are usually of physiological pH. Tris-buffered saline (TBS) and phosphate buffered saline (PBS) are frequently used and can be supplemented with detergents to aid in reducing non-specific binding (NSB).

12.5.5 Blocking of Non-specific Reaction Sites

The blocking stage in an immunosorbent assay functions to reduce NSB. An initial step in many immunoassays involves coating the surface of the receptacle in which the assay will take place (e.g. a microtitre plate) with a protein (often an antibody or a protein conjugate). The coating protein never fully achieves total surface area coverage, thus leaving areas that could potentially bind to reagents added later during the assay (e.g. capture antibody, detection antibody, biotin, avidin, or the enzyme substrate). Naturally reactive endogenous substances or autoantibodies may also bind to the assay surface or the capture antibody. This can result in the observation of falsely positive or falsely negative results [4]. The blocking of non-specific reactions results in a situation where ideally only the required specific antibody–antigen reaction occurs.

Several blockers should be tested when developing a novel immunoassay. The blocker which produces the best signal to noise ratio should be chosen for the assay [46].

Examples of blockers include:

- Bovine serum albumin (BSA), 1–5% (w/v) in 10–150 mM PBS, pH 7.
- Dilute non-fat dried milk powder, 0.1–5% (w/v) (may contain biotin, which will interfere with an experiment if biotin is incorporated). This can be purchased 'off-the-shelf', e.g. Marvel.
- Casein (main component of non-fat dried milk, and therefore lacks major impurities).
- Fish gelatin (1–5%, (w/v), works better in Western, Northern and Southern blots than in ELISAs); it functions to reduce protein-protein interactions; therefore, it may be more applicable for use in washing buffers.
- Animal serum, 5–10% (v/v), reduces cross-reactivity; however, it should be noted that horse serum contains endogenous peroxidases that may interfere with detection systems that involve peroxidase. Serum works well as a blocking agent due to its high diversity of proteins.
- Protocols that may encounter naturally occurring endogenous peroxides (e.g. immunohistochemistry that involves liver or kidney samples). This may be blocked before the addition of signalling enzyme by adding 3–10% (v/v) H_2O_2.

In addition to biological blockers, detergents are also used as blocking agents. Detergents are not as efficient as protein blockers but in some cases may be more suitable. Detergent blockers disrupt ionic and hydrophobic biomolecular interactions and strip loosely bound molecules from the surface. The most commonly used blockers are non-ionic and include Tween, Triton and Non-ident P-40. Non-ionic detergents act to prevent the hydrophobic adsorption of protein onto the solid phase, and also prevent the aggregation of macromolecules. Ionic detergents such as sodium dodecyl sulphate (SDS) have inhibitory effects on the antibody/antigen interaction, and zwitterionic detergents, such as CHAPS, can be used in combination with mixed proteins as blocking agents.

Noteworthy point:

If background signal remains high, include a protein blocker in the wash steps (as well as the blocking step and the antibody application steps).

12.5.6 Checkerboard Titration for Optimisation of ELISA Components

To obtain the optimal dilution of detection antibody and 'tracer' a 'checkerboard' enzyme-linked immunosorbent assay (ELISA) can be carried out (Protocol 12.10). A checkerboard ELISA involves the titration of different dilutions of each component against each other identifying optimal dilution values (Fig. 12.3). Each ELISA format may differ in the constituent parts that require titration. A direct ELISA requires the titration of antigen against antibody, indirect ELISAs require the titration of antigen, sample antibody and enzyme-linked anti-species antibody, while competitive ELISAs require the titration of adsorbed analyte against 'tracer'.

Protocol 12.10
Checkerboard ELISA: identify optimal reagent concentrations

Reagents required:

- Coating antigen or capture antibody at desired concentration in capture buffer (1–10 μg in PBS or bicarbonate/carbonate buffer; see Table 12.2)
- Detection antibody (enzyme-conjugated antibody) at desired concentration
- Coating buffer (for examples see Table 12.2)
- Washing buffer (for examples see Table 12.2)
- Blocking reagent (for examples see Table 12.2)
- Reagent diluent (see Table 12.2)
- Colour producing substrate
- Stop solution (e.g. 2 M H_2SO_4)

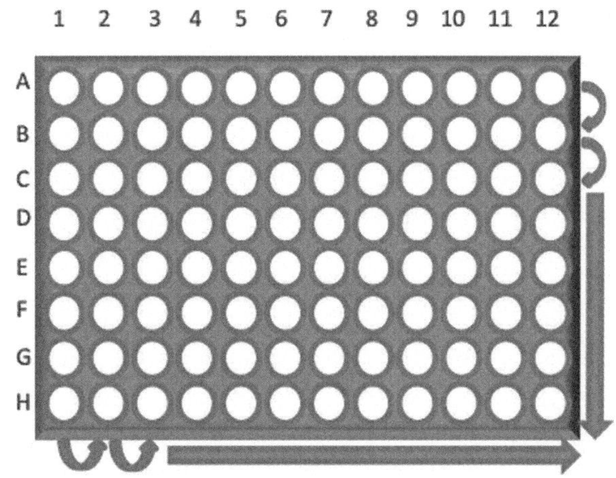

Figure 12.3 The checkerboard ELISA is used to determine optimal concentrations of, firstly, coating antigen/antibody and, secondly, enzyme-conjugated antibody on a 96-well microtitre plate.

Experimental

(1) Coating buffer (100 μL) is added to each well of a 96-well plate. Then, using an 8-channel multichannel pipette, add 100 μL of the sample antigen into each well in column 1. The solution is pipetted up and down 8 times to mix. Using new tips, add 100 μL from each well in column 1 to column 2.

(2) Repeat the procedure by pipetting up and down 8 times and adding 100 μL from each well in column 2 into column 3, this process is repeated until column 11 is reached.

(3) Column 12 acts as a control.

(4) Upon reaching column 11 there will now be 200 μL of mixture in column 11, discard 100 μL so that only 100 μL of the mixed solution remains.

(5) Allow the antigen to bind to the plate (incubate the plate at 4°C overnight, room temperature for 2 hours or at 37°C for 1 hour).

(6) The volume of blocking solution should be three times the volume used for coating. Incubate for 2 hours at room temperature, or 4°C overnight, or 37°C for 1 hour.

(7) Wash the plate with 3XPBST (300 μL) per well, 3XPBS (300 μL) per well. Blot plate on dry clean tissue.

(8) The second stage of the checkerboard ELISA requires the optimisation of the enzyme-conjugated detection antibody. The enzyme-conjugated antibody is sequentially diluted in reagent diluent. The antibody is diluted down the multi-titre plate (see Fig. 12.3), from row A to G.
(9) Add 100 μL reagent diluent to all wells in a 96-well plate. Dilute the conjugated antibody in a separate tube before adding to the plate.
(10) Pour diluted antibody into a reservoir and using a multichannel pipette, pipette the diluted antibody into row A (100 μL per well).
(11) The solution should be mixed up and down 8 times.
(12) From each well in row A, 100 μL is taken and placed into row B. This is now mixed using pipetting action 8 times, and the procedure is repeated (changing the tips each time) until row G is reached.
(13) Row H acts as a negative control.
(14) The plate is incubated and washed. A suitable enzyme substrate is added, a signal is generated, and the colour development stopped using stopping solution. The absorbances of the solution in the wells of the plate are read on a spectrophotometer at the appropriate wavelength.

12.5.7 Introduction of Appropriate Positive and Negative Controls into the Assay Protocol

The inclusion of appropriate positive and negative controls into the immunoassay will serve to validate the result. Upon completion of an experiment, a signal from a **positive control** indicates that the experiment has worked. The accompanying absence of signal from wells containing the negative control indicates that the assay appears to be working correctly. In the case of immunoassays, a previously determined 'known' sample can be used as a positive control.

A **negative control** is a sample that is known not to contain any of the protein or antibody you wish to detect. Inclusion of a negative control in the assay will test for the presence of non-specific binding. If the negative control contains a signal, then the experiment has not worked optimally and non-specific binding is occurring. Therefore, some false positive results may be observed in the sample wells.

12.5.7.1 Use of a spiked control

A spiked control contains a known quantity of sample in an appropriate sample matrix (e.g. blood, plasma, urine, cell lysates, sea-water etc.). The inclusion of a spiked control in sample matrix will give an indication of the assay performance under relevant conditions.

12.5.7.2 Standard curve

For accurate concentration quantification, a standard curve that spans the dynamic detection range of the binding analyte must be included. The concentration of the sample analyte may require optimisation; for instance, the sample analyte may require dilution. Standard curve concentrations should always be determined in triplicate.

12.5.8 Immobilisation Strategies for Biomolecules onto Solid Surfaces

Choosing the most suitable immobilisation strategy is critical in the development of any assay, as it must allow the ligand to retain its activity and also ensure that the appropriate binding sites are exposed to the binding partner (such as an antibody) [47]. Immobilisation of proteins to any surface can be achieved using physical, covalent or bio-affinity strategies.

Physical adsorption exploits ionic, hydrophobic and polar intermolecular reactions that can occur between a protein and select surfaces [48]. Physical adsorption is an inexpensive and simple biomolecule binding method. However, it can result in the random orientation of the protein onto the surface, and may result in the reduced exposure of critical sites. It should be noted, that physically adsorbed proteins can be easily removed by washing with buffers containing detergent.

Covalent immobilisation can be carried out by directly linking chemical groups (e.g. NH_2–COOH or –SH) or by chemically functionalising the biomolecule to enable linkage [48] (Table 12.3). Pierce Thermo Scientific provide a range of immobilisation strategy kits [16].

Before starting the immobilisation process for a protein the following points should be addressed and/or optimised:

- Select either a direct or capture immobilisation strategy.
- Establish the purity and concentration of the protein.
- Find the optimum buffer pH for the immobilisation reaction.
- Identify residues in the proteins amenable for immobilisation, e.g. cysteine, lysine.
- Determine the ideal reaction time.
- Decide the optimal ionic strength reaction buffer.
- Identify the most appropriate coupling technique depending on the groups available and the need for a linker (or not).
    - Amine
    - Carboxyl
    - Thiol
    - Aldehyde
    - Pegylation
    - Maleimide

Bioaffinity immobilisation involves the use of biologically derived binding molecules. They can aid in the gentle immobilisation of specifically orientated molecules, maintaining their structural integrity and functionality [48]. The biotin/avidin bond occurs readily and is unimpeded by exposure to varying pH, temperature and organic solvents. Disadvantages relating to the use of avidin are associated with its glycosylation and a pI of 10.5 at neutral pH. Streptavidin is a biotin-binding molecule derived from *Streptomyces avidinii* that does not have any associated glycosylation and has an acidic pI of 5. A recombinant avidin molecule known as NeutrAvidin™ is also a deglycosylated form of native avidin. It has a more neutral pI (NeutrAvidin's pI is 6.3 compared to 10.5 for avidin) and forms less non-specific interactions. The biotin/avidin

Table 12.3 Covalent immobilisation methods

Coupling group	Activation reagents	Reacts with the following on the surface	Makes use of the following residues/groups on the ligand	Conditions of reaction	Ref.
Amine (-NH_2)	EDC/NHS to form active esters	• activated carboxyl derivatives to form an amide bond, • aldehydes to form an imine, • isothiocyanate to form thiourea. NHS ester reacts with primary amide on ligand/protein surface	Lysine and unblocked N-terminal amino acid residues	Not compatible with Tris buffer or sodium azide as they compete with the ligand for coupling; used at pH 7.2 to 8.5.	[47–49]
Carboxyl (–COOH)	Carbodiimide (EDC) activates carboxylates (–COOH)	Amines (–NH_2)	Aspartic acid and glutamic acid.	Acidic conditions pH 4.5 to 5.5 in MES buffer or pH $\leq$ 7.2	[48]

(*Contd.*)

Table 12.3 (*Continued*)

Coupling group	Activation reagents	Reacts with the following on the surface	Makes use of the following residues/groups on the ligand	Conditions of reaction	Ref.
Thiol (–SH) ligand	EDC/NHS to form active esters and PDEA to introduce reactive disulphide bonds	Maleimide, disulphide bonds, haloacetyl groups	Cysteines	pH 6.5–7.5 (maleimide) pH 7 and above (high pH provides more reactive thiolate (S^-) groups)	[49, 50]
	EDC/NHS to form active esters, DTT or DTE to introduce thiol groups	Carboxyl or amine groups	Disulphide groups that have been introduced onto the ligand's carboxyl groups using PDEA or SPDP (amine groups)		[49, 51]
Pegylation	Amine, sulfhydryl or carboxy reactive polyethylene glycol	Primary amines (–NH_2), sulphydryls (–SH), carboxy groups.	Lysine Cysteine Carboxylates	Conditions vary for each pegylation	[16, 48]

EDC: *N*-ethyl-*N′*-(3-(dimethylamino)propyl)carbodiimide; PDEA: 2-(2-pyridinyldithio) ethaneamine hydrochloride; NHS: *N*-hydroxysuccinimide; DTE: dithioerythritol; DTT: dithiothreitol; SPDP: *N*-succinimidyl-3-(2-pyridyldithio)-propionate.

interaction can facilitate protein attachment to a variety of solid supports.

12.6 What Type of Immunoassay to Choose?

Equipped with the information already supplied in this chapter on how to prepare for an immunoassay, the next step is to decide what type of immunoassay to use to best address each analytical measurement requirement. Different types of immunoassay format will be discussed.

12.6.1 Enzyme-Linked Immunosorbent Assay (ELISA)

Enzyme-linked immunosorbent assay (ELISA) is a very widely used method to detect the presence of analyte in a sample. It is often the 'gold standard' to which other immunoassays are compared. It is a rapid, sensitive, specific and reproducible method based on the ability of an immunoglobulin to detect a specific antigen. The ELISA can be used in multiple formats, with different read-outs. The format chosen depends on the detection requirements of the assay, the concentration of the analyte, the structure and size of the analyte and whether the analyte is soluble or membrane bound. ELISA has rapidly increased in popularity due to its high-throughput capabilities, where it is capable of measuring many samples in a relatively short period of time.

The next section of this chapter describes in more detail the fundamentals of direct, indirect, sandwich and competitive ELISA.

12.6.1.1 Binding of capture protein/antibody to the surface

The development of solid phase ELISAs was made possible by the findings of Catt and Tregear in 1967 who found that proteins readily adhere to plastic surfaces, thus providing a solid-phase attachment surface and an appropriate means of separating bound from unbound reactants [52]. The selection of a suitable solid-phase/surface in the development of immunoassays is key, as it facilitates the binding of the first stage reagent. A more detailed description of surfaces used in immunoassays is described in Chapter 3 of this book. The binding of reagent to the solid surface mainly occurs through a process known as passive adsorption but other methods of binding can also be used such as the use of covalent binding, immunochemical adsorption or bio-affinity binding [1, 9, 53]. The process of passive adsorption should always be considered first as it is the most inexpensive and straight forward. The principle of passive adsorption relies on hydrophobic interactions between non-polar elements and the hydrophobic surface of the plate. It should be noted that during the binding/capture process, a certain percentage of the proteins will become denatured, as a result of internal hydrophobic residues accessing the surface of the protein and interacting with the surface of the plastic plate. This in turn causes the partial denaturation of the binding protein, which may lead to a reduction in available antigenic epitopes or a decrease in biological activity [53]. Immunochemical adsorption relies on the initial adsorption of a reactant-specific capture antibody followed by the application of the required reactant.

Immunochemical adsorption can be useful as it serves to physically move the target analyte away from the plastic surface, where it may become somewhat denatured. A further binding alternative takes advantage of the high affinity of avidin, streptavidin or neutrAvidin for biotin. Either avidin or biotin is covalently bound to the plastic surface and the respective biotin- or avidin-conjugated carrier protein is applied.

Depending on the read-out signal of the assay a specific plate must be chosen. Clear plastic polystyrene flat-bottomed plates are used for colourimetric assays, black polystyrene flat-bottomed plates are used for fluorescence-based assays and white polystyrene flat-bottomed plates are used for chemiluminescence-based assays. Key factors that influence ELISA efficiency are displayed in Table 12.4.

12.6.2 Commonly Used ELISA Protocols

The following section describes detailed protocols for direct, indirect, sandwich and competitive ELISAs.

Table 12.4 Factors influencing ELISA efficiency. Adapted from Thermo Fisher piercenet.com ELISA guide [16]

Factor	Influencing factors
Assay Surface	Material (polystyrene and polydimethylsiloxane), well shape and pre-activation
Binding buffer (capture buffer)	Composition and pH
Capture antibody	Specificity, titre, affinity, incubation time and temperature used
Blocking buffer	Composition, concentration and cross-reactivity.
Target antigen	Concentration, stability, availability of epitopes, aggregation, purity, presence of contaminants in associated matrix
Detection antibody	Specificity, titre, affinity, incubation time, temperature and cross-reactivity
Enzyme conjugate	Type of enzyme, type of conjugate, activity, concentration and cross-reactivity
Washes	Buffer composition, volume, duration and frequency
Substrate	Sensitivity, stability, self-quenching at high concentrations
Signal Detection	Imaging, instrument exposure time, availability of appropriate wavelength filters, sensitivity, speed of signal generation, matrix interference

Protocol 12.11
Direct antigen ELISA

Note 1: *The simplest ELISA format involves the direct coating of antigen onto a solid-phase plastic surface (microtitre plate or polystyrene test tube). The sample analyte is incubated, followed by washing, where any unbound analyte is washed away. Each sample well is then blocked to reduce non-specific binding. The presence of the analyte sample is then detected with an enzyme-linked antibody. The concentration of sample analyte present is directly proportional to the signal level.*

Note 2: *Controls: Negative – (a) no antigen, (b) no primary detection antibody, (c) PBS/media alone and (d) no secondary labelled antibody. Positive – (e) known concentrations of antigen for preparation of standard curve.*

Note 3: *Some of the buffer recipes used in this protocol have been obtained from Refs* [44, 45].

Reagents required:

- Antigen (1–10 μg mL^{-1}) in coating buffer (for examples see Table 12.2)
- Blocking buffer (Table 12.2)
- Detection antibody (enzyme-conjugated antibody) in reagent diluent (Table 12.2).
- Wash buffer (e.g. PBS-Tween see Table 12.2)
- Enzyme substrate (Table 1.3)
- Stopping solution (e.g. 2M H_2SO_4)

Experimental

(1) Apply 1–10 μg mL^{-1} pure antigen (in coating buffer, see Table 12.2) or crude (sample analyte) to each well of a clean, colour appropriate, plastic/PVC microtitre plate. Incubate overnight at 4°C, room temperature for 2 hours or 37°C for 1 hour.

(2) Use serially diluted antigen at known concentration to generate a standard curve; preferably, each concentration in the appropriate range should be added in triplicate, and must be incubated for exactly the same length of time as the analyte.

(3) Remove the contents of the well and add blocking solution to each well at three times the volume used for coating. Incubate for 2 hours at room temperature, or 4°C overnight, or 37°C for 2 hours.

(4) Wash with 3XPBST (300 μL/well) and then blot on clean dry tissue; then wash with 3XPBS (300 μL/well) and blot plate on clean dry tissue.

(5) Add a pre-determined concentration of enzyme-labelled detection antibody diluted in reagent diluent. Incubate at room temperature for 1–2 hours.

(6) Wash with 3XPBS, (300 μL/well). Blot plate on clean dry tissue.

(7) For detection and generation of signal, add 50 μL of enzyme substrate and incubate for between 5–30 minutes, monitor signal and select suitable time for subsequent ELISAs.
(8) The reaction must then be stopped; this is often achieved by changing the pH, for example, by the addition of acid. Add 50 μL of stopping solution after the optimal development time period.
(9) Read the absorbance on a colourimetric plate reader or fluorescence on a fluorimeter and generate a standard curve from the serial dilution of standards. Place the concentration on the X-axis (log scale), and absorbance/fluorescence on the Y-axis (linear scale). Interpolate the concentration of sample from the standard curve.

Protocol 12.12
Indirect ELISA

Note 1: *Indirect ELISAs are commonly used to detect antibodies in a sample that bind to a particular antigen.*
Note 2: *Controls: Negative controls: (a) pre-bleed taken from animal before immunisation, (b) no primary antibody, (c) primary antibody replaced with isotype-matched, non-specific antibody. Positive control (d) positive sample from previously run experiments (or coat a well with known antigen).*

Reagents required:

- Antigen (1–10 μg mL^{-1}) in coating buffer (for examples see Table 12.2)
- Blocking buffer (Table 12.2).
- Capture antibody (antigen-specific)
- Detection antibody (enzyme-labelled species-specific antibody) in reagent diluent (Table 12.2)
- Wash buffer (e.g. PBS-Tween see Table 12.2)
- Enzyme substrate (Table 1.3)
- Stopping solution (e.g. 2M H_2SO_4)

Experimental

(1) Apply 1–10 μg mL^{-1} pure antibody/analyte (in coating buffer, see Table 12.2) to each well of a clean, colour appropriate, plastic, PVC microtitre plate. Use 100 μL/well and incubate

overnight at 4°C, room temperature for 2 hours or 37°C for 1 hour.

(2) Use serially diluted antibody/antigen of known concentration to generate a standard curve. Preferably, each standard sample should be prepared in triplicate and must be incubated for exactly the same length of time.

(3) Remove the contents of the wells and add a suitable blocking solution (Table 12.2) to each well at three times the volume used for coating. Incubate for 2 hours at room temperature, or 4°C overnight, or 37°C for 1 hours.

(4) Wash with 3XPBST (300 μL/well) and then blot on clean dry tissue, then wash with 3XPBS (300 μL/well) and blot plate on clean dry tissue.

(5) Add 50 μL of serum (blood, urine, ascites fluid etc.) containing antibody, diluted in reagent diluent and incubate for 1–2 hours at room temperature.

(6) Wash with 3XPBST (300 μL/well) and then blot on clean dry tissue. Wash with 3XPBS (300 μL/well) and blot plate on clean dry tissue.

(7) Add a pre-determined concentration of enzyme-labelled detection antibody diluted in reagent diluent. Incubate at room temperature for 1–2 hours. The antibody used must be directed against the species of the primary antibody (present in serum) used.

(8) Wash with 3XPBST, (300 μL/well) and then blot on clean dry tissue, then wash with 3XPBS (300 μL/well) and blot plate on clean dry tissue.

(9) For detection and generation of signal, add 50 μL enzyme substrate and incubate for between 5–30 minutes, monitor signal and select suitable time for subsequent ELISAs.

(10) The reaction must then be stopped; this is often achieved by changing the pH, for example, by the addition of acid. Add 50 μL of stopping solution after the optimal development time period.

(11) Read the absorbance on a colourimetric plate reader or fluorescence on a fluorimeter and generate a standard curve from the serial dilution of standards. Place the concentration on the X-axis (log scale), and absorbance/fluorescence on the

Y-axis (linear scale). Interpolate the concentration of sample from the standard curve.

Protocol 12.13
Sandwich ELISA

Note 1: *The key principle that separates sandwich ELISAs from other types of ELISAs is that sandwich ELISAs use two antibodies, the first to capture the target antigen and the second signal its presence.*

Note 2: *A number of experimental controls must be included. Negative controls: (a) capture antibody alone, (b) detection antibody alone, (c) PBS/media alone. Positive control: (d) include standards containing serially diluted analyte of known concentrations.*

Reagents required:

- Capture antibody (1–10 μg mL^{-1}) (antigen-specific) in coating buffer (see Table 12.2)
- Blocking buffer (Table 12.2)
- Sample antigen (appropriately diluted)
- Detection antibody (antigen-specific enzyme-labelled) in reagent diluent (Table 12.2)
- Wash buffer (e.g. PBS-Tween see Table 12.2)
- Enzyme substrate (Table 1.3)
- Stopping solution (e.g. 2M H_2SO_4)

Experimental

(1) Apply 1–10 μg mL^{-1} of pure capture antibody to each well of a clean, colour appropriate, plastic, PVC microtitre plate. Use 100 μL/well and incubate overnight at 4°C, room temperature for 2 hours or 37°C for 1 hour.

(2) Add a suitable blocking solution to each well at three times the volume used for coating. Incubate for 2 hours at room temperature, or 4°C overnight, or 37°C for 1 hour.

(3) Wash with 3XPBST (300 μL/well) and then blot on clean dry tissue, then wash with 3XPBS (300 μL/well) blot plate on clean dry tissue.

(4) Use 100 μL of sample analyte in blood, urine etc. diluted in reagent diluent and incubate for 1–2 hours at room temperature. Serially diluted standards of known concentration should also be added to the plate, generate a standard curve. Preferably, each standard sample should be prepared in triplicate and must be incubated for exactly the same length of time as the samples. The concentration of analyte in the standard curve must span the dynamic range of the sample analyte.

(5) Wash with 3XPBST (300 μL/well), blot on clean dry tissue, then wash with 3XPBS (300 μL/well) and blot plate on clean dry tissue.

(6) Add a pre-determined concentration of enzyme-labelled detection antibody diluted in reagent diluent (100 μL/well).

(7) Wash with 3XPBST (300 μL/well), blot on clean dry tissue, then wash with 3XPBS (300 μL/well) and blot plate on clean dry tissue.

(8) For detection and generation of signal, add 50 μL of enzyme substrate and incubate for between 5–30 minutes, monitor signal and select suitable time for subsequent ELISAs.

(9) The reaction must then be stopped; this is often achieved by changing the pH, for example, by the addition of acid. Add 50 μL of stop solution after the optimal development time period.

(10) Read the absorbance on a colourimetric plate reader or fluorescence on a fluorimeter and generate a standard curve from the serial dilution of standards. Place the concentration on the X-axis (log scale), and absorbance/fluorescence on the Y-axis (linear scale). Interpolate the concentration of sample from the standard curve.

Protocol 12.14
Competitive ELISA

Note 1: *Competitive immunoassays are commonly used for the detection of small molecules such as drugs, toxins and hormones, because, due to their small size, they may be only have one epitope available for antibody recognition. A* ***competitive ELISA*** *requires an antigen-specific antibody and a 'tracer' (enzyme-*

conjugated analyte). The assay allows the determination of the concentration of free analyte in an analytical sample. The fundamental principle of the competitive immunoassay is that the unknown concentration of analyte competes with a pre-titrated 'tracer' labelled-analyte of known concentration for available binding sites on the surface-adsorbed specific antibody. A competitive curve is generated. The higher the concentration of analyte in the sample, the lower the signal generated, conversely, the lower the concentration of analyte the higher the signal generated. The amount of signal generated is thus inversely proportional to the concentration of analyte present.

Note 2: *Controls: Negative control (a) a blank sample – PBS/media alone and (b) positive control, a positive reference standard should be included.*

Reagents required:

- 1–10 μg mL^{-1} antigen (small molecule covalently linked to larger carrier protein) in coating buffer (Table 12.2)
- Blocking buffer (Table 12.2)
- Sample antigen (appropriately diluted)
- Detection antibody (enzyme-labelled and antigen specific) in reagent diluent (Table 12.2)
- Wash buffer (e.g. PBS-Tween; see Table 12.2)
- Enzyme substrate (Table 1.3)
- Stopping solution (e.g. 2M H_2SO_4)

Experimental

(1) Apply 1–10 μg mL^{-1} of pure antigen in coating buffer (Table 12.2) (small-molecule covalently linked to a larger protein, e.g. BSA ('tracer')) to each well of a clean, colour appropriate, plastic, PVC microtitre plate. Use 100 μL/well and incubate overnight at 4°C, room temperature for 2 hours or 37°C for 1 hour.

(2) Add a suitable blocking solution to each well at three times the volume used for coating. Incubate for 2 hours at room temperature, or 4°C overnight, or 37°C for 1 hour.

(3) Wash with 3XPBST (300 μL/well), blot on clean dry tissue, then wash with 3XPBS (300 μL/well) and blot plate on clean dry tissue.

(4) A pre-titrated concentration of specific antibody (in a 50 μL volume) is added to 50 μL of sample analyte diluted in reagent diluent. This mixture is added to the plate. The added sample analyte and surface bound analyte compete for antibody binding sites. The samples are incubated at room temperature for 1–2 hours. Serially diluted standards should also be added to the plate, in appropriately labelled wells for the generation of a standard curve.

(5) Wash with 3XPBST (300 μL/well), and blot on clean dry tissue, then wash with 3XPBS (300 μL/well) and blot plate on clean dry tissue.

(6) Add a pre-determined concentration of enzyme-labelled detection antibody diluted in reagent diluent (100 μL/well). The antibody used must be directed against the species of the primary antibody used.

(7) Wash with 3XPBST (300 μL/well), and blot on clean dry tissue, then wash with 3XPBS (300 μL/well) and blot plate on clean dry tissue.

(8) For detection and generation of signal, add 50 μL enzyme substrate and incubate for between 5–30 minutes, monitor signal and select suitable time for subsequent ELISAs.

(9) The reaction must then be stopped; this is often achieved by changing the pH, for example, by the addition of acid. Add 50 μL of stop solution after the optimal development time period.

(10) Read the absorbance on a colourimetric plate reader or fluorescence on a fluorimeter and generate a standard curve from the serial dilution of standards. Place the concentration on the X-axis (log scale), and absorbance/fluorescence on the Y-axis (linear scale). Interpolate the concentration of sample from standard curve.

(11) It is also feasible to have a competitive assay where the analyte-specific antibody is immobilised on the plate. Labelled (tracer) analyte (added in known amounts) competes with unknown

amounts of analyte (from the samples being analysed) for binding to the enzyme immobilised on the plate. If the label is an enzyme or is fluorescent it can be detected as outlined in steps 8–10.

12.6.3 Fluorescence-Linked Immunosorbent Sandwich Assay (FLISA)

Fluorescent immunoassays or FLISAs use the same basic steps as standard ELISAs but differ in that the enzyme (e.g. alkaline phosphatase (AP), β-galactosidase or peroxidase) conjugated to the detection antibody use substrates that produce a product that emits fluorescence instead of colour. Alternatively, a fluorescently labelled antibody can be used as the detection entity.

Similarly to ELISA, the fluorescence units emitted are proportional to the amount of analyte present. However, it is important to note that the fluorescence-based ELISA is only slightly more sensitive than a colourimetric ELISA, but the dynamic range in which the signal can be read is much wider.

Many fluorescent substrates can be found on the market today. Thermo Scientific produces a Quanta Red Enhanced chemifluorescent HRP substrate, which claims to provide sensitivity comparable to enhanced chemiluminescence readouts. All fluorescence-based assays should be carried out in opaque black plates to minimise background fluorescence.

The production of a fluorescent signal is influenced by many different parameters including pH, temperature, ion concentration, drying, light scattering, quenching and bleaching [54, 55]. To avoid negative impacts on the signal, some considerations can be made:

- *Limit light scattering*
  - Reagents and diluents should be as pure as possible.
  - Filter reagents through 0.45 μm filter membrane before use.
  - Use black opaque plates for reading signals.
  - Remove any bubbles when reading signals.

- *Reduce background fluorescence/autofluorescence*
    - Limit the presence of cellular debris.
    - Limit dust or fingerprints on the plate.
    - Ensure plate used is of high quality.
    - Carefully choose reagents for immobilisation, e.g. glutaraldehyde [56].
- *Limit quenching effects*
    - Quenching effects can be exasperated by the presence of oxygen in the buffers; to alleviate, degas the reagents prior to use.
- *Reduce bleaching effects*
    - Some of the reagents used may be light sensitive; reduce the effects of bleaching by carrying out the immunoassay process in the dark.

12.6.4 Time-Resolved Fluorescence Immunoassay

Time-resolved fluorescence (TRF) assays use metals from the lanthanide series in the periodic table as antibody labels. Metals from the lanthanide series have fluorescent properties and compared to traditional fluorescence molecules, the lanthanides have much longer emission lifetimes and larger Stokes shifts. TRF assays take advantage of these properties and benefit from a reduction in background fluorescence and an increased sensitivity over traditional fluorescence assays. TRF assays give more information about the molecular environment of the fluorophore as the fluorophore is influenced by its surroundings over time. TRF immunoassays are similar to ELISAs in their format as they can be carried out as sandwich or competitive immunoassays [57]. The rare earth metal Europium is one of the most commonly used lanthanides for TRF immunoassays. It acts as an energy donor providing longer life-time fluorescence. It can be conjugated to an antibody or antigen for use in sandwich or competition immunoassays [58, 59]. A protocol that describes a time resolved fluorescence-based sandwich immunoassay is described in Protocol 12.15.

Protocol 12.15
Time-resolved fluorescence sandwich immunoassay

Note 1: *All buffers used in this assay can be purchased from Perkin Elmer at www.perkinelmer.com. Time-resolved fluorescence can be measured using a 1234 DELFIA research-fluorimeter and counts can be processed by Multicalc software (Perkin Elmer).*

Note 2: *Antibodies can be Europium-labelled by amine functionalisation using Europium-labelling kits from companies like Abnova (www.abnova.com) or can be purchased from Perkin Elmer.*

Note 3: *Include a standard curve using known concentrations of analyte and an uncoated plate as a control to account for any background fluorescence that might arise from the plate.*

Reagents required:

- DELFIA wash buffer (Perkin Elmer)
- DELFIA assay buffer (Perkin Elmer)
- Europium-labelled antibody (or Europium-labelled analyte)
- DELFIA enhancement solution (Perkin Elmer)

Experimental

(1) Coat microtitre plate (compatible with fluorescence measurements) with (100 μL/well) antigen (1–2 μg mL^{-1}), diluted in suitable assay buffer at suitable pH.
(2) Cover and incubate at 4°C overnight.
(3) Wash four times in suitable wash buffer.
(4) Dilute serum samples (containing unknown concentrations of antibody of interest) in assay buffer; include a standard curve diluted in identical assay buffer.
(5) Include an uncoated microtitre plate as a control to account for any non-specific fluorescence activity.
(6) Incubate at room temperature for 2 hours, place on an orbital shaker at 125 rpm.
(7) Wash four times.
(8) Dilute Europium-labelled anti-human IgG (or other appropriate antibody) in assay buffer and add 100 μL into each well.

(9) Incubate for 1–2 hours at room temperature on an orbital shaker at 125 rpm.
(10) Wash four times.
(11) Add 100 μL enhancement solution to each well.
(12) Shake the plates for up to 15 minutes at room temperature in the dark.
(13) Fluorescence can be read using a fluorimeter.
(14) Counts can be processed using Multicalc software (Perkin Elmer).
(15) The concentration can be interpolated onto the standard curve and expressed as mIU L^{-1}.

12.6.5 Fluorescence Polarisation Immunoassay (FPIA)

Fluorescence polarisation (FP) was first described in 1926 by F. Perrin [60]. Fluorescence polarisation immunoassays (FPIA) are homogenous assays (i.e. do not require the removal of bound analyte). During FPIA a molecule binds to a fluorescent partner molecule (fluorescently bound antibody or antigen) and is excited by plane polarised light. It then emits parallel and perpendicular light, the ratio of which is based on the size of the molecule. In solution, small molecules rotate more rapidly than larger molecules due to Brownian motion. A fluorescent antibody that binds to its antigen will change its size thereby changing the ratio whereby emitted light is polarised (Fig. 12.4) [61]. A photomultiplier tube amplifies the signal strength, and it is measured using a fluorescence spectrophotometer.

Polarised light is used to excite fluorescent molecules, and when excited, they emit light in the vertical and horizontal planes. The degree by which the vertical light moves to the horizontal light depends on the size and the degree of rotation of the molecule. A small molecule will rotate more than a large molecule, therefore, with small molecules there will be more horizontal light.

FP is most often used for the detection of small molecules, as the rate of Brownian motion (tumbling) when a fluorescent small molecule competes for binding to a larger molecule (e.g. antibody) is much greater than when two larger molecules bind, i.e. the relative change in tumbling between two larger molecules compared to one

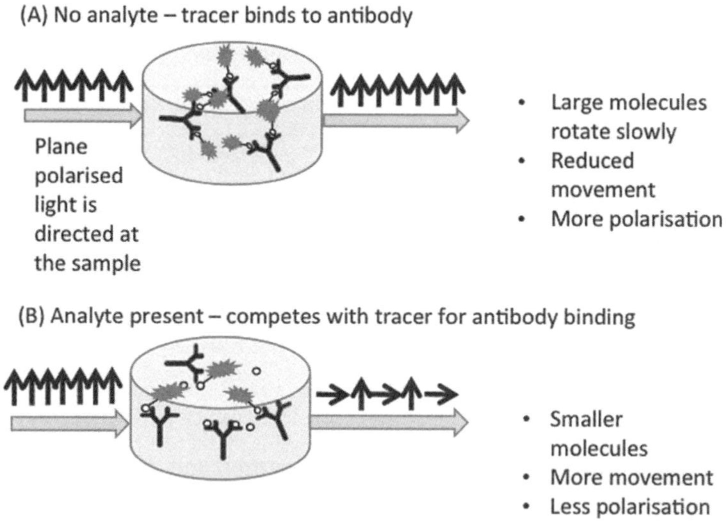

Figure 12.4 Schematic representation of fluorescence polarisation. Plane polarised light is directed at each sample. The sample in (A) does not contain analyte, and so antibody binds to tracer forming large slowly rotating complexes, emitting polarised light. The sample in (B) contains analyte that competes with the tracer for antibody binding sites, thus the fluorescent tracer does not bind antibody, with less complex formation in the sample there is more movement and lower emission of plane polarised light.

small and one large is much less. Additionally, larger molecules are not ideal for use in FP due to the longer time they take to rotate [62].

Dyes used for FP such as BODIPY (4,4-difluoro-4-bora-3a,4a-diaza-s-indacene) can be purchased from Life Technologies Corporation and other companies. BODIPY dyes have longer excited-state lifetimes than fluorescein and rhodamine dyes rendering the FP sensitivity of BODIPY more sensitive to binding interactions over a larger molecular weight range. A protocol that describes the use of fluorescence polarisation in an immunoassay is described in Protocol 12.16.

A disadvantage in the use of FPIA is the requirement of expensive dedicated equipment, which may limit its use. A more economical alternative to FPIA may be fluorescence resonance energy transfer (FRET), which is discussed in the next section of this chapter.

Protocol 12.16
Fluorescence polarisation Immunoassay (FPIA)

Note 1: *This protocol is adapted from published protocols* [61, 63].

Reagents required:

- Antibody directed against target analyte diluted to pre-titrated concentration in reagent diluent (Table 12.2)
- Analyte of known concentration to be used in standard curve preparations
- Fluorescein-labelled analyte diluted in reagent diluent

Experimental

(1) Dilute sample material in suitable buffer and add to a black, round-bottom, polystyrene 96-well plate containing at least 50 μL sample volumes.
(2) Incubate the samples at room temperature for 2 minutes and take a blank fluorescent reading in the fluorescence polarisation analyser.
(3) To each well, add serially diluted competing ligand (include at least 8 serial dilutions), carry out each sample in triplicate and include positive and negative controls.
(4) To each well, add a previously titrated (known) amount of fluorescence-conjugated analyte (tracer).
(5) Incubate for 15 minutes in the dark at room temperature, while gently shaking the plate at 30 rpm.
(6) Centrifuge at 300 g for 2 minutes at room temperature.
(7) Take a second fluorescence reading.
(8) Measure parallel intensities ($I\|$) and perpendicular intensities ($I\perp$).
(9) Analyse results.

12.6.6 Fluorescence Resonance Energy Transfer (FRET) Immunoassay

Fluorescence resonance energy transfer (FRET) occurs when energy is transferred from a molecule in an excited state (donor) to a second molecule (acceptor) (Fig. 12.5). When the two molecules come

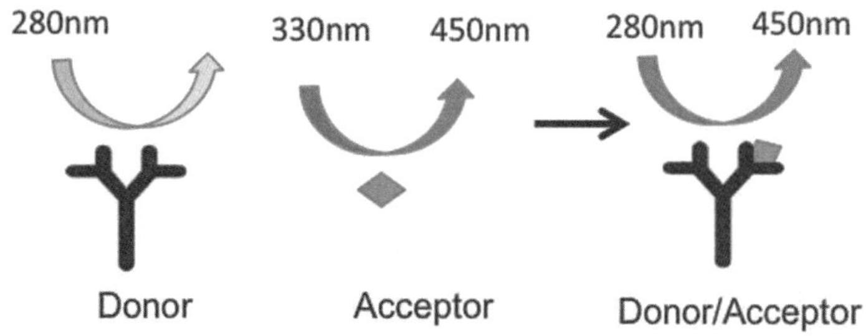

Figure 12.5 Schematic representation of fluorescent resonance energy transfer using antibodies. In this case, the antibody molecule is acting as a donor molecule and the analyte is acting as an acceptor molecule.

within close enough proximity (1–10 nm) energy is transferred between the two molecules [64].

FRET immunoassays can be used in competitive or sandwich immunoassay formats. The presence of tryptophan (Trp) in antibodies imparts intrinsic fluorescent properties, having excitation and emission wavelengths of 280–290 nm and 340 nm, respectively. Due to these inherent fluorescent properties, antibodies can be used in 'label-free' experiments.

A limitation attributed to FRET immunoassays is the occurrence of autofluorescence that may arise during the detection of larger molecules [62]. FRET is a cheaper alternative to FPIA in that it uses a simple fluorimeter for detection. FRET can also be used to readily detect small and large molecules [62].

12.7 Surface Plasmon Resonance Protocols

Surface plasmon resonance (SPR) is an optical signal transduction method that is used to measure biomolecular interactions. It identifies changes in mass that occur when two biomolecules interact at the interface between a solid-gold surface and liquid. Plane polarised light is directed onto the gold-surface/water interface at a specific angle to cause total internal reflection (TIR), an evanescent wave is produced that moves exponentially along the gold surface exciting **plasmons** (electron charged density waves). This reduces the reflected light being detected at the photo diode detector. When a biomolecular interaction occurs (i.e. antibody binds to its analyte) a change in mass occurs. This changes the refractive index between the liquid and the solid gold surface and thus changes the angle at which SPR occurs. This is measured by a photo diode detector and is displayed on a sensorgram in real-time.

A number of initial steps need to be taken to carry out a SPR immunoassay including pre-concentration and immobilisation of ligand on the sensor surface and optimising regeneration solutions. All of these steps require pre-planning. For instance, the method of immobilisation (e.g. amine, carboxyl or thiol coupling) must be carefully considered to ensure that the immobilised ligand maintains its activity and functionality.

Please refer to Chapter 11 of this book for a more detailed description of SPR. The proceeding sections in this chapter outline some useful protocols for developing SPR-based immunoassays.

Protocol 12.17
Pre-concentration of ligand onto sensor chip surface

Note 1: *The function of the pre-concentration step is to concentrate the protein on the dextran matrix to high levels (>100 mg mL^{-1}), thereby facilitating the coupling reaction* [51] *and reducing the amount of protein required. Preconcentration is an important step in SPR-based immunoassay development as it controls the immobilisation level of ligand onto the sensor chip. The immobilisation onto the sensor chip is largely based on the isoelectric point of the protein. The isoelectric point (pI) of a protein is the point where the protein or molecule has no net charge at a certain pH. In a buffer with a pH less than the pI of the protein, the net charge of the protein will be positive, while in a buffer with pH greater than the pI, the net charge of the protein will be negative. Therefore, it is important to use a buffer with a pH less than the pI of the protein to ensure immobilisation as the principle behind electrostatic pre-concentration exploits the tendency of the electropositive proteins to be attracted to the electronegatively charged carboxylated dextran matrix.*

Note 2: *A preconcentration study should first be carried out to determine the optimal pH of a protein to achieve an electropositive charge. A buffer at a range of various pHs should be tested.*

Reagents required:

- Immobilisation ligand (high concentration e.g. 25 μg mL^{-1}, the purity of ligand should be above 95%)
- 10 mM sodium acetate (with varying pHs e.g. 4, 4.5, 5, 5.5).
- Biacore chip (e.g. CM sensor chip)
- 20 mM NaOH

Experimental

(1) Immobilisation ligand is diluted in a buffer of low ionic strength (i.e. 10 mM sodium acetate), with a pH below the isoelectric point (pI) of the protein (typically 0.5–1 pH units below the pI of the protein). This will give the protein a net positive charge thus facilitating the electrostatic binding to the electro-negatively charged carboxyl groups on the chip surface.
(2) Pass this range of buffers over an underivatised chip surface and the degree of electrostatic binding should be monitored.
(3) The highest pH at which preconcentration occurs should be chosen, as it must be kept in mind that in the later stages the coupling occurs more readily at a higher pH, because activated carboxyl groups react better with uncharged amino groups.
(4) Prepare 25 μg mL^{-1} of immobilisation ligand (final volume 100 μL) in low ionic strength buffer (e.g. 10 mM sodium acetate) at varying pH increments (e.g. pH 4, 4.5, 5, 5.5).
(5) Inject each sample over flow-cell 2 of a preconditioned CM sensor chip for 30 seconds at a flow rate of 10 μL min^{-1}.
(6) Some ligands may have a tendency to non-specifically stick to the dextran surface, 20 mM of NaOH may be injected for 15 seconds after each preconcentration step if necessary.
(7) Determine the slope of preconcentration response and assess whether the required ligand density has been achieved.
(8) Choose the pH value that achieved the best ligand immobilisation for subsequent assays.

Protocol 12.18
Determining optimal regeneration conditions

Note 1: *Regeneration involves the removal of analyte at the sensor surface before the next round of SPR analysis is initiated. This must be achieved without damaging the bound ligand* [49, 65]. *Consideration of the regeneration solution to ensure compatibility with the running buffer must be undertaken to avoid the production of aggregates or salts (as these would block the equipment lines and give inaccurate results):*

Possible regeneration solutions/additives:

- High ionic strength buffers (1–2 M NaCl, 1–4 M $MgCl_2$)
- Ethylene glycol (up to 100%, v/v)
- SDS (low concentration 0.05%, w/v)
- 20–100 mM NaOH in 50% (v/v) acetonitrile

Experimental

(1) Prepare regeneration buffers.
(2) Inject/flow 60 μL of analyte over the previously immobilised ligand at 30 μL min^{-1}.
(3) Starting with the mildest buffer; inject 15 μL of the regeneration buffer at 30–50 μL min^{-1} over a short period of time (e.g. 1 min).
(4) Repeat steps 2 to 3 five times and then change to the next buffer.
(5) Monitor both the baseline and binding levels.

Protocol 12.19
Ligand coupling onto sensor surface

The method of coupling chosen for ligand immobilisation onto the sensor surface depends on the ligand to be immobilised. Amine coupling is the most frequently used as it employs the use of primary amines (of which there are many) on the protein surface. Thiol coupling can be considered when the orientation of a ligand is important or if the active site of the protein contains a reactive amine group. The number of thiol immobilisation points is generally limited, and this reduces the number of ligand orientations that can occur.

Protocol 12.19 (A)
Amine coupling of ligand onto the sensor surface

Note 1: *Amine coupling is one of the most commonly employed methods to covalently immobilise ligand onto a SPR-sensor surface. Carboxyl groups on the sensor surface are activated using an EDC/NHS (1-ethyl-3-(3-dimethylaminopropyl)-carbodiimide/N-hydroxysuccinimide) mixture and bind to primary amine groups present on the surface of the protein.*

Note 2: *This protocol has been modified from the* Biacore Surface Sensor Handbook [49].

Performing immobilisation on a Biacore chip surface:

- Duration should take less than 30 minutes.
- Use a flow rate 5 to 10 μL min^{-1}.
- Select a concentration of ligand from 1 to 100 μg mL^{-1}.
- The purity of any ligand chosen for use should be above 95%.

Reagents required:

- Ligand to be coupled; 120 μL of protein at 20–50 μg mL^{-1} in suitable pre-concentration buffer
- 1:1 mixture of EDC (0.4 M) in water and NHS (0.1 M) in water; 120 μL. Do not make up until just before proceeding with coupling
- Ethanolamine/HCl (1 M), pH 8.0, 120 μL
- Regeneration solution

Experimental

(1) Set the flow rate to 10 μL min^{-1}.

(2) Activation of carboxymethyl groups with a 1:1 mixture of EDC and NHS produces highly reactive succinimide esters which react with amines and other nucleophilic groups on proteins [51]. Activation time should take between 1 and 10 minutes. This can be varied depending on the immobilisation levels required. As a general rule, injection of EDC/NHS onto the sensor chip surface for 7 minutes at a flow rate of 10 μL min^{-1} should suffice.

(3) The ligand (diluted in preconcentration buffer at previously established pH) is injected into the instrument, and flows over the sensor surface at 10 μL min^{-1} for 7 minutes (70 μL used in total). This functions to concentrate the ligand on the matrix and helps to drive the coupling reactions.
(4) A blocking step is incorporated to block any remaining activated carboxymethylated groups, thereby reducing non-specific binding. This is achieved by injecting high concentrations of ethanolamine (1M) (flow rate 10 μL min^{-1}, 7 minutes).
(5) A regeneration step can now be carried out if desirable. Inject 30 μL regeneration solution using previously established regeneration buffer(s).
(6) The structural integrity of the bound ligand should be assessed. This can be carried out either by the addition of a specific antibody, or if binding analyte is available, testing the binding capabilities of the analyte for the ligand.
(7) View the sensorgram to confirm that the immobilisation is homogenous.

Protocol 12.19 (B)
Ligand thiol coupling on sensor chips

Note 1: *Ligand thiol coupling involves the introduction of disulphide groups onto the sensor chip surface (dextran matrix) first by activating with EDC/NHS followed by the addition of a disulphide group using 2-(2-pyridyldithio)ethylamine (PDEA). Coupling occurs via a thio-disulphide exchange.*

Note 2: *This protocol has been modified from the Biacore Surface Sensor Handbook* [49].

Reagents required:

- 1:1 mixture of EDC (0.4 M) in water and NHS (0.1 M) in water; total volume 100 μL. Do not make up until just before proceeding with coupling
- 80 mM PDEA in 0.1 M sodium borate, pH 8.5. It is recommended to use this solution within 1 hour of preparation
- 50 mM cysteine and 1 M NaCl in 0.1 M sodium acetate, pH 4.3
- Ligand at 10–50 μg mL^{-1} in immobilisation buffer
- 15 mg mL^{-1} PDEA in 0.1 M MES buffer

Experimental

(1) Activate the surface with EDC/NHS creating reactive succinimide esters on the sensor chip surface. Use a 1:1 mixture of EDC/NHS; 10 μL min^{-1} for 2 minutes contact time.
(2) Flow PDEA (which contains an active disulphide bond) over the sensor surface. This introduces reactive disulphide groups onto the surface of the sensor chip. Inject PDEA at 10 μL min^{-1} for 4 minutes.
(3) Inject ligand containing –SH (thiol) group (10 μL min^{-1} for 7 minutes).
(4) Deactivate the excess reactive groups by adding 50 mM cysteine, 1 M NaCl and 0.1 M sodium acetate (5 μL min^{-1} for 4 minutes).

Protocol 12.19 (C)
Surface thiol coupling onto dextran surface

Note 1: *Surface thiol coupling operates in the reverse to ligand-thiol coupling. Thiol groups are introduced onto the sensor surface (dextran matrix) and disulphide groups are introduced onto the ligand. Thiol groups are added to the surface, and disulphide groups are added to the ligand.*
Note 2: *This protocol was modified from* Biacore Surface Sensor Handbook [49].

Reagents required:

- 1:1 mixture of EDC (0.4 M) in water and NHS (0.1 M) in water; total volume 100 μL. Do not make up until just before proceeding with coupling
- 0.04 M cystamine dihydrochloride in 0.1 M sodium borate, pH 8.5
- 0.1 M dithioerythritol (DTE) in 0.1 M sodium borate, pH 8.5 (DTT may also be used)
- PDEA/NaCl: 20 mM PDEA and 1 M NaCl in 0.1 M sodium acetate, pH 4.3
- Immobilisation ligand at 10–50 μg mL^{-1} in immobilisation buffer
- 0.1 M morpholinoethanesulfonic acid (MES) buffer, pH 5.0

Experimental: modify the ligand with PDEA

(1) Prepare 0.5 mg of ligand in 0.5 mL 0.1 M MES buffer at 25°C.
(2) Add 250 μL of 15 mg mL^{-1} PDEA (which introduces reactive disulphide groups onto carboxyl residues on the ligand) in 0.1 M MES buffer (with a final concentration of mix of 22 mM).
(3) Add 25 μL of 0.4 M EDC (final concentration equals 13 nM).
(4) Mix and incubate for 10 minutes at 25°C; if this is thought to have a negative effect on the integrity of the ligand, carry out the procedure on ice for 1 hour.

Experimental: immobilisation procedure

(1) Set the flow rate to 10 μL min^{-1} for the addition of all reagents during this procedure.
(2) Activate the surface using EDC/NHS mixture for 2 minutes. Introduce disulphide groups onto the dextran surface using cystamine for 3 minutes.
(3) The disulphide bonds are then reduced to thiol groups using dithioerythritol (DTE) (0.1 M DTE in 0.1 M sodium borate, pH 8.5) for 3 minutes.
(4) Inject immobilisation ligand (10–50 μg mL^{-1}) for 7 minutes.
(5) Deactivate the remaining excess reactive groups using PDEA-NaCl (20 mM PDEA and 1 M NaCl in 0.1 M sodium acetate, pH 4.3) for 4 minutes.

12.8 Trouble Shooting

Some issues that may arise during immunoassay development are covered in the following section. An attempt has been made to identify possible causes and solutions are given that may resolve the problems encountered.

12.8.1 Binding of Protein to Surfaces

Pre-treatment of proteins in buffer at pH 2–3 can increase hydrophobicity. This works by altering the shape of the protein, thus exposing some hydrophobic residues. This will serve to increase the binding of the protein to the solid surface but may result in altered conformational structure and reduced binding affinity for the ligand [50].

12.8.2 ELISA Trouble Shooting

(1) *Presence of a high background signal.*

Possible cause

- Too high a concentration of detection antibody or substrate.

Solution

- Use a lower concentration of detection antibody or lower concentration of enzyme detection substrate.

Possible cause

- Insufficient washing of plate.

Solutions

- Increase the number of plate washes.
- Include some surfactants in wash buffer.
- Change or increase the concentration of blocking solution.
- After washing the plate, thoroughly blot the plate dry before proceeding to the next step of the ELISA.

(2) *Signal disappearing too rapidly.*

Possible cause

- May be due to too high a concentration of enzyme-conjugate using up all of the substrate.

Solutions

- Decrease the concentration of enzyme-conjugate.
- Dilute the antigen.

(3) *The immunoassay read-out signal is poor.*

Possible causes

- Insufficient concentration of analyte or antibody.
- Antibody has lost binding capacity.

- Lack of sufficient antigen (or antibody depending on assay format) immobilised on plate.
- Incorrect detection settings e.g. filters, gain.
- Emission/excitation wavelengths.

Solutions

- Increase the concentration of analyte and/or antibody.
- The detection antibody may need to be replaced.
- Check the detection settings on the assay reader.

12.9 Summary

This short compilation of immunoassay protocols, while not exhaustive, aims to provide a starting point for their development. Depending on the reagents available for the assay, i.e. the type, size and availability of analyte, the matrix, antibody format, etc. will impact on the type of assay that can be used. Each technique must be thoroughly research and optimised, and suitable controls included to achieve the best assay format feasible.

References

1. Ayyar, B.V., et al., Affinity chromatography as a tool for antibody purification. *Methods*, 2012. **56**(2):116–129.
2. Chiu, M.L., et al., Matrix effects—a challenge toward automation of molecular analysis. *JALA*, 2010. **15**(3):233–242.
3. Berthiller, F., et al., Masked mycotoxins: a review. *Mol Nutr Food Res*, 2013. **57**(1):165–186.
4. Tate, J., and G. Ward, Interferences in immunoassay. The clinical biochemist. *Clin Biochem Rev*, 2004. **25**(2):105–120.
5. Gagnon, P., *Purification Tools for Monoclonal Antibodies*. 1 ed. Validated Biosystems, Inc., 1996.
6. Chambers, E., et al., Systematic and comprehensive strategy for reducing matrix effects in LC/MS/MS analyses. *J Chromatogr B Analyt Technol Biomed Life Sci*, 2007. **852**(1–2):22–34.
7. Antibody purification handbook. 2015; Available from: http://www.gelifesciences.com/protein-purification.

8. Exalpha buffer formulations. 2015; Available from: http://www.exalpha.com/protocols/buffers.
9. Arora, S., B.V. Ayyar, and R. O'Kennedy, Affinity chromatography for antibody purification. *Methods Mol Biol*, 2014. **1129**:497–516.
10. Björk, L., and B. Åkerström, *Bacterial Immunoglobulin Binding Proteins*, ed. M.B.P. Boyle. Vol. 1. 1990: Academic Press, London.
11. Affinity Chromatography: Principles and Methods. 2015; Available from: http://www.gelifesciences.com.
12. Ma, H., and R.J. O'Kennedy, The purification of natural and recombinant peptide antibodies by affinity chromatographic strategies. *Peptide Antibodies: Methods and Protocols*, ed. H. Gunnar. Vol. 1. Estimated to be published September 2015: Wiley, Chichester.
13. Delves, P.J., *Antibody Production*. Essential Techniques Series, ed. D. Rickwood. Vol. 1. 1997, John Wiley & Sons, Chichester, Sussex.
14. Lefkovits, I., *Immunology Methods Manual: The Comprehensive Sourcebook of Techniques*. Vol. 1. 1997, Academic Press, Inc. London.
15. Vashist, S.K., et al., Effect of antibody immobilization strategies on the analytical performance of a surface plasmon resonance-based immunoassay. *Analyst*, 2011. **136**(21):4431–4436.
16. Thermo Scientific Pierce Protein Biology. 2015; Available from: http://www.piercenet.com.
17. Procedure for Conjugation of Alkaline Phosphatase to Antibodies and Other Proteins Conjugation 201505.08.2015; Available from: http://www.sigmaaldrich.com/life-science/metabolomics/enzyme-explorer/analytical-enzymes/alkaline-phosphatase/conjugation.html.
18. Harlow, E., and D. Lane, *Antibodies: A Laboratory Manual*. Vol. 1. 1988: Cold Spring Harbor Laboratory Press (Cold Spring Harbor, NY).
19. Javois, L.C., *Immunocytochemical Methods and Protocols*. Methods in Molecular Biology. Vol. 115. 1999, Humana Press Inc.
20. Michalet, X., et al., Quantum dots for live cells, in vivo imaging, and diagnostics. *Science*, 2005. **307**(5709):538–544.
21. Medintz, I.L., et al., Quantum dot bioconjugates for imaging, labelling and sensing. *Nat Mater*, 2005. **4**(6):435–446.
22. Xing, Y., et al., Bioconjugated quantum dots for multiplexed and quantitative immunohistochemistry. *Nat Protoc*, 2007. **2**(5):1152–1165.
23. Goldman, E.R., I.L. Medintz, and H. Mattoussi, Luminescent quantum dots in immunoassays. *Anal Bioanal Chem*, 2006. **384**(3):560–563.

24. Avidin-Biotin Technical Handbook. 2009; Available from: http://www.isibang.ac.in/~library/onlinerz/resources/technicalhandbook.pdf.

25. Tully, E., S.P. Higson, and R. O'Kennedy, The development of a 'labeless' immunosensor for the detection of *Listeria monocytogenes* cell surface protein, Internalin B. *Biosens Bioelectron*, 2008. **23**(6):906–912.

26. Bondos, S.E., and A. Bicknell, Detection and prevention of protein aggregation before, during, and after purification. *Anal Biochem*, 2003. **316**(2):223–231.

27. Fink, A.L., Partially-folded intermediates and protein aggregation. *Federation of American Societies for Experimental Biology Journal*, 1997. **11**(9):A871.

28. Fink, A.L., Protein aggregation: folding aggregates, inclusion bodies and amyloid. *Fold Des*, 1998. **3**(1):R9–R23.

29. Kreilgaard, L., et al., Effect of Tween 20 on freeze-thawing- and agitation-induced aggregation of recombinant human factor XIII. *J Pharm Sci*, 1998. **87**(12):1597–1603.

30. Chaudhuri, J.B., B. Batas, and A.D. Guise, Improving protein refolding yields by minimizing aggregation. *Ann NY Acad Sci*, 1996. **782**:495–505.

31. Hamada, H., T. Arakawa, and K. Shiraki, Effect of additives on protein aggregation. *Curr Pharm Biotechnol*, 2009. **10**(4):400–407.

32. Arakawa, T., et al., Suppression of protein interactions by arginine: a proposed mechanism of the arginine effects. *Biophys Chem*, 2007. **127**(1–2):1–8.

33. Neagu, A., M. Neagu, and A. Der, Fluctuations and the Hofmeister effect. *Biophys J*, 2001. **81**(3):1285–1294.

34. Urh, M., K. Simpson, and K. Zhao, Affinity chromatography: general methods, in *Methods in Enzymology*, 2009, Elsevier. pp. 417–38.

35. Samuel, D., et al., Proline inhibits aggregation during protein refolding. *Protein Sci*, 2000. **9**(8):1604.

36. Tsumoto, K., et al., Practical considerations in refolding proteins from inclusion bodies. *Protein Expr Purif*, 2003. **28**(1):1–8.

37. Yancey, P.H., Organic osmolytes as compatible, metabolic and counter-acting cytoprotectants in high osmolarity and other stresses. *J Exp Biol*, 2005. **208**(15):2819–2830.

38. Street, T.O., D.W. Bolen, and G.D. Rose, A molecular mechanism for osmolyte-induced protein stability. *Proc Acad Natl Sci USA*, 2006. **103**(38):13997–14002.

39. Kerwin, B.A., et al., Effects of Tween 80 and sucrose on acute short-term stability and long-term storage at -20 degrees C of a recombinant hemoglobin. *J Pharm Sci*, 1998. **87**(9):1062–1068.
40. Arakawa, T., and Y. Kita, Protection of bovine serum albumin from aggregation by Tween 80. *J Pharm Sci*, 2000. **89**(5):646–651.
41. Timasheff, S.N., Control of protein stability and reactions by weakly interacting cosolvents: the simplicity of the complicated. *Adv Protein Chem*, 1998. **51**:355–432.
42. Yin, Y., et al., Colorimetric immunoassay for detection of tumor markers. *Int J Mol Sci*, 2010. **11**(12):5077–5094.
43. Technical guide for ELISA. Available from: http://www.kpl.com.
44. Bio-rad. Buffer formulations. 2015; Available from: http://www.bio-rad.com/webroot/web/pdf/lsr/literature/Bulletin_6199.pdf.
45. Abcam. General procedure and tips for direct ELISA. 2015; Available from: http://www.abcam.com/index.html?pageconfig=resource&rid=11388.
46. Vogt, R.F., et al., Quantitative differences among various proteins as blocking-agents for ELISA microtiter plates. *J Immunol Methods*, 1987. **101**(1):43–50.
47. Jason-Moller, L., M. Murphy, and J. Bruno, Overview of Biacore systems and their applications. *Curr Protoc Protein Sci*, 2006: John Wiley & Sons, Inc.
48. Rusmini, F., Z. Zhong, and J. Feijen, Protein immobilization strategies for protein biochips. *Biomacromolecules*, 2007. **8**(6):1775–1789.
49. *Biacore Sensor Surface Handbook (web)* G. Healthcare, ed., GE Healthcare. pp. 1–100.
50. Wild, D., ed. *The Immunoassay Handbook*. Vol. 3. 2005, Elsevier.
51. van der Merwe, P.A., ed. Surface plasmon resonance. In *Protein-Ligand Interactions: Hydrodynamics and Calorimetry*. Practical Approach Series, 2001, eds. S.E. Harding, and B.Z. Chowdhry. New York: Oxford University Press.
52. Catt, K., and G.W. Tregear, Solid-phase radioimmunoassay in antibody-coated tubes. *Science*, 1967. **158**(3808):1570–1572.
53. Butler, J.E., Solid supports in enzyme-linked immunosorbent assay and other solid-phase immunoassays. *Methods*, 2000. **22**(1):4–23.
54. Brand, L., and M.L. Johnson, eds. Fluorescence spectroscopy. *Methods in Enzymology*. Vol. 480. 2008, Academic Press.

55. Albani, J.R., ed. *Principles and Applications of Fluorescence Spectroscopy.* 2007, Wiley-Blackwell.

56. Lopez-Gallego, F., J.M. Guisan, and L. Betancor, Glutaraldehyde-mediated protein immobilization. *Methods Mol Biol*, 2013. **1051**:33–41.

57. Maple, P.A.C., C.S. Jones, and N.J. Andrews, Time resolved fluorometric immunoassay, using Europium labelled anti-human IgG, for the detection of human tetanus antitoxin in serum. *J Clin Pathol*, 2001. **54**(10):812–815.

58. Maple, P.A., et al., Performance of a time-resolved fluorescence immunoassay for measuring Varicella-zoster virus immunoglobulin G levels in adults and comparison with commercial enzyme immunoassays and Merck glycoprotein enzyme immunoassay. *Clin Vaccine Immunol*, 2006. **13**(2):214–218.

59. Diamandis, E.P., Immunoassays with time-resolved fluorescence spectroscopy: principles and applications. *Clin Biochem*, 1988. **21**(3):139–150.

60. Perrin, F., Polarization of light of fluorescence, average life of molecules in the excited state. *Journal de Physique et le Radium*, 1926. **7**:390–401.

61. Rossi, A.M., and C.W. Taylor, Analysis of protein-ligand interactions by fluorescence polarization. *Nat Protoc*, 2011. **6**(3):365–387.

62. Ueda, H., and J. Dong, From fluorescence polarization to Quenchbody: Recent progress in fluorescent reagentless biosensors based on antibody and other binding proteins. *Biochim Biophys Acta*, 2014. **1844**(11):1951–1959.

63. Nielsen, K., et al., Fluorescence polarization immunoassay: detection of antibody to *Brucella abortus*. *Methods*, 2000. **22**(1):71–76.

64. Gordon, G.W., et al., Quantitative fluorescence resonance energy transfer measurements using fluorescence microscopy. *Biophys J*, 1998. **74**(5):2702–2713.

65. Andersson, K., M. Hamalainen, and M. Malmqvist, Identification and optimization of regeneration conditions for affinity-based biosensor assays. A multivariate cocktail approach. *Anal Chem*, 1999. **71**(13):2475–2481.

Index

absorbance 223, 273, 282, 369, 390, 399, 400, 402, 404
ACS *see* acute coronary syndrome
acute coronary syndrome (ACS) 166, 276, 351
acute myocardial infarction (AMI) 147, 165, 351
adsorption 67, 68, 396
affinity chromatography 46, 60, 364, 367, 369, 370, 380
affinity maturation 46, 259
AFP *see* alpha-fetoprotein
agarose 366, 370, 371
aliquots 97, 110, 111, 366, 371–373
alpha-fetoprotein (AFP) 25, 163, 179, 311
AMI *see* acute myocardial infarction
amino acids 45, 52, 67, 79, 145, 265, 383, 384
amnesic shellfish poisoning (ASP) 235, 236, 238
ASP *see* amnesic shellfish poisoning
assay 78, 89–92, 95–100, 107–113, 131–136, 209–211, 230–234, 238, 239, 241, 242, 280, 296, 297, 316, 317, 351, 352, 386, 387, 390, 391
  automated 112
  bead-based 280
  biobarcode 268, 269
  biochemical 317
  biosensor-based 140
  chemiluminescence-based 225
  chemiluminometric 173, 174
  competition 228
  cytometry-based 178
  dip-stick 199
  fluorescence-based 396, 405
  heterogeneous 128, 297
  homogenous 408
  immunodiagnostic 150
  microfluidic 149
  nanoparticle-based 143
  protease 280
assay sensitivity 77, 106, 108, 128, 130, 131, 133–136, 142, 149, 207, 269
assay step 23, 28, 97, 209, 361
assay time 23, 201, 211, 230, 231
azaspiracid 235, 236

Bacillus anthracis 138, 195, 200, 203
bacteria 6, 9, 24, 26, 45, 168, 170, 193, 205, 222, 226, 262, 264, 329
  gram-negative 262
  gram-positive 262
bacterial cell 38, 39, 127, 134, 136–138, 140, 261
bacterial pathogen 136, 137, 150, 222, 227
BAW *see* bulk acoustic wave

bead 128, 134, 142, 280, 367
acceptor 281
chitin-coated 77
polystyrene latex 15
bias 45, 47, 98, 99, 101, 103
binding 7–9, 12, 13, 26, 27, 73, 75, 259, 261, 293–295, 299, 328, 330, 335, 336, 338, 343, 344, 395, 396
antigen–antibody 266
bio-affinity 396
biomolecular 336
cleft 51
electrostatic 413
hapten 50, 51
methotrexate 50
streptavidin 340
bioluminescence 15, 18–20
biomarkers 147, 148, 161, 162, 209, 225, 232, 278
human 43
prognostic 180
biosensors 53, 60, 93, 134, 225, 227, 234, 279, 295, 306, 330, 342
biotin 133, 303, 305, 347, 379–381, 386, 387, 396
biotinylated antibodies 131, 227, 281, 299, 379–381
blood 91, 96, 100, 109, 118, 145, 147, 162, 165, 167, 180, 277–281, 315, 316, 400, 402
BNP *see* brain natriuretic peptide
bovine serum albumin (BSA) 38, 298, 299, 308, 309, 342, 372, 373, 385, 387, 403
brain natriuretic peptide (BNP) 76, 166, 334
BSA *see* bovine serum albumin
buffers 71, 75, 93, 96, 97, 100, 366, 369, 371, 375, 385, 386, 388, 391, 406, 407, 412, 413, 417, 418
inorganic 18
neutralisation 370, 371
physiological 336
sodium carbonate 375
bulk acoustic wave (BAW) 25

calibration model 92, 97, 98
camelids 50, 52, 77
cancer 148, 174, 179–183, 310, 316
breast 181–183
colorectal 182
hepatocellular 181
medullary thyroid 182
pancreatic 181
uterus 183
carcinoembryonic antigen (CEA) 181, 182, 304, 306, 311, 334
cardiac markers 165, 276, 279, 334
cardiovascular disease 117, 145, 165, 167, 278
causative agent 132, 133, 135, 137, 142, 191, 192, 195, 198, 205, 232
CBD *see* chitin-binding domain
CDR *see* complementarity determining region
CEA *see* carcinoembryonic antigen
cells 37, 133–137, 223, 313, 329, 338, 340, 363
immune 271
insect 262
insulin-secreting beta 173
mouse myeloma 256
multi-flow 297
tumour 148
centrifugation 364, 366, 370, 371, 382
CFP *see* ciguatera fish poisoning
CFU *see* colony-forming unit
chemical vapour deposition (CVD) 71, 117, 121, 145, 148, 305, 309, 343

chemiluminescence 14, 15, 18, 19, 256
CHF *see* congestive heart failure
chip 124, 129, 138, 295, 337, 340
  allyl-mercaptane-modified 341
  carboxymethyl-coated 340
  commercial 311
  film-based SPR 342
  matrix-free 340
  microarray 63
  waveguide-coupled SPR 333
chitin-binding domain (CBD) 77
ciguatera fish poisoning (CFP) 235
circulating tumour cell (CTC) 148, 149
CK *see* creatine kinase
clones 4, 41, 47, 263, 346
  antibody-producing 4
  antigen-binding 47
  B-cell 2
  high-affinity 47
colony-forming unit (CFU) 134, 136, 223, 226
complementarity determining region (CDR) 43, 45, 62, 129
congestive heart failure (CHF) 147, 276
conjugates 63, 79, 95, 234, 292, 397
  antibody-drug 79
  antibody-enzyme 270
  chimeric 269
  hapten–carrier 95
conjugation 53, 60, 76, 78, 79, 142, 207, 351, 363, 374, 380
  chemical 52
  fluorescein 376
contaminants 109, 221–223, 225, 227, 235, 239, 242, 243, 397
  bacterial 316
  environmental 221
  haptenic 51
cortisol 19, 20, 163, 174, 175
coupling 61, 78, 333, 335, 347, 374, 377, 393, 413–417
  amine–carboxylic acid 378
  carboxyl–amine 377
  covalent 347, 376
  glutaraldehyde 142, 143
  ligand-thiol 417
C-reactive protein (CRP) 145–148, 352
creatine kinase (CK) 147, 148, 165, 166, 179
CRP *see* C-reactive protein
CTC *see* circulating tumour cell
Cushing's disease 174, 175
Cushing's syndrome 174, 175
CVD *see* chemical vapour deposition

deep vein thrombosis 276
detection 21, 130–136, 138, 142, 144–148, 178, 179, 182, 183, 206, 209–211, 222, 223, 225–232, 238, 239, 266–268, 271–273, 295, 296
  bacterial 135
  biological 25
  bioterrorism 193
  cardiac marker 148
  chemiluminescent 144
  immunologically-based 293
  immunomagnetic 133
  laser-based 138
  malarial 200
  multiplex 127, 140, 226–228, 231, 241, 242
  oligonucleotide 27
  on-site 142, 241
  on-slide 225
  optical 119, 128, 266, 314
  optical fibre-based 128
  protein 59
  ultrasensitive 268

detection antibody 9–12, 140, 268, 270, 386, 388, 397–399, 401, 403, 419, 420
  enzyme-conjugated 390
  enzyme-labelled 398, 400, 402, 404
  enzyme-linked 12
  fluorescent 126
  goat anti-biotin 133
detection mechanism 23, 134, 143
detection methods 134, 266, 267, 269, 271, 273, 284, 350
detection systems 14, 18, 26, 28, 95, 255, 273, 387
detergent 349, 386–388, 391
devices 25, 119, 125, 127, 128, 132, 196–198, 209, 210, 212, 257, 275, 277, 278, 315–318, 351
  flow-injection 310
  fourth-generation 197
  immune-diagnostic 81
  integrated multiplexed 212
  lab-on-a-chip 122, 277
  live-saving 212
  microfluidic-based single-use 277
  miniaturised 183, 242
  multi-fluorescent 280
  non-instrumented 212
  potentiometric 300
dextran matrix 337, 340, 343, 348, 412, 416, 417
DFA *see* direct fluorescent antibody
diabetes mellitus (DM) 167, 173, 178, 179
diagnosis 22, 162–166, 169–173, 176–178, 180, 193, 197–200, 206, 212, 232, 259, 275–277
diarrheic shellfish poisoning (DSP) 141, 235, 236, 238
direct fluorescent antibody (DFA) 169
disease 90, 109, 161, 164, 169, 174, 177–180, 182, 191, 193, 195, 198, 209, 232, 233, 272, 273
  animal 232
  autoimmune 173
  cerebrovascular 167
  chronic inflammatory multisystem 176
  chronic kidney 280
  chronic skeletal muscle 166
  diagnosing cardiac 166
  foot-and-mouth 233
  interstitial lung 179
  lysosomal storage 280
  paraneoplastic 182
  rheumatological 177
  thyroid 173, 174
  urinary tract 162
  vaccine-preventable 193
disease markers 24, 145, 147, 164, 183
display technology 208, 259, 260, 282
  eukaryotic 262
  in vitro 263
  phage 6, 7, 261
  recombinant antibody 259
display
  bacterial 259, 262
  cell 260
  in vitro 260, 261
  mRNA 259, 263, 264
  phage 42, 49, 96, 259, 260, 262, 282
  ribosome 259, 263, 264
  yeast 80, 259, 262
DM *see* diabetes mellitus
drugs 2, 9, 12, 38, 108, 109, 162, 175, 229, 259, 334, 350, 363, 402
  antiprotozoal 230
  biological 258
  growth-enhancing 231
  performance-enhancing 162

DSP *see* diarrheic shellfish poisoning

EIS *see* electrochemical impedance spectroscopy
electrochemical immunoassays 267, 292–297, 299, 314–317
electrochemical impedance spectroscopy (EIS) 24, 139, 203, 204
electrode 25, 136, 137, 279, 295–297, 299, 301, 304, 307, 310, 314
  carbon paste 302, 306
  glassy carbon 143, 302, 305
  gold nanoparticle 303
  indium tin oxide 305
  microarray 308
  polyaniline 308
  pyrolytic graphite 305
  screen-printed graphite 303
  sol-gel-coated 302
electro-osmotic flow (EOF) 119, 121
ELISA *see* enzyme-linked immunosorbent assay
enzyme 9, 10, 14, 18, 19, 147, 256, 292, 295, 296, 298, 305, 313, 329, 374, 397, 402, 405
  isothermal 272
  liver 179
  non-proofreading 264
  peroxidase 14
enzyme immunoassay 169, 197
enzyme-linked immunosorbent assay (ELISA) 8, 176, 178, 211, 212, 222, 234, 238, 239, 270, 292–294, 296, 362, 363, 387, 388, 395, 399–402, 404–406
enzyme substrate 11, 386, 398, 399, 401–403
EOF *see* electro-osmotic flow
epitopes 2, 8, 11, 12, 38, 73–75, 133, 206, 230, 281, 293, 301, 352, 397, 402
evanescent wave 328, 330–332, 411

FACS *see* fluorescence activated cell sorting
fast protein liquid chromatography (FPLC) 368
FFD *see* fluid-force discrimination
FLISA *see* fluorescence-linked immunosorbent sandwich assay
fluid-force discrimination (FFD) 128
fluorescence 15, 18–21, 28, 74, 78, 211, 223–225, 273, 274, 282, 311, 399, 400, 402, 404, 408, 410
  supercritical angle 74, 149, 273
  time-resolved 211, 362, 406, 407
  total internal 273
  total internal reflection 74, 328
fluorescence activated cell sorting (FACS) 78, 262, 263
fluorescence-linked immunosorbent sandwich assay (FLISA) 16, 203, 223, 224, 362, 405
fluorescence polarisation immunoassay (FPIA) 7, 362, 408–411
fluorescence resonance energy transfer (FRET) 22, 362, 409–411
fluorescence signal 21, 272
fluorimeter 329, 399, 400, 402, 404, 408, 411
fluorophore 9, 12, 20, 21, 256, 267, 271–274, 375, 406
Fourier transform 23, 68

FPIA *see* fluorescence polarisation immunoassay
FPLC *see* fast protein liquid chromatography
FRET *see* fluorescence resonance energy transfer
fungal toxins 140, 142, 144
fungi 193, 205, 262

GFP *see* green fluorescence protein
glycol 67, 394
  ethylene 70, 372, 386, 414
  polyethylene 4, 67, 70, 74, 363
gold colloid 207, 210, 211
gold electrode 299, 306
gold film 294, 331, 340
gold nanoparticle 23, 74, 133, 210, 211, 268, 269, 280, 301–303, 306, 351
  antibody-coated 225
  citrate-modified 302
  colloidal 15
  dextran-capped 341
GOS *see* graphene oxide sheet
graphene oxide sheet (GOS) 342
green fluorescence protein (GFP) 20

HAMA *see* human anti-mouse antibody
haptens 37, 38, 96, 338
haptoglobin 232
HBV *see* hepatitis B virus
HCR *see* hybridisation chain reaction
HCV *see* hepatitis C virus
hepatitis B virus (HBV) 11, 195, 211
hepatitis C virus (HCV) 11, 195
high-performance liquid chromatography (HPLC) 175, 230, 238, 350, 363
HIV *see* human immunodeficiency virus
horse radish peroxidase (HRP) 14–16, 23, 133, 136, 143, 297, 313, 374
HPLC *see* high-performance liquid chromatography
HRP *see* horse radish peroxidase
human anti-mouse antibody (HAMA) 93, 209
human immunodeficiency virus (HIV) 10, 11, 48, 193, 195, 197, 199, 203, 210, 276
hybridisation chain reaction (HCR) 271, 272
hybridoma technology 4, 39, 258–260, 282
hydrophilicity 64, 69, 121, 122, 131
hydrophobicity 44, 65–67, 120, 418

IDL *see* intermediate density lipoprotein
IEC *see* ion-exchange chromatography
immobilisation 21, 52, 59–61, 63, 72, 73, 77, 80, 130, 300, 343, 347, 350, 406, 412, 416
  covalent 306, 347, 348, 392
  direct DNA 74
  high-density 66
  ligand 413
immune repertoire 39, 41, 44, 49, 80
immune response 3, 38, 44, 258, 259
immune system 2, 3, 38, 40, 43, 197, 198
immunoassays 1, 2, 6–8, 14, 16–24, 89–92, 117–119, 161–168, 178–183, 212, 221–223, 228–234, 255, 256, 314–317, 361–364, 394–410

apolipoprotein 167
automated 256
commercial 167, 230
direct antibody 9
fluorescent polarisation 362
impedance-based 68
lab-on-a-chip 119, 120, 133, 134, 144, 147, 149, 162
lateral flow 23, 196, 223, 226, 227, 238, 241, 362
microfluidics-based 128
multiplexed 280
nanoparticle-based 25
reverse-indirect 10
salivary cortisol 163
sandwich-type 303
urine 162
immunoassay sensitivity 63, 125, 226, 283
immunoassay system 60, 279, 315, 316
immunoglobulin 1–3, 49, 364, 366, 367, 395
immunosensor 142, 204, 238, 239, 293, 295, 296, 299–304, 306, 309, 310, 350
incubation 125, 226, 312
infection 133, 168–171, 193, 197, 200–202, 205, 206, 273
anthrax 210
drug-resistant 198
malarial 199, 200, 207
parasitic 200
sexually transmitted 193, 195
sporadic 201
upper respiratory tract 169
viral 49
infectious disease 191–193, 195–197, 199, 201, 202, 209, 212, 213, 232, 258, 276, 281
inflammation 145, 176, 181, 232, 278, 352
influenza 170, 171, 195, 201, 204, 276, 281
insulin 14, 173, 334
interaction 60, 61, 72, 78, 98, 128, 140, 207, 292, 294, 341, 344–346, 383, 388, 392, 395
analyte–ligand 344
antibody–antigen 118, 267, 277, 295, 344, 384
bacterial-receptor 367
biological 294
bio-molecular 328, 330
electrostatic 62
hydrophobic 65, 72, 383, 386, 396
intramolecular 383
molecular 332, 333, 345
non-covalent 379
protein-protein 330, 387
intermediate density lipoprotein (IDL) 167
ion-exchange chromatography (IEC) 364, 366, 369

keyhole limpet hemocyanin (KLH) 38
KLH *see* keyhole limpet hemocyanin

label-free immunosensor 299, 300
LAMP *see* loop-mediated isothermal amplification
lateral-flow assays 231, 293, 296, 315, 316
LBA *see* ligand binding assay
ligand binding assay (LBA) 97, 98, 102
light chains 2, 5, 40, 48, 62, 266, 367
universal 43

limit of detection (LOD) 97, 104, 106–108, 211, 226, 230, 233, 234, 238, 239, 299, 306, 351
lipoproteins 167, 168
Listeria monocytogenes 137, 195, 222, 299
liver 145, 171, 179, 200, 232, 387
LLOQ *see* lower limit of quantification
localised surface plasmon resonance (LSPR) 268, 334
LOD *see* limit of detection
loop-mediated isothermal amplification (LAMP) 272, 273
lower limit of quantification (LLOQ) 97, 100, 101, 103, 104, 108, 111
LSPR *see* localised surface plasmon resonance

macromolecule 38, 102, 387
malaria 176, 193, 199, 200, 203, 207
marine toxins 141, 235, 238, 241
markers 145, 147, 148, 165, 176, 177, 179, 181, 269, 270, 292, 293
  diagnostic 182, 183
  fluorescent 374
  inflammation-related 232
  stroke 316
  tumour cell surface 38
maximum residue limits (MRL) 229, 230, 243, 264
microarrays 63, 74, 130, 307–309, 311
  fabricated 309
  fluorescence-based 77
  multiplex 241
microbes 222, 243
micro-cantilevers 26, 27
microchannels 120, 125, 126, 128, 136, 140, 142
microcystins 239, 240, 242, 316
microelectrodes 136, 307, 311–313, 315
microfluidic channels 119, 126, 127, 136, 137, 142
microfluidic chips 144, 241
microfluidic devices 26, 125–127, 133, 137, 149, 268
  eight-channel 140
  non-instrumented 209
microfluidic immunoassays 133, 137, 140, 142, 145
microfluidic systems 136, 148, 209, 276, 328
microtitre plates 11, 63–65, 125, 293, 297, 386, 389, 397, 398, 407
monoclonal antibodies 4, 39, 96, 142, 205, 228, 239, 256, 258, 260, 309, 364, 368
  enzyme-conjugated anti-OA 235
  fluorescent liposome-labelled 241
  hybridoma-derived 38
MRL *see* maximum residue limits
myocardial infarction 147, 165, 351
myoglobin 26, 146, 148, 165, 166

neuron specific enolase (NSE) 309, 314
neurotoxic shellfish poisoning (NSP) 235, 238
non-specific binding (NSB) 6, 7, 10, 12, 13, 28, 131, 293, 305, 328, 336, 340, 343, 384, 386, 390, 391, 397
NSB *see* non-specific binding
NSE *see* neuron specific enolase

NSP *see* neurotoxic shellfish poisoning
nucleic acid amplification method 269, 271, 272

OA *see* okadaic acid
okadaic acid (OA) 141, 235, 236, 238, 242
oxidation 61, 71, 143, 211, 313, 350

paralytic shellfish poisoning (PSP) 235, 237, 238
parasitic disease 191, 192, 195, 205, 207
pathogens 132, 134, 136–138, 140, 147, 150, 222, 223, 225–227, 269, 316
  enteric 281
  foodborne 222, 225
  fungal 117, 132, 142, 144
  life-threatening human 137
  suspected 132
  viral 140
patients 43, 49, 108, 164, 167, 169, 172–180, 182, 191, 201, 258, 259, 269, 273, 275, 276, 279
  chronic care 280
  diseased 112
  immunocompromised 169
  selected 181
PCR *see* polymerase chain reaction
PE *see* pulmonary embolism
peptide 38, 337, 338, 383
photolithography 123, 145, 307
phycotoxins 140–142, 235
plasma 67, 91, 162, 232, 234, 278, 391
platforms 96, 138, 140, 143, 144, 148, 202–204, 209, 212, 266, 267, 269, 271, 273, 276, 282, 300
  automated detection 24
  battery-operated diagnostics 280
  diagnostic 197
  four-channel SPR sensor 241
  immunoanalysis 118
  lab-on-a-chip 118, 130, 136
  microfluidic-based 148
  miniaturised 130, 135, 138
  multicomponent 138
  multiplex 60
poisoning 235–237
  amnesic shellfish 235
  diarrhetic shellfish 235
  neurotoxic shellfish 235
  paralytic shellfish 235
polarised light 329, 331, 332, 408, 409, 411
polyclonal antibody 3, 39, 75, 208, 210, 229, 230, 234, 380
polyelectrolyte 62, 69, 70
polymerase chain reaction (PCR) 46, 170, 200, 222, 227, 264, 266, 269, 270
polymers 62, 64, 72, 119, 120, 122, 299, 334
  amino acid 70
  conductive 295, 304
  conjugate 78
  cycloolefin 68
  insulating 307
  non-toxic 120
polymyositis 166, 178
PPI *see* protein phosphatase inhibition
prostate specific antigen (PSA) 23, 24, 180, 269, 281, 305, 306, 309, 334
protease inhibitor 372, 373
protein blocker 387, 388
protein immobilisation 71, 391

protein phosphatase inhibition (PPI) 241
proteins 3, 59–61, 68, 77–80, 95, 337, 338, 342, 343, 347, 348, 363, 364, 367, 368, 382–387, 390–392, 395, 396, 412–415, 418
  antibody-binding 367
  avidin-conjugated carrier 396
  capsid 261
  contaminating 375
  cysteine-rich 131
  cytoplasmic 179
  electropositive 348, 412
  endogenous 9
  human 3
  hybrid 262
  immunoglobulin 2
  mammalian 39
  stroke marker 314
  total serum 3
  transmembrane 337
protocol 97, 112, 361, 363, 364, 367–370, 374, 375, 377, 378, 380, 381, 388, 396–399, 401, 402, 406, 407, 409, 410, 412, 414–417
  bioassay 279
  radioimmunoassay 292
PSA *see* prostate specific antigen
PSP *see* paralytic shellfish poisoning
pulmonary embolism (PE) 70, 147, 172
purification 3, 46, 263, 282, 364–371, 373, 375, 377, 379, 381
  high-resolution 366, 368

QCM *see* quartz crystal microbalances
QD *see* quantum dot
quantum dot (QD) 15, 21, 22, 75, 76, 147, 210, 225, 267, 296, 330, 374, 376–379
quartz crystal microbalances (QCM) 25, 74, 203, 204, 239

RA *see* rheumatoid arthritis
radioimmunoassay 172, 174, 175, 256, 293
radiolabels 12, 14, 256
rapid diagnostic tests (RDT) 200, 205, 206, 209, 212
RDT *see* rapid diagnostic tests
reaction 18, 19, 292, 294, 313, 379, 381, 393, 394, 399, 400, 402, 404
  allergic 229
  biological 19
  biotinylation 381
  chemiluminescent 19
  hypersensitivity 170
  immunological 297
  intermolecular 331
  silver enhancement 25
reagent 69, 71, 95, 97, 208, 209, 211, 351, 369, 370, 374, 375, 377, 378, 380, 381, 393, 394, 398, 399, 405–407, 415–418
  analytical 117, 122, 126
  biotinylation 380
  kosmotropic 384
  polyclonal 208
recombinant antibodies 2, 5, 6, 53, 59, 73, 76, 80, 199, 208, 259, 262, 265, 341, 361, 368
refractive index (RI) 27, 140, 223, 328, 329, 331–333, 335, 336, 350, 412
response 42, 44, 49, 90, 101, 104, 176, 202, 307, 315, 317, 335
  acute-phase 147
  allergic 171

antibody 3
humoral 39
immunological 232
inflammatory 176
response units (RU) 42, 335, 336
rheumatoid arthritis (RA) 48, 175, 176, 178
RI *see* refractive index
RU *see* response units

SAF *see* supercritical angle fluorescence
saliva 145, 162, 163, 174, 280, 363
SAMs *see* self-assembling monolayers
scanning electron microscopy (SEM) 23, 229, 230, 307
SCLC *see* small cell lung cancer
screen-printed carbon electrode (SPCE) 142, 143, 225, 230, 298
SDA *see* strand displacement amplification
SEB *see* Staphylococcus enterotoxin B
self-assembling monolayers (SAMs) 61, 62, 74, 340, 341
SEM *see* scanning electron microscopy
sensing layer 149, 330, 350
sensor chip 329, 332, 336, 337, 340, 348, 351, 412, 413, 416, 417
sensors 24, 296, 299–302, 305, 306, 309, 310, 328, 329
acoustic 25
acoustic wave 26
Au-film-based 342
cantilever-based 27
fibre-optic 334, 335
glucose 308
label-free capacitative 300
label-free impedimetric 300
sandwich-based SPR 342
screen-printed 305
single-shot 295
surface acoustic waves 26
serum 3, 38, 52, 91, 96, 162, 163, 165, 167, 173–175, 180, 181, 232, 292, 363, 364, 370, 400
animal 387
horse 387
human 210, 302
sexually transmitted infection (STI) 193, 195
signal 2, 9–14, 26, 98, 106, 227, 228, 267, 269–271, 283, 295, 307, 311, 384, 390, 399–405
bridging 351
fluorescent 11, 21, 210, 271, 405
lab-on-a-chip platforms 150
oscillating 26
signal amplification 138, 225, 269–271, 277
signal detection 144, 273, 277, 380, 397
signal generation 14, 15, 17, 19, 21, 257, 266, 397, 399, 400, 402, 404
Sjögren's syndrome (SS) 176–178
skeletal muscle 147, 166, 178
SLE *see* systemic lupus erythymatosus
small cell lung cancer (SCLC) 182, 183
SOP *see* standard operating procedure
SPCE *see* screen-printed carbon electrode
species 3, 80, 206, 231, 301, 313, 347, 370, 400, 404
electroactive 313
legionella 169
redox-active 298
SPR *see* surface plasmon resonance

SPRI *see* surface plasmon resonance imaging
SS *see* Sjögren's syndrome
standard operating procedure (SOP) 97, 113
Staphylococcus enterotoxin B (SEB) 131, 138, 139, 228
STI *see* sexually transmitted infection
Stokes shift 20, 22, 225, 406
strain 133–135, 168, 227, 239, 265
  antibiotic-resistant 229
  bacterial mutator 265
  infective bacterial 168
strand displacement amplification (SDA) 269
substrate 10, 12–14, 18, 21, 119, 121, 124, 126, 127, 292, 295, 297, 299, 304, 306, 307, 419
  analytical 149
  chromogenic 14
  electroactive 295
  enzyme detection 419
  fluorescent 21, 405
  photoresist-covered 122
  platinum 309
  polymer 66
supercritical angle fluorescence (SAF) 74, 149, 273, 274
surface plasmon resonance (SPR) 41, 74, 148, 231, 268, 294–296, 327, 330–336, 340, 350, 352, 353, 362, 411–413, 415, 417
surface plasmon resonance imaging (SPRI) 334, 350
systemic lupus erythymatosus (SLE) 176–178

TB *see* tuberculosis
TBG *see* thyroxine binding globulin
TDM *see* therapeutic drug monitoring
technology 23, 27, 38, 42, 60, 118, 148, 149, 193, 196, 212, 268, 275, 278–280, 282, 333
  electronic 316
  high-speed flow cytometry 262
  lab-on-a-chip 28, 144, 164
  lateral-flow immunoprecipitation 222
  monoclonal antibody 258
  oligonucleotide 45
  optical microscopy 340
  optical signalling 327
  portable cartridge 279
therapeutic drug monitoring (TDM) 350
thyroxine binding globulin (TBG) 174
time-resolved fluorescence (TRF) 15, 211, 362, 406, 407
TIR *see* total internal reflection
tissue 108, 109, 161, 166, 167
  damaged 166
  diseased 162
  exocrine 171
  fruit 143
  neoplastic prostate 180
  soft 175
total internal reflection (TIR) 74, 273, 274, 328–332, 411
toxin detection 142, 144, 147, 239, 241, 242, 329
toxins 2, 9, 12, 117, 118, 127, 132, 138, 140–142, 144, 222, 227, 228, 235, 236, 239–242, 269, 329
  botulinum 127, 227
  cholera 138, 305
  dinophysis 235
  hydrophilic 235
  lipophilic 235
tracer 8, 9, 12, 13, 211, 230, 388, 402–404, 409, 410

treatment 69, 73, 108, 164, 169, 179, 197, 259, 316
TRF *see* time-resolved fluorescence
tuberculosis (TB) 193, 194, 198–200, 203, 273

urine 91, 145, 162, 168, 174, 363, 391, 400, 402

virus 2, 9, 11, 24, 26, 193, 195, 197, 201, 205, 206, 222, 340
  dengue 211
  respiratory 281
  rubella 149

yeast 76, 77, 262